A Compassionate Calling

This book will help open minds and heart to the real-world issues—the drawbacks and the joys—of the veterinary profession and the real risks to those who practice it when the pressures and the heartache overwhelm.

—Grant Hayter-Menzies, author of *Freddie: The Rescue Dog Who Rescued Me*

A Compassionate Calling offers an unflinching and deeply personal look into the realities of the veterinary profession.

Dr. Marie Holowaychuk, a veterinary specialist with experience in academia, emergency and referral hospitals, and general practice, weaves candid personal stories with evidence-based insights from published research. In 40 concise and thought-provoking chapters, she explores the hidden curriculum of veterinary school, the toll of on-call work, the emotional impact of euthanasia, the challenges of practicing during a pandemic, and many other important topics. Marie also tackles pressing issues like diversity, equity, inclusion, and the evolving dynamics of pet insurance and corporatization in veterinary medicine.

Despite nearly 90% of pet owners viewing their animals as family members, few truly understand the challenges veterinarians face daily. This book pulls back the curtain to address questions such as:

- Why don't more veterinarians recommend the profession to others?
- How do distressing events, like euthanasia and moral stress, affect veterinarians' mental health?
- What do veterinarians wish pet owners knew about the emotional and mental toll of caring for their animals?

With its blend of heartfelt storytelling and practical insights, *A Compassionate Calling* is essential reading for pet owners, aspiring veterinarians, and anyone curious about the veterinary profession. Practicing veterinarians will also find comfort and connection in the honest exploration of the joys and struggles of veterinary life.

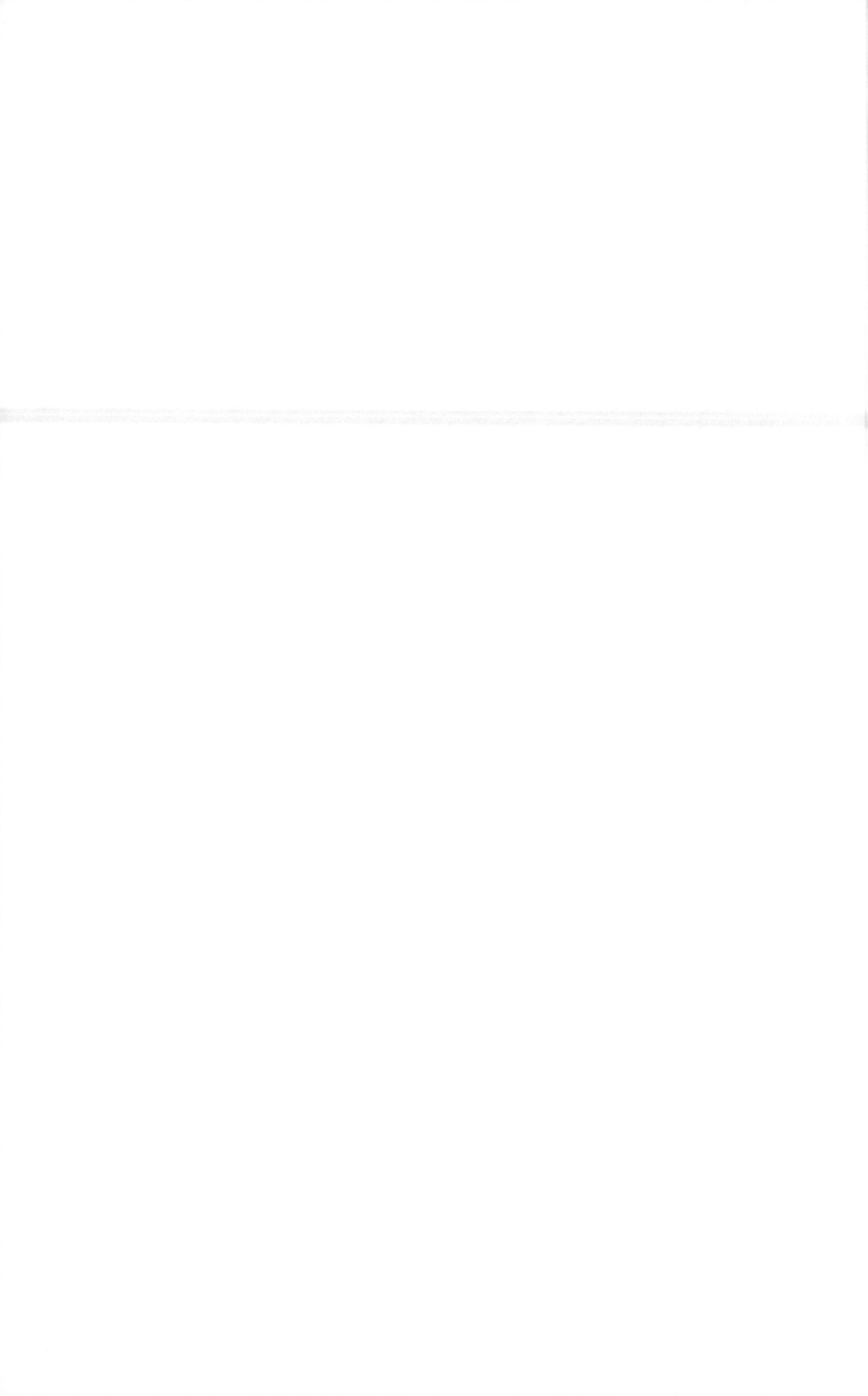

A Compassionate Calling

What It Really Means to Be a Veterinarian

Marie Holowaychuk

CRC CRC Press
Taylor & Francis Group
Boca Raton   London   New York

CRC Press is an imprint of the
Taylor & Francis Group, an **informa** business

Front cover design by Samantha Fung samanthafung.com

First edition published 2026
by CRC Press
2385 NW Executive Center Drive, Suite 320, Boca Raton FL 33431

and by CRC Press
4 Park Square, Milton Park, Abingdon, Oxon, OX14 4RN

CRC Press is an imprint of Taylor & Francis Group, LLC
© 2026 Marie Holowaychuk

ISBN: 9781032389059 (hbk)
ISBN: 9781032389035 (pbk)
ISBN: 9781003347385 (ebk)

DOI: 10.1201/9781003347385

Typeset in Minion Pro
by Deanta Global Publishing Services, Chennai, India

Dedication

To my parents, Drs. Bob and Elly Holowaychuk, whose dedication to veterinary medicine inspired my own path in this incredible profession.

To my daughter, Bethany, who reminds me every day why I'm proud to be a veterinarian.

Contents

Preface

One of my earliest memories is sitting on the couch in my mom's veterinary clinic office, waiting for her to finish work and take me home. After school, my dad often brought me there, where I helped by emptying garbage or cleaning exam rooms while he handled repairs or cleaning, and my mom wrapped up her appointments. The bookshelves in her office were filled with textbooks on medicine, surgery, anatomy, and physiology, alongside the works of James Herriot, the British veterinarian who authored *All Creatures Great and Small*, *If Only They Could Talk*, and *Let Sleeping Vets Lie*. Although too young to read them then, I saw in these books stories from a veterinarian's perspective that profoundly influenced public perception of our profession.

James Herriot's books have sold millions globally and have been adapted into movies and TV series. Growing up in the 1980s, the cartoonish covers of Herriot's books intrigued and puzzled me, portraying a veterinary world different from what I witnessed daily in my mom's practice. Today, over 50 years since Herriot's first publication, veterinary medicine has evolved significantly. Women now dominate the profession, transforming it from rural mixed practices to urban companion animal care. Specialty hospitals dot cityscapes, and technology has revolutionized our daily practices. Despite this evolution, veterinary medicine faces challenges, with job satisfaction ratings among the lowest in professional fields.

Fifteen years into my veterinary career, I was startled by a study in the *Journal of the American Veterinary Medical Association* that revealed less than half of veterinarians would recommend this profession, particularly those under 35. This revelation made me reflect deeply. When people learn I'm a veterinarian, they often express dreams for their children to follow this path. I smile, yet silently question whether they truly grasp the demands of our profession. Students often enter veterinary medicine idealistically, driven by love for animals or a desire to help pet owners. They may overlook the realities: long hours, modest incomes compared to human healthcare providers, and challenging client interactions. Contrary to popular belief, veterinary work isn't just cuddling puppies and kittens. It demands resilience, compassion, and a deep sense of responsibility.

My journey into veterinary medicine has taken me through competitive pre-vet education, four years of veterinary school, a one-year internship, a three-year residency program, five years in academia, and more than a decade working as a veterinary specialist, consultant, speaker, researcher, and advocate. Even so, I am only beginning to truly understand the profession's complexity. There are challenges, moments of healing, life-saving surgeries, and connection with dedicated pet owners that bring immense satisfaction. Yet, the profession's realities—nontraditional hours, financial constraints, and ethical dilemmas—demand transparency.

Embarking on the journey of writing this book over three transformative years—spanning the challenges of a global pandemic and the joys of becoming a mother—was profound. Some days, the words flowed effortlessly from my experiences and reflections; other days, I grappled with the responsibility of portraying veterinary medicine authentically. As someone deeply passionate about this profession, I felt compelled to weave together personal narratives with rigorous research, offering a comprehensive view that celebrates its triumphs and acknowledges its challenges. In doing so, I made a concerted effort to include perspectives and research from around the world, primarily the United States, the United Kingdom, and Australasia, despite my training and working primarily in Canada and the United States.

Growing up in a household where both parents dedicated their lives to veterinary practice—my mother a seasoned small animal veterinarian and my father immersed in regulatory medicine—I was steeped in the realities and aspirations of veterinary care from an early age. These experiences uniquely positioned me to witness the evolution of veterinary medicine firsthand, from its traditional roots to its modern complexities. This intimate perspective, combined with years of clinical practice and academic inquiry, fueled my commitment to write a book that not only captures the essence of veterinary medicine but also sparks meaningful conversations about its future.

This book is for everyone connected to veterinary medicine—whether you're a seasoned practitioner navigating the complexities of modern practice, an aspiring veterinarian eager to understand what lies ahead, or a supporter who values the dedication and sacrifices of those in the field. It aims to bridge our shared experiences, shedding light on the multifaceted roles veterinarians play in society today. Through research-backed anecdotes and a balanced portrayal of its joys and struggles, I hope this journey enriches your understanding of veterinary medicine and inspires collective action toward a sustainable and fulfilling future for our profession.

I invite you to join me in exploring these pages, where personal stories intertwine with scholarly insights, offering a compassionate and insightful perspective on the challenges and triumphs that define our veterinary community. May this book not only inform but also ignite conversations and foster a deeper appreciation for the vital role veterinarians play in the wellbeing of animals and the communities they serve.

PART ONE

Journey of a Veterinary Critical Care Specialist

1

Pursuing a Lifelong Calling

Even after 31 years of practice, I still tell young bright minds that it is a wonderful profession that I love and highly recommend. If that is their passion, do not let anyone dampen their dream.

—Caroline Heffernan, BSc, DVM
(Small Animal General Practitioner)

I cannot recall a time in my life when I did not want to be a veterinarian. Like most vets I have known or worked with over the years, my desire to practice veterinary medicine started at a very young age. Given that I grew up with two veterinarians as parents, this is perhaps unsurprising; I was immersed in veterinary practice from the moment I was born. Many veterinarians choose their career because they grow up with a menagerie of pets, but, aside from my brief encounters with cows on the family farm, the cats and fishes in my mom's clinic, and the various other companion animals I saw at my mom's practice, we shared our house only with dogs. Because of my mom's allergies, we tended toward non-shedding breeds such as Sealyham Terriers, Miniature Poodles, and then Standard Poodles, still my favorite today.

Although many children aspire to be veterinarians, most do not follow through with this plan. I've lost track of the number of people who, when I reveal my profession, have said to me: "I always wanted to be a veterinarian." They also share that they inevitably gave up because their grades were not high enough or they were put off by the idea of having to do surgery or put animals to sleep. A 2020 survey of more than 2,100 adults in the United States asked about their career aspirations as children. Veterinarian was ranked number 3 as the dream job in elementary school (Box 1) and was ranked number 2 specifically among girls. Among children surveyed in 2016, veterinarian remains one of the top career aspirations among those aged 4–11 years old.[1] I briefly contemplated other careers (including professional basketball!), but my fondness for animals and helping the families who love them kept pulling me back to veterinary medicine.

DOI: 10.1201/9781003347385-2

Box 1: Did You Know?

Top 10 Career Aspirations among United States Elementary School Students[1]
Professional athlete (13.8%)
Teacher (13.7%)
Veterinarian (13.5%)
Doctor (12.9%)
Astronaut (12.3%)
Scientist (8.3%)
Artist (7.8%)
Actor/actress (6.4%)
Musician/singer (5.7%)
Police officer/detective (5.7%)

Some of my earliest memories are of helping my mom in her suburban companion animal practice outside of Edmonton, Canada. I began emptying garbage, cleaning kennels (the ones I could reach), and, when I was tall enough, wiping exam room tables and vacuuming. I remember feeling triumphant when I was finally able to change the mop water without having to ask someone else for help! As I matured and had the confidence to speak to clients, I started taking on tasks such as vaccine reminder phone calls and updating the client rolodex. This was an era before email, text messaging, and computer files. Eventually I was working at the reception desk admitting clients, answering the phone, and scheduling appointments after school, on Saturdays, and throughout the summer months. I loved my hours working in the practice. Spending time with my coworkers (many of whom had known me since birth) and getting to help care for the dogs, cats, ferrets, rabbits, birds, and random reptiles remain some of my fondest childhood memories.

My dad also influenced my affection for animals and my faithfulness to veterinary medicine. His veterinary career was devoted to animal welfare and regulatory medicine in his decades-long roles with the Canadian Food Inspection Agency and Alberta Agriculture. Many weekends during my early childhood involved my dad taking us to his parents' farm, where we sometimes tended to beef cattle that needed pregnancy checks, ear tagging, deworming, and other preventative veterinary care. I loved spending that time outdoors and away from suburbia.

My parents both attended veterinary school at the University of Saskatchewan's Western College of Veterinary Medicine (WCVM), less than a decade after the first class graduated in 1969. They were one year apart in school (my dad was ahead of my mom), and they often joked about how my mom was "the devoted student" and my dad was "the class clown," an unlikely match. But they dated for just under a year before they decided to get married.

In 1975, my dad graduated from WCVM and started working for Agriculture Canada as a meat inspection veterinarian in Saskatoon. My mom's graduation followed in 1976, after which they moved to a town outside of Edmonton where she did locums before officially opening her practice, Mills Haven Veterinary Clinic, in a newly built shopping center on March 1, 1977. By 2001 they were outgrowing the clinic, so my parents purchased land nearby to build a new 4,000-square-foot building that remains today. My dad retired in 2013 after his tireless devotion to food safety, and my mom retired in 2018 after more than four decades in companion animal practice.

Veterinary school in the 1970s was vastly different from what it is today. The curriculum was heavily focused on farm animals, including cows, sheep, chickens, and horses. The graduating classes were relatively small and predominantly (or solely) male (Box 2). While attitudes toward dogs and cats were changing, companion animal practice did not grow until the mid-1970s and early 1980s. After that, class sizes slowly increased, and, decades later, they shifted toward a predominantly female class. At the time, Canada had three veterinary schools that served applicants from their respective geographic regions. Residents from British Columbia, Alberta, Saskatchewan, and Manitoba were admitted to WCVM, whereas students in central and eastern Canada went to the Ontario Veterinary College. The only French-speaking veterinary school in North America was in Saint-Hyacinthe and admitted applicants primarily from Quebec. Each province had an allotment of seats in every class related to the amount of government funding that was contributed to the veterinary school. This was based on the presumption that those veterinarians would return to their home province to work after graduation.

Box 2: Did You Know?

The Western College of Veterinary Medicine's first class graduated in 1969 and was the only class with no female graduates. Fifty years later, the Class of 2019 had just 13 men among its 78 graduates.[2]

As I grew up and spent more time in my mom's practice, I became more conscious of the demands of veterinary medicine. Even though the pressures of veterinary practice in the 1980s and 1990s were vastly different from what they are today, I could see that being a veterinarian was not always easy. As a practice owner, my mom worked long days and was often home hours after we had eaten dinner. Even when she was not in the clinic, she was very often doing something work-related: balancing the practice's ledger, preparing for tax payments, and writing staff cheques. She spent evenings taking phone calls from clients who were given her home phone number for emergencies. When animals were very sick or needed surgery, my mom went into the clinic, and

I often accompanied her to help hold an animal or clean up when everything was done. What these early memories taught me was that veterinary medicine was not a "regular job" but was more of a unique calling. When pets and their families needed my mom's help, she was always there. And she never complained.

My decision to apply for the pre-veterinary medicine program at the University of Alberta in the Faculty of Agriculture therefore felt preordained. I was lucky to have been awarded a $10,000 Louise McKinney scholarship that paid for my tuition and, because the university was just a 25-minute drive away, I lived at home and carpooled with my older brother, who was enrolled in chemical engineering. Despite being archrivals at school (there's a longstanding battle between the "aggies" and "geers"), we spent hours in the evening studying together and taking turns with power naps or breaks.

In the late 1990s, it was still possible to load the pre-veterinary program to incorporate all the necessary veterinary school prerequisites into a two-year program. This meant taking four or five classes per semester, many of which were science classes and included weekly four-hour labs. The schedule was demanding, but I thrived, enjoying university life and the freedom of self-directed study. In fact, I continued to work at the clinic on Saturdays. My favorite classes were ecosystem health and animal science, and my least favorite were biochemistry and physics. Why we needed physics as a prerequisite for veterinary school still boggles my mind!

I decided to apply for veterinary school at the end of my first semester of second year. Back then, the application process involved submitting high school and university transcripts, providing two veterinarian references, and writing a letter of intent. At the time, letters of references were presented to me in sealed and signed envelopes and letters of intent were written by hand. Typed submissions were not allowed, presumably to limit the chance of a person copying or submitting someone else's ideas. Everything was sent to the veterinary school's admissions office by mail and then the wait began. For more on the arduous and competitive journey of getting into veterinary school, including evolving pathways like international programs and the persistent challenges faced by aspiring veterinarians, see Chapter 9, where I explore the intricacies of the admissions process and its impact on the profession.

It was after my second semester of the second year of my pre-veterinary program was complete that my final transcripts were submitted and I learned that I had passed the first part of the admissions process. The next step was to complete an interview with members of the veterinary school admissions committee. I recall showing up to my interview in my carefully selected blouse and khaki pants, seeing another interviewee in a full pants suit and immediately questioning whether I had misjudged the entire thing! Nevertheless, I made it past a panel of three interviewers, two of whom were current WCVM faculty members and the other a practicing veterinarian. They asked me questions about my experience, post-veterinary school aspirations, and whether I felt

I was ready. It was an unnerving experience, but I left feeling I had done the best I could. Beyond that, it was out of my hands.

Approximately one month later I received a letter from the University of Saskatchewan, which I opened in front of everyone in my mom's practice. We celebrated together as I read "Congratulations—we are pleased to tell you that you have been accepted into the Class of 2004 Doctor of Veterinary Medicine program at the Western College of Veterinary Medicine." It was truly one of the proudest and happiest moments of my life: I wasn't yet 20 years old, and I was already well on my way to achieving my lifelong dream.

2

Between Pre-Vet and Practitioner

> One of the most complicated relationships in my life is with veterinary school. Getting in wasn't easy, but staying in was almost impossible—I nearly left twice. I don't often share this, not wanting to burden veterinary hopefuls with my challenges, but my biggest triumph is that I stayed and made it through.
>
> —Jill Girgulis, DVM
> (Small Animal General Practitioner)

Veterinary school was more difficult than I could have imagined, both academically and emotionally. You'd think an A+ student with extensive veterinary experience would transition seamlessly but that was definitely not the case for me. Living away from home for the first time, managing an intense classroom and laboratory schedule, taking classes in subjects that were entirely new to me, and memorizing anatomical and physiological concepts—it was all much harder than I anticipated.

I was admitted to veterinary school at the age of 19 (Box 1) and it was after my 20th birthday that I moved to my neighboring province to attend the Western College of Veterinary Medicine at the University of Saskatchewan. Saskatoon was a small city in a primarily agricultural area, although still about five times the size of the suburb where I grew up. I felt quickly at home in the city, known for its beautiful riverside trails and 319 days of sunshine per year. The people were incredibly friendly, so navigating everyday tasks such as driving to school, buying groceries, and interacting with my neighbors was easy.

Box 1: Did You Know?

According to the American Association of Veterinary Medical Colleges, the mean age of first-year veterinary students has changed over the years. In 1975, it was 22.4, then in 1995 it increased to 24.9, and in 2018 it decreased again to 23.3 years of age.[1]

DOI: 10.1201/9781003347385-3

My parents purchased a two-bedroom condominium that I rented throughout my four years in Saskatoon and was a short five-minute drive from the veterinary school. I used the tiny second bedroom as my study space, squeezing in a desk and computer, complete with dial-up internet. With no space for a roommate, I took one of the family dogs as my housemate, a Standard Poodle named Ronnie (short for Veronica). At the time, my parents had begun breeding Standard Poodles and Ronnie was in one of their first litters named entirely after characters from the Archie Comics. She had an outgoing personality from puppyhood and was considered the most confident and show-worthy in her litter. After she obtained her Canadian and American championships, she returned home to have two litters of puppies before officially retiring, getting spayed, and becoming our family dog.

Devastatingly, shortly before I was planning to move with her to Saskatoon, she developed a life-threatening disease called immune-mediated hemolytic anemia. This autoimmune disease results in the body attacking its own red blood cells, which led to Ronnie experiencing severe anemia, weakness, and lethargy. Thankfully she responded to immunosuppressive therapy and her red blood cell count rebounded in time for the move. I was able to wean her off the medications on the advice of my mom throughout the first months of veterinary school and she was lucky to never have a relapse afterward.

My initial few weeks of veterinary school were among the loneliest I had felt in my life. Despite a class size of nearly 70 students, I felt challenges connecting with classmates and spent most of my lunch breaks studying in the

Figure 2.1
Marie and Ronnie in their home in Saskatoon after moving to attend veterinary school at the University of Saskatchewan Western College of Veterinary Medicine.

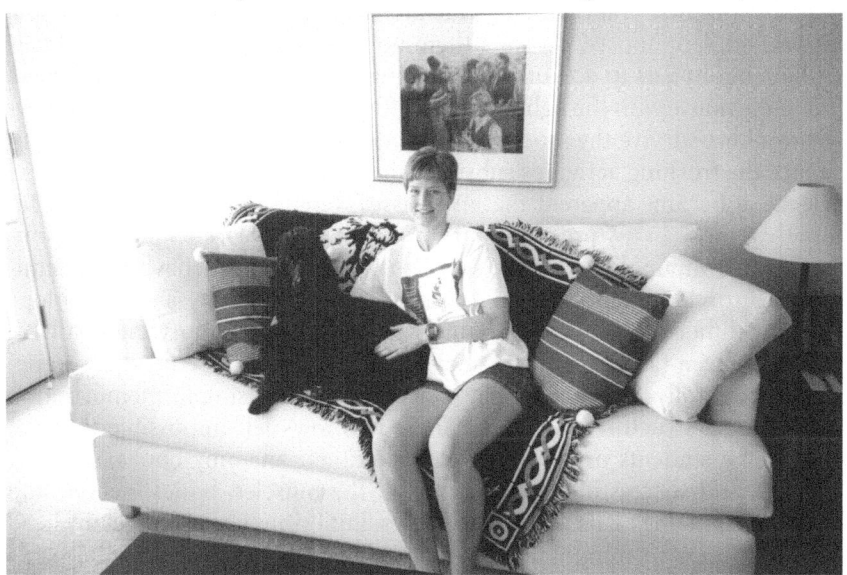

library. Ronnie got me through those trying times with her spunky personality, incessant energy, and relentless presence. We enjoyed our walks around the neighborhood, trips to the off-leash parks, and eventually classes that included fly-ball and agility. Her athleticism and desire to please were a perfect combination for these competitive sports. I felt grateful each and every day to have her as my steadfast furry companion.

Making friends in Saskatoon was daunting, as I only recognized a couple of students from my pre-veterinary program. But, ultimately, I became close with other classmates from Alberta, some of whom had grown up near me, and, over time, I built friendships with others in my class, including those from British Columbia, Saskatchewan, and Manitoba. Despite these friendships, I felt intensely lonely at times. Living alone (well, without another human) often felt isolating, especially given that most of my classmates had roommates or lived with family. And while we all shared a common interest in veterinary medicine, it was difficult to connect over hobbies or interests outside of school. Eventually I joined a competitive basketball league with non-veterinary students and embraced intramural sports like floor hockey. Unfortunately, the big vet school sports were ice hockey and curling, neither of which I had the skills to play or the equipment and confidence to start to learn. Moreover, as someone who struggled with social anxiety (an affliction we had no name for back then), I avoided the social aspects of these events like the plague.

Nonetheless, I felt a strong kinship toward several of my classmates, some of whom remain my closest friends today. As for those social events, there were no shortage throughout my four years, from "happy hours" during all the major holidays (that involved drinking alcohol at the school!) to nights out at the local bars and pubs. Activities were always being planned and everyone was invited, although whether I chose to attend was another story! I remember our first year froshing, which involved the upper years going to the first-year student houses, dressing them up in embarrassing outfits, and taking them out to bars to do humiliating things. On the night this was planned, I hid in my house with the lights off and refused to answer my doorbell, knowing I wouldn't survive the mortifying experience!

Once the froshing activities subsided and we settled into our first-year experience, it became apparent that my classes were going to challenge me far more than those in my pre-veterinary program. First year included anatomy, physiology, immunology, histology, animal welfare and behavior, epidemiology, neuroscience, and veterinary skills. I found anatomy and physiology especially difficult, given the amount of studying and memorizing involved. I've always been (and continue to be) someone who only remembers something once I fully understand the concept, meaning simple memorization of anatomical structures and physiologic pathways felt impossible to me. I recall seeing students in the library coloring their anatomy books, studying skeletons, and successfully memorizing all the muscles, bones, nerves, and blood vessels of dogs, cats, horses, and cows. But I simply couldn't get my head around the massive amount of data I needed to commit to memory.

Figure 2.2
Marie with a calf during her first-year herd health class in veterinary school.

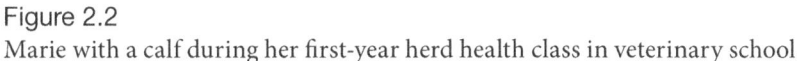

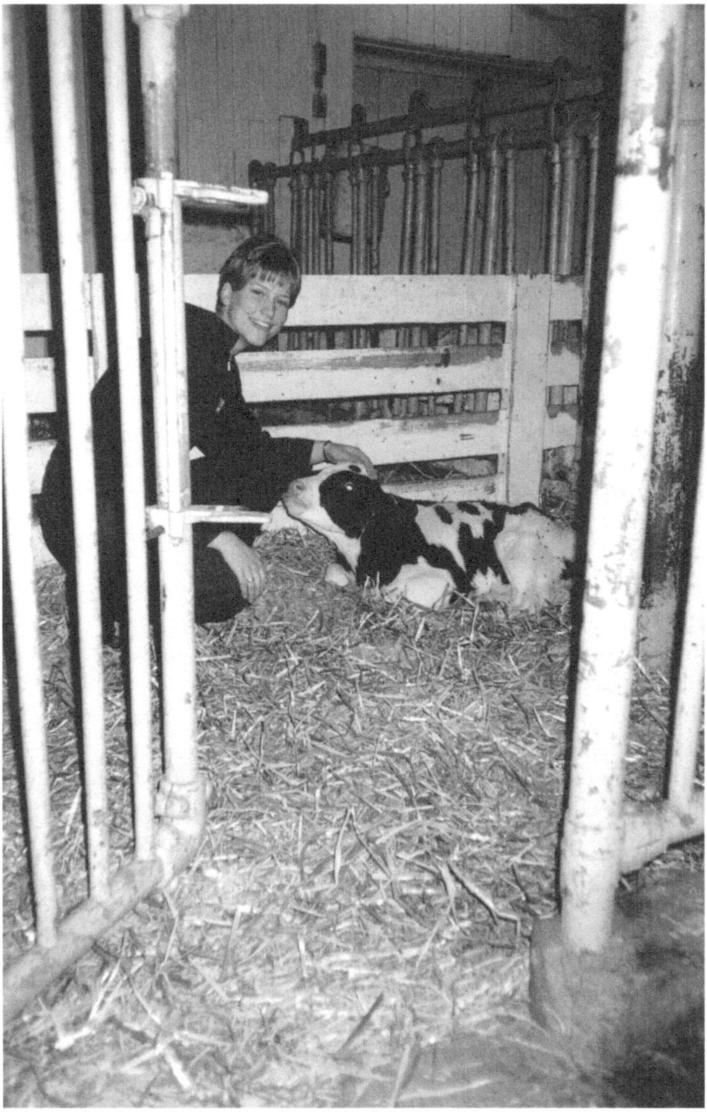

Not surprisingly, I nearly failed my first anatomy exam. I'll never forget seeing the 57% score on my paper; I'd never in my entire life received a grade so low! One of our anatomy professors showed me how on the multiple-choice questions I had consistently narrowed down the answers to two, one of which was correct—and almost always selected the incorrect one! It didn't help that I hated the anatomy lab; the smell of the formaldehyde made me sick to my stomach and I resented having to study and dissect the same dog for an entire year. I was almost always the last student to arrive and the first one to leave after the tasks were completed. I felt guilty that my anatomy partner (my best friend) got stuck with such an absent study buddy!

My experience with physiology was similar and confounded by the fact that most of my classmates had taken a physiology class before veterinary school, so were already familiar with many of the concepts. Everything was brand new for me and, once again, required tremendous memorization and application. I remember my cardiovascular physiology exam, which I felt wholly unprepared for (fast forward two decades and this is now one of my favorite subjects!). A friend suggested I "pull an all-nighter" with two bottles of Jolt Cola to get me through. As a non-coffee-drinker, this was more caffeine than I'd ever had in my life. I stayed awake, but my heart was beating so hard I thought it would jump out of my chest! Needless to say, the quality of my study time was poor; I was too jittery to rest at all and was exhausted and unfocused the next day during the exam. This time my score was not so low that I had to meet with the professor, but it was another wake-up call to the amount of work that veterinary school was demanding of me.

In hindsight, I was starting to experience some of the first symptoms of depression and anxiety that I would officially be diagnosed with later in life. I felt tremendous guilt and pressure about being admitted to veterinary school so young when others in my class had applied several times prior to getting in. That awareness, coupled with my struggle in classes like anatomy, left me feeling dejected, worried, and, at times, worthless. Sometimes I had trouble concentrating and my sleep was all over the place. There were times in class when I felt so restless and anxious about memorizing the concepts that I thought I might jump out of my seat. Thankfully I was able to manage most of my symptoms by socializing with friends, exercising regularly, and walking with Ronnie, but I have no doubt that my mental health problems impeded my learning and relationships at times (Box 2). For an in-depth look at the often-overlooked mental health challenges faced by both veterinary students and professionals, turn to Chapter 24, where I underscore the critical need for stronger support systems and healthier workplace cultures to safeguard both practitioners and patients.

Box 2: Did You Know?

Research performed at Kansas State University shows that symptoms of anxiety and depression are prevalent among veterinary students, especially those in their second and third years. Factors associated with anxiety and depression symptoms include difficulty fitting in, heavy workload, homesickness, unclear expectations from instructors, and perceived poor health.[2]

Throughout this time, I was doing my best to remember what one of the faculty told us during our orientation. That as A+ students, we would have to accept the fact that in veterinary school some of us would move to average, and some to below average, compared to our classmates. Of course, just like everyone else, I told myself I'd most definitely stay in the above-average category. Until my first series of midterm exams landed me solidly in the average to below-average portion of the class! As difficult as that was, I tried to remember that I'd worked hard to get here, that I'd survived difficult classes before (including physics!), and that I would without a doubt get through this as well.

Second year proved every bit as challenging with its onslaught of "-ology" classes, including pharmacology, toxicology, virology, parasitology, bacteriology, clinical pathology, and systemic pathology. However, these classes, and those that were more clinical such as anesthesia and analgesia, medical imaging, diagnostic medicine, and surgical principals, felt more familiar to me. Despite having to memorize new words and theory, the application to veterinary practice was much more tangible. I was able to recall cases I'd seen in my years working in my mom's practice, helping me to apply and thus remember the concepts. Perhaps surprisingly, given the heaviness of the class schedule and the overwhelming volume of information we were learning, my grades improved in my second year, and I settled into a routine similar to what I had anticipated going into veterinary school.

My grades and experiences improved again during my third and final pre-clinical year, when I really hit my stride. All the concepts learned had application to clinical practice, including food animal production medicine, equine medicine and surgery, companion animal theriogenology, exotic animal medicine and surgery, ophthalmology, and small animal medicine and surgery. We also had clinical skills and surgical exercises where we had hands-on exposure and experience performing the many different physical examination, procedural, and surgical skills that we'd need as veterinarians in practice. I really enjoyed getting to work with live animals (so long anatomy cadavers!), and I started to see the light at the end of the veterinary school tunnel.

After the first three pre-clinical years consisting of lectures and laboratories, the final year was (and still is) almost entirely spent in the veterinary teaching hospital working alongside faculty clinicians, residents, interns, technicians, and other staff. Close to the end of third year we went through what was then called "The Draft": a half-day event whereby each student in the class would choose their desired clinical rotations for fourth year. I still remember the anticipation leading up to this day. Those students who were focused on post-graduate internships wanted to frontload their schedule with the rotations that would give them the most favorable reference letters for their applications. Other students with unique interests such as equine or exotic medicine wanted to grab spots for those less often offered or limited enrollment rotations.

The tension on Draft Day was palpable, yet I mainly remember feeling excited to define what my fourth and final veterinary school year would look like. Ultimately, I got nearly every rotation I wanted: these were companion animal-focused and included small animal medicine (4 weeks), surgery (4 weeks), exotics (1 week), nutrition (1 week), radiology (2 weeks), clinical pathology (1 week), anatomic pathology (2 weeks), and anesthesia (4 weeks), among others. At the time we were still required to take some large animal rotations, so I stuck with cows (my large animal of choice) and took a summertime bovine rotation (when we'd be looking after calves with scours) and a field service rotation in the freezing cold month of January. There were definitely some rotations that were more favorably timed than others(!) but, overall, I was pleased with my selections.

Figure 2.3
Ronnie and Marie in her veterinary school graduation photo.

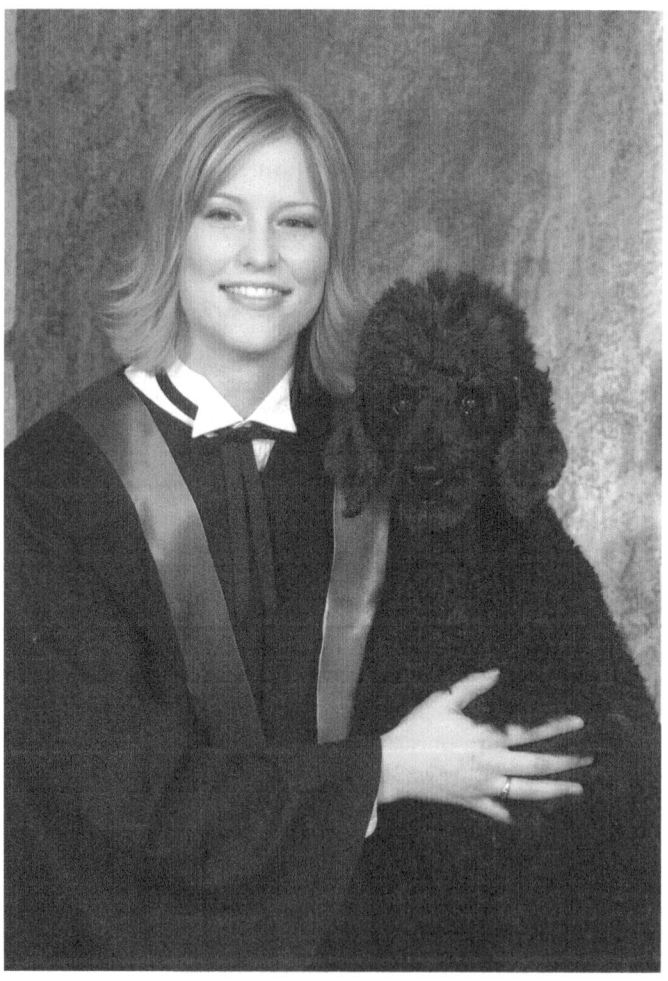

As I anticipated, my fourth year garnered me the best experience (and grades) of veterinary school. I felt like I was in my element in the clinical learning environment, with practical and seamless application to real-life cases and the opportunity to work within a team, something I'd always enjoyed in my mom's practice. I thrived on developing a rapport with clients, problem-solving difficult cases, administering patient treatments, and writing up medical records. Whether the patients were cows, dogs, cats, ferrets, or hamsters, I enjoyed every single one and felt a renewed sense of awareness that I'd absolutely chosen the right career path.

This isn't to say that my final year of veterinary school was all rainbows and butterflies (or perhaps more appropriately, puppies and kittens). I had many moments of sleep deprivation after nights sleeping in the on-call dorms, self-doubt when I was unable to sort through the ins and outs of a case, and even tears when I felt overwhelmed with the emotion of having to euthanize a patient of mine for the first time. Nevertheless, I felt with newfound certainty that my learning journey was not over. Another year of clinical mentorship during an internship program was exactly what I wanted and needed.

3

The Path to Veterinary Specialization

Whoever said "If you love what you do, you'll never work a day in your life" clearly was not a veterinarian. More appropriately, the expression should go something along the lines of "if you love what you do, you'll be willing to work more hours than you thought were possible, to achieve your dreams." This expression is twice as true for those of us who want to pursue additional training through internships and residencies.

—Danny Sack, DVM
(Surgery Resident, Small Animal Veterinarian)

Telling my mom I wouldn't be joining her veterinary practice after graduation was one of the toughest decisions I've made, but it led to one of the most rewarding steps in my career. Opting for an internship over immediately joining my mom's practice allowed me to explore the vast array of opportunities beyond general companion animal practice. While I cherished my time in my mom's clinic, forming lasting bonds with families and their pets, I was drawn to academia's enriching teaching environment and the chance to provide cutting-edge care through specialty medicine.

Entering veterinary school, my passion for animals and desire to help pet owners was unquestionable. I thrived on problem-solving, relishing the technical aspects of procedures and surgeries, and I found fulfillment in recommending ways to enhance the lives of both pets and their owners. Yet the routine of general practice left me questioning the fate of cases referred to specialty facilities. When a locum veterinarian broached the idea of applying for an internship, it was a revelation for me.

Alongside my clinical rotations at my veterinary school, I managed to arrange two additional externship weeks in dermatology and ophthalmology at other hospitals. These experiences shed light on the breadth of services specialists could offer, from diagnosing chronic skin conditions to performing sight-saving surgeries. It was a pivotal time that shaped my veterinary career trajectory, setting me on a path toward specialization and deeper fulfillment in my profession.

I vividly remember the day that I told my mom I wouldn't be returning to work in her practice. It had always been expected that I would assume ownership of the clinic after her retirement, so my mom was incredibly upset and

DOI: 10.1201/9781003347385-4

disappointed by the news. Some not-so-nice words were exchanged, and my mom didn't speak to me for weeks afterwards, leaving me feeling horribly guilty. Yet I also felt relief, knowing I'd made the right choice for my veterinary career path.

And so began my journey of applying for an internship. Navigating to VIRMP.org, the platform hosted by the American Association of Veterinary Clinicians, I meticulously noted key dates for accessing the program database, submitted my applications with transcripts and references, ranked preferred programs, and eagerly awaited the match results. For more on the demanding journey to becoming a veterinary specialist, including insights into the competitive VIRMP matching process, board certification, and the rising demand for specialists, turn to Chapter 12, where I explore the evolving landscape of veterinary specialties and the critical shortage impacting patient care.

Opting for a small animal rotating internship, I aimed to delve into various specialties, particularly emergency, medicine, and surgery. Despite the plethora of options—over 100 programs at veterinary schools and specialty practices—I narrowed my focus to academic institutions. Enthusiastic about the prospect of cage-side rounds and collaborative learning in a teaching hospital environment, I sought to continue my veterinary education in a setting dedicated to fostering student, intern, and resident training.

In a move I wouldn't necessarily recommend today, I applied to programs without consulting current or past interns. Placing my trust in the academic pedigree of these institutions, I ranked programs based on instinct and proximity to home, prioritizing those with robust emergency rotations, a highlight of my clinical year in veterinary school. Additionally, I favored schools known to be receptive to Canadian applicants. Ultimately, I was thrilled to match with my top choice, Washington State University (WSU) College of Veterinary Medicine.

Situated in the picturesque college town of Pullman, Washington, WSU boasts the distinction of being the fifth oldest veterinary school in the United States. As my internship commenced on July 1, 2004, I journeyed by car from British Columbia into the heart of the Palouse region, where I joined fellow interns hailing from WSU, University of Florida, and University of Georgia, with the later addition of a fifth intern from Europe. Amidst the newly constructed teaching hospital and the warm camaraderie of faculty and peers, receiving my security access card marked the beginning of an enriching chapter in my professional journey. WSU's dress code required men in my internship class to wear ties, while I ensured my wardrobe of dress pants and blouses complied. Walking the crimson, grey, and white Cougar-crested hallways, I felt a sense of pride in fully embracing the professionalism expected in our clinical environment.

During orientation we also created our rotation schedule, allocating time for the services and within the specialties that most interested us. We all had to complete a minimum number of rotations within emergency, medicine, and surgery, but my schedule was heavily weighted toward my primary interests: emergency and internal medicine. I was also able to schedule additional core rotations, including community practice and neurology, as well as elective rotations such as behavior, critical care, oncology, and radiology.

I hit the ground running during my internship, beginning with an emergency rotation over the Fourth of July weekend. Notorious for being the only emergency hospital in the southeastern region of Washington State at the time, the emergency service could be exceptionally busy, especially during holidays and weekends. I saw no less than 20-something cases over the weekend with the help of my faculty backup and residents who took over the care of the surgery, medicine, or neurology referrals. To say that I was overwhelmed was an understatement. I remember sobbing after my first 24 hours. I'd never been the primary veterinarian for a single case before (let alone more than a dozen cases), and I felt like I was spinning my wheels.

Needless to say, the schedule wasn't conducive to emotional or mental wellbeing. During orientation we were given the option to continue "as it always had been," which was to start the emergency rotation during cage-side rounds at 4 p.m. on Friday and then work until 8 a.m. Monday. This schedule was meant to accommodate naps when the service was not busy, as well as sleep overnight after the patients were tended to. Of course, this did not account for busy weekends or holidays when the cases kept coming in, even overnight. One might wonder who in their right mind would agree to such a schedule! The flipside was that we'd have weekends off when we weren't rotating on emergency, rather than having to cover for one another to allow our intern mate to sleep.

As interns, not only were we seeing cases that presented to the hospital outside of regular business hours, but we were also responding to pages from the answering service (to speak to owners or referring veterinarians and determine whether the animal should be seen), checking patients in or out, setting up files, and completing paperwork. Essentially, we were functioning as doctors, receptionists, and client care representatives. It was a lot for a new veterinarian to shoulder and understandably led to overwhelm. Thankfully, the following year WSU changed its intern rotation schedule to ensure that the emergency intern would be able to go home to sleep during the day rather than spending the entire weekend in the hospital. Small mercies!

I had several emergency rotations during which I slept only one to two hours over a 24-hour period. Despite having a single bed in the intern office and the option to turn off the lights and shut the door, I was a magnet for emergencies and was constantly busy taking care of patients or finishing up my medical records. When the opportunity presented itself to rest or nap, I felt guilty and instead dedicated my time to teaching the fourth-year students who were rotating through the emergency service at night. These students functioned as technicians for in-hospital patients since the hospital was unable to staff a full-time overnight technician team. So, rather than get some much-needed shut eye, I opted to round with the fourth-year students on blood gas interpretation, transfusion medicine, and a plethora of other interesting emergency topics.

Unsurprisingly, there were mornings when I drove home and felt drunk behind the wheel. Studies have shown that exhaustion is like intoxication when it comes to driving (Box 1), but I hadn't experienced this firsthand until my internship. One morning I was pulled over by a police officer for turning right illegally, in my exhausted stupor, and received a warning.

Box 1: Did You Know?

Being awake for 17 hours is like having a blood alcohol concentration (BAC) of 0.05 (the level some countries use for impaired driving violations). Being awake for 24 hours is like having a BAC of 0.10 (above the United States impaired driving level of 0.08).[1]

Luckily my apartment was only a five-minute drive from the veterinary school. I had moved to WSU with my four-legged housemate Ronnie, but finding affordable housing that would accommodate an intern salary (and allow dogs) was challenging. Of course, I had to sign a lease sight unseen, and my choices were limited to a sketchy trailer rental or student-family housing. I opted for the latter and rented a one-bed apartment with no on-site laundry. It was nice enough as far as student housing went and within the restricted budget of my $18,500 USD annual salary (Box 2). This experience underscores a significant issue in our profession: the financial pressures that many veterinary students and early-career veterinarians face. In Chapter 10, I delve into the substantial impact of educational debt on the veterinary profession, analyzing how rising tuition costs juxtaposed with stagnant starting salaries create burdens that affect our financial wellbeing and career choices.

Box 2: Did You Know?

The average annual salary disclosed by the American Association of Veterinary Medical Colleges for academic internship positions secured through the Veterinary Internship and Residency Matching Program for the 2020–2021 training year was $28,372 USD.[2] A recent study comparing internship program salaries with regional living wages found that, on average, intern salaries may not meet the minimum income standard for a living wage, with mean income surpluses before taxes averaging $5,829 USD.[3]

Transitioning from the familiar environment of my mom's companion animal practice to the demanding pace of an internship program was both daunting and exhilarating. While it provided invaluable hands-on experience and exposure to diverse specialties, it also presented challenges such as long hours and overwhelming caseloads. Another unexpected hurdle was the abrupt shift from being a student to suddenly assuming a teaching role. I found myself navigating my own steep learning curve while simultaneously guiding and mentoring students. This involved sharing cases, reviewing their medical records entries, and facilitating client communications. Despite the irony of having been a student myself just months before, I embraced the opportunity to contribute to the education and clinical experience of students. It was immensely rewarding to be able to deepen my understanding of veterinary medicine while imparting knowledge to future practitioners.

During my internship, one of the most memorable experiences was my rotation in the oncology service, where I witnessed groundbreaking treatments, including radiation therapy for brain tumor patients. Remarkably, one French Bulldog undergoing treatment at WSU was a patient at my mom's practice, located 675 miles away! This firsthand exposure underscored the vital role of specialty medicine in delivering cutting-edge care to animals. I also delved into a plethora of journal articles and research papers with enthusiasm. My intern mates often teased me about the pile of papers on my desk, joking that if a student had a question, "Marie has a paper for that." Engaging with the latest advancements in veterinary medicine not only broadened my knowledge but also sharpened my critical thinking and research skills. Furthermore, it inspired me to author and submit three research papers to peer-reviewed journals before the conclusion of my internship, no small feat given the strenuous working hours of the program.

It wasn't uncommon for us to admit exotic or wildlife species to the hospital during our emergency rotations. In an agricultural community with no other out-of-hours wildlife services, clients frequently brought raptors, rodents, and other wild creatures to the university for care. Amidst these encounters, one incident stands out vividly. Returning home from the end of a demanding shift, I was greeted by a rooster perched on my apartment doorstep. It was Thanksgiving and most students had returned home to see family for the holiday, so perhaps the rooster knew that I was the only person in the building! Not seeing any obvious injuries but recognizing he wasn't in good condition, I found a box, scooped him up, and promptly returned with him to the veterinary school. I'd become adept at administering fluids to birds and knew how to assess the rooster's hydration and offer subcutaneous fluid replenishment. We named him Roy and he stayed with the exotics and wildlife service for several weeks, his comb and waddle turning a deep red color, indicating his return to health. He was eventually adopted by one of the faculty members to live out his life on their farm, likely narrowly avoiding his previous life's fate of becoming somebody else's dinner!

   Reflecting on my internship, I'm deeply grateful for the experiences that reinforced my love for teaching, research, and emergency medicine. Each unique case sharpened my appreciation for veterinary medicine and solidified my commitment to advancing the field and mentoring future veterinarians. It's a path that continues to inspire me every day.

Figure 3.1
Ronnie and Marie during her internship at Washington State University.

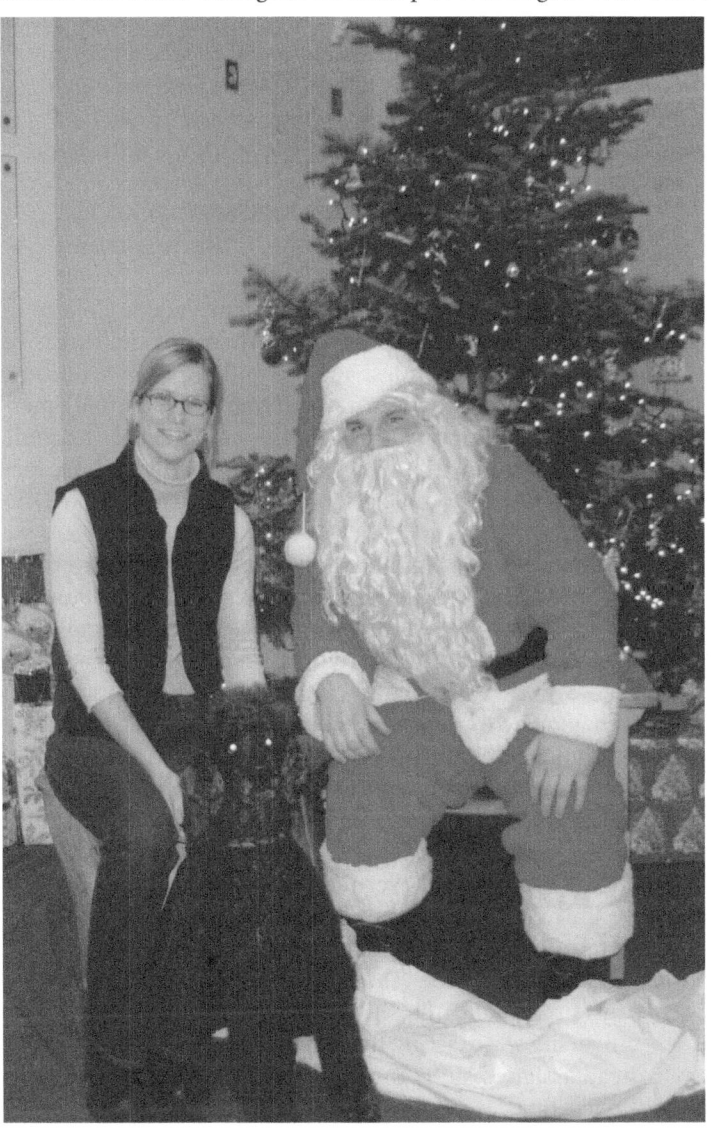

4

The Challenges and Realities of a Residency

I made $28,000 in Connecticut for my internship, and then took a pay cut when I moved to New York City to start my residency. I got a raise each year but by the end of the 4-year program I was only making $32,000. After I paid rent in my hospital owned cheap studio apartment, I only took home $800 a month. In NYC. It was brutal.

—Allison Sande, DVM, DACVIM (SAIM), DACVECC
(Staff Criticalist)

Embarking on my residency at North Carolina State University's College of Veterinary Medicine, I found myself thrust into a whirlwind of challenges I'd never imagined. Sleep deprivation, relentless anxiety, and imposter syndrome became unwelcome companions in my journey through small animal emergency and critical care (ECC). With only the anecdotes of a mentor to guide me, I dove headfirst into the unknown, leaving behind the familiar landscapes of my Canadian upbringing for the complexities of life below the Mason-Dixon line.

I packed up my life in a week and embarked on a cross-country adventure to Raleigh, North Carolina, with Ronnie and my then boyfriend. Stops at landmarks like the Corn Palace and Mount Rushmore offered glimpses of the vastness of the American landscape. Arriving in North Carolina, I was greeted not only by the warm climate but also by the rich tapestry of southern culture, from the tantalizing flavors of grits and barbecue to the idiosyncrasies of southern hospitality and colloquialisms (bless her heart!).

My residency program was a bit of a nightmare in the beginning. I was the second of two residents in a newly established program and my resident-mate was starting her second year. She'd already spent a year working in the ICU at the university, as well as evening and overnight shifts, without mentorship, at a local emergency clinic. A week into my residency, I received my clinic schedule and realized that I wouldn't be able to fulfill my credential requirements with so much unmentored time. Thankfully, my mentors agreed that the schedule wasn't sustainable and the shifts at the local emergency clinic were removed. The university was starting their own emergency service at the time, so we were instead assigned shifts there, where we'd maintain access to specialists for advice regarding case management.

DOI: 10.1201/9781003347385-5

Figure 4.1
Ronnie and Marie at the beach during her residency at North Carolina State University.

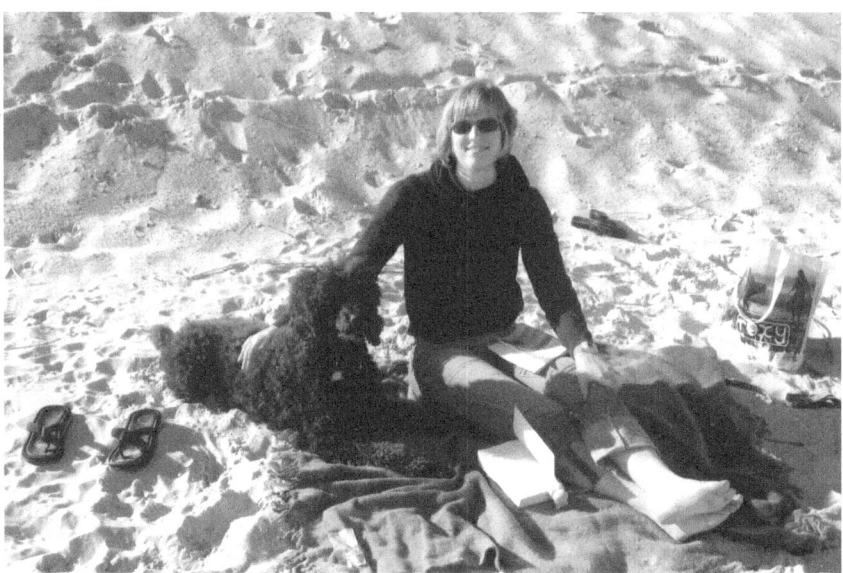

Unfortunately, not only did my program lack appropriate scheduling of clinic rotations, but structured teaching in the form of rounds and journal review were limited. We participated in cardiology rounds when we would review electrocardiograms (ECGs), as well as intern-resident rounds that rotated between critical care, cardiology, and neurology topics. We also met with our ECC mentors at a local coffee shop once weekly to review two recent journal articles, but my reading list for my board certification exam far surpassed that. At that pace, I'd never be able to review and comprehend all that was expected of me prior to finishing my residency. So, I fervently made a weekly rounds schedule to accommodate the previously established rounds, as well as case-based physiology rounds with the internal medicine residents, journal club when we'd cover at least two to three recently published articles, and book rounds when we'd read and review a chapter from a required physiology textbook. Naturally, I dreaded intern-resident rounds the most. The thought of being quizzed in front of residents from various specialties filled me with anxiety. A wrong answer would confirm their suspicions that I wasn't cut out for the residency program. I constantly battled imposter syndrome, always lurking in the background, undermining my confidence at every turn.

And so, I trudged along, rotating from week to week between services that included primarily critical care (with direct mentorship) and emergency (with direct or indirect mentorship), as well as internal medicine, surgery, cardiology, and anesthesia as my other required rotations. I was also permitted two elective weeks per residency year that included radiology, neurology, ophthalmology, and clinical pathology. My elective weeks usually felt like a vacation compared to my critical care and emergency rotations. They rarely required me to have primary case responsibility, which meant my hours in the clinic were limited to weekday daytimes. In contrast, my emergency shifts were usually swing (4 p.m. to 12 p.m.) or overnight (10 p.m. to 8 a.m.) and often continued hours longer.

When I was rotating through the intensive care unit (ICU) for my critical care weeks, I was scheduled on days, but, because there was no overnight ICU resident at the time, I was required to stay as long as I was needed. This meant some days finishing after 5 p.m. cage-side rounds and other days close to or after midnight (a total of more than 16 hours), especially if there was a ventilator or other challenging case in ICU (Box 1). And, of course, when rotating on ICU I was required to be on call, meaning that once I went home, if a critical patient was transferred into the ICU, I was required to answer questions or come back to help in person. The thought of being called in led to stress, so those nights I slept poorly regardless. And because there was usually only one resident rotating on ICU at a time, we also covered the weekends. For more insights into the high-stakes world of veterinary ICUs, including stories of critical cases and the emotional highs and lows of ICU work, turn to Chapter 13, where I explore the complexities of treating the most vulnerable patients and the dedication it requires.

Box 1: Did You Know?

According to a recent survey of more than 300 veterinary interns and residents, most work 11 to 13 hours on a typical weekday and approximately one-third have clinical duties seven days per week.[1]

To add to the struggle of this period, after the first year of my residency ended, my steadfast furry companion, Ronnie, now ten years old, developed severe neck pain. Despite trying a handful of different medications on the advice of several specialists in the hospital, it would not subside. As a last resort, we hospitalized her in the ICU for a constant IV infusion of pain relievers, but she developed aspiration pneumonia, a common complication in old or debilitated patients. She went into septic shock and nearly died. I remember spending the night in the ICU with her, wishing and praying that she would stay with me longer. I couldn't imagine finishing my residency without my best friend, who'd been steady at my side from pre-veterinary school. Ronnie did survive that night, but she went on to develop seizures, either as an adverse reaction to her antibiotics or secondary to whatever condition was causing her undiagnosed neck pain. I begged my parents to pay for an MRI so that we could try to figure out what was happening, but even that didn't reveal any obvious diagnosis. That night I took Ronnie home and spent the night

Figure 4.2
Ronnie and Marie during her second year of veterinary school during a fundraising event.

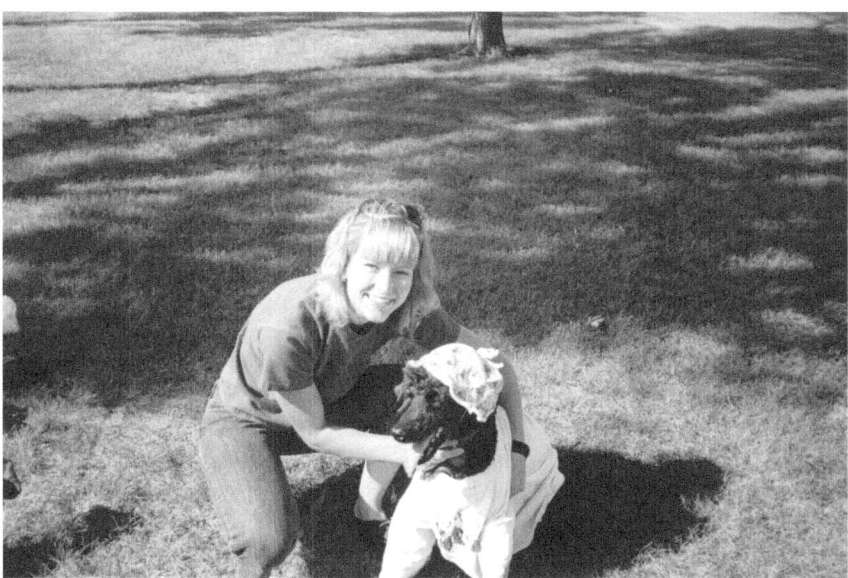

with her on the floor of my apartment. She couldn't jump on the bed, and she continued to have short seizures throughout the evening, so it was the safest place for us. The next day, I made the agonizing decision to euthanize her. Retelling this story still brings up emotions to this day.

After that, I had difficulties coping with everything in my residency and I fell into a deep depression. I became more frustrated with my program and couldn't see how I could possibly meet all my requirements and pass my board certification exam at the end. Perhaps unjustly, I blamed my mentors and didn't believe that anybody cared enough to ensure my success in the residency. I recall writing a letter to the department that oversees the residency training programs describing my feeling of being unsupported. I felt that my mentors needed a wake-up call to the realities of my experience and the need for more guidance and supervision. My mentors were surprised by this feedback and received a warning from the department. One was very hurt, letting me know that she wished I had spoken to her first. I regret not doing so and, while I do believe that my program was lacking in some aspects, in retrospect I appreciate that most of my angst came from my depression and the feelings of helplessness and hopelessness that accompanied it. Thankfully, my mentors acknowledged the program's shortcomings, changes were made, and, eventually, my grief and depression subsided.

During my third year, I visited the University of California–Davis veterinary school, where I did weeklong elective rotations in clinical nutrition and hemodialysis. At the time of my residency, the American College of Veterinary Emergency and Critical Care had little in the way of Residency Training Guidelines aside from the amount of direct and indirect emergency and critical care supervision, other core rotations, and permitted electives. Years later, due, in part, to large discrepancies in the quality of different training programs, the college devised comprehensive guidelines that detailed program requirements. These include the amount of time spent in-clinic with different forms of supervision, as well as requirements for didactic learning (classroom-style, conference seminars, or course work), or teaching (hands-on and classroom). The guidelines also include a skills and experience checklist and training benchmarks that are designed to verify and reinforce the knowledge and skills required for board certification. These annual requirements serve to ensure consistency of mentorship and training among emergency and critical care residency programs.

Once my clinic rotations came to an end, I focused my time on preparing for my board certification exams, the last step to becoming a recognized veterinary specialist. When I wrote my boards in 2008, the exam was a three-day endeavor. The first day was the written clinical exam, consisting of short answer, long answer, and list-type questions pertaining to cases. The second day was the general multiple-choice exam that included everything from respiratory, cardiovascular, and renal physiology to pharmacology, toxicology, and fluid therapy. The third and final day was also a multiple-choice exam that focused on scientific articles that had been published within the last three years pertinent to emergency and critical care. In preparation, I spent countless hours reading textbooks and taking notes, preparing flash cards of important calculations, photocopying pertinent scientific articles and highlighting them, and completing practice questions and mock exams provided by my mentors. Once my clinic rotations were done, I spent most of my days studying in the library.

Unfortunately, during those two months of exam prep, I had some of the most difficult times of my residency since losing Ronnie. Two things happened that resulted in tremendous distraction and overwhelm. First, my internship mentor had relocated to Auburn University and had asked me to enroll dogs in a study that she was performing to investigate stress hormones, like cortisol, in dogs after trauma, infection, or surgery. Each time a case was enrolled, the dog had to undergo hormone testing that took approximately four hours. I enrolled nearly a dozen dogs and thus spent almost 50 hours performing tests, recording data, and processing the samples that were to be shipped and analyzed at Auburn. Horrifyingly, I learned that the frozen blood samples I'd shipped to the veterinary school had thawed during transport. This meant they were no longer viable for a portion of the study tests. To say that the loss of all this time and effort, including obtaining consent from the pet owners to retrieve the blood samples, was distressing would be an understatement. Thankfully, some tests were still able to be performed and most of the data was ultimately published in a scientific paper years later.

The second situation was the diagnosis of potentially pre-cancerous cells during my routine PAP test. I was notified by student health of the atypical results and a colposcopy (scope) and biopsy of my cervix was recommended. Unfortunately, I couldn't make an appointment with an OB-GYN (obstetrician-gynecologist) prior to my exam (just weeks away at that point), so I decided to put this on hold until after. Consequently, the abnormal results nagged at my mind while I was studying, despite my attempts to push them aside in the hope that all would be well in the end. Which, thankfully, it was.

Almost comically, the drama around my board certification exams didn't end when I finished studying. In fact, the real drama began days before I traveled to Phoenix, where the exams were being held. This was in September of 2008, and I had a flight from Raleigh to Phoenix, connecting in Houston. At that very same time Hurricane Ike was making its way toward the Texas coastline and was projected to make landfall in Houston as a Category 2 storm. So, it's not surprising that my flight was canceled. I frantically managed to re-route through Chicago, arriving 48 hours before my exam was set to start.

Due to the expense of taking the exam ($1,000 USD), traveling to Phoenix, and registering for the conference (mandatory for all residents taking the exam), I was on a budget. I'd therefore chosen one of several "satellite hotels" close enough to walk to the conference. Upon landing at the Phoenix airport, I asked my cab driver to take me to my hotel, to which he responded, "which location?" It hadn't occurred to me that there was more than one hotel with the same name! When we arrived, I immediately realized I'd booked the wrong place: the lobby was a ghost town, far from anything that resembled a conference center and with no signage or information pertinent to the meeting. I panicked. It quickly became apparent that the cab ride downtown to where the conference center was located would take at least 45 minutes during rush-hour traffic. My upcoming three-day, eight hours per day exam that was going to validate the last three agonizing years of my life was about to be derailed by traffic and a cab ride I couldn't afford. After a few hours of tears, futile attempts to study, and several desperate phone calls, one of my residency mentors offered to share her room with me (and my three binders of study notes) on a promise that we wouldn't speak a word about the exam.

Thankfully I got through three grueling days of exams, and, months later, I received my passing results to become a proud board-certified member of the American College of Veterinary Emergency and Critical Care. Not bad considering less than half of the residents who wrote the same year passed and all that I went through in the months leading up to the exam. To this day, those results embody one of the biggest moments of simultaneous joy and relief I've experienced.

In the more than 15 years that have passed since I wrote my board certification exam, individuals have sought to investigate the mental health and wellbeing of veterinary residents and what can be done to better support them. Several stressors unique to house officers (interns, residents, and fellows) have been identified with survey research (Box 2).[2] This led the American Association of Veterinary Medical Colleges (AAVMC) to administer a survey to interns and residents in United States veterinary colleges, as well as private and corporate practices. The survey revealed large proportions of the respondents expressing concerns about aspects of their physical and mental wellbeing, access to mental health resources, workload, and learning environment. Overall, symptoms of moderate-to-severe depression impacted more than half of respondents and nearly one-third were reporting post-traumatic stress disorder (PTSD) symptoms or thoughts of suicide (Box 3).[3]

Box 2: Did You Know?

A survey of veterinary interns, residents, and fellows in 2017–2018 revealed their most common stressors were finances, mental and emotional impact of the work environment, organizational skills, patient management, relationships, research, teaching, time management, and work–life balance.[2]

Box 3: Did You Know?

A 2020 survey[3] of more than 470 house officers, representing about 25% of the total population of interns and residents, revealed that

- 85% reported experiencing depressive symptoms within the previous two weeks
- 60% felt emotionally drained from work a few times a week or every day
- 54% screened positive for moderate-to-severe depression
- 53% disagreed or strongly disagreed that there was enough faculty/clinical and staff support provided for their program
- 52% experienced problems with debt
- 35% felt their program offered adequate mental health support services
- 30% reported having some measure of suicidal ideation over the past two weeks

---

Additionally, certain characteristics of the training program trended among those who were satisfied or dissatisfied with their experience. Respondents who reported overall satisfaction in their programs had programs with characteristics such as quality mentoring; structured scheduling and protected time off; dedication to teaching; supportive workplace culture; adequate staffing; accessible mental health and wellbeing supports; and affirming, professional feedback. Conversely, respondents who reported lower satisfaction in their program shared that their programs had characteristics such as poor communication; a lack of structured learning opportunities; unprofessional workplace culture; unsuitable workload, hours, or scheduling; a lack of psychosocial support; poor mentorship; and inconsistencies within the program experience.[3]

Perhaps unsurprisingly, residents in emergency and critical care had lower physical wellbeing scores, more severe PTSD scores, lower access to mental health resources, higher burnout scores, and lower workload satisfaction scores compared to those in other specialties. Interestingly, the survey also revealed that if you were female or single, like me, you were more likely to have less desirable scores for physical wellbeing, depression, burnout, workload satisfaction, or social support.[3] These findings mirror those of a more recent survey of residents in more than 20 specialty programs, which revealed that those in emergency and critical care residencies had the lowest quality of life scores across the domains of physical and psychological health, social relationships, and environment.[4]

Henceforth, many changes have since been made to residency programs like mine, with the intention of reducing the stress and workload of residents and allowing time and space for studying and self-care. These changes stem from the findings from the AAVMC study, as well as recommendations from the AAVMC House Officer Wellbeing Task Force guidelines for internship and residency programs published in 2022 (Box 4).[5] A significant change that has happened in my residency program since I completed my training is the addition of more residents to provide 24/7 ICU and ER coverage that allows for breaks and reprieve as necessary between shifts. This included the addition of an overnight ICU shift, which was prompted by concerns about resident fatigue due to increasing caseloads and overnight phone calls. This shift is designated "Super" and is taken by a resident who oversees both ICU and ER caseloads overnight.

Faculty availability has also improved, with dedicated oversight for daytime ER and ICU and an on-call ICU faculty overnight. Additionally, board preparation has been revamped with a structured three-year cycle, dividing topics among faculty members and incorporating mandatory readings, PowerPoint lectures, and occasional guest speakers. Residents now benefit from scheduled four-day shifts followed by dedicated "reading days," introduced in the second half of the first year. These changes aim to enhance resident education and wellbeing, while maintaining high standards of patient care amidst a very busy caseload.

Box 4: Did You Know?

The American College of Veterinary Medical Colleges devised Guide-lines for Veterinary Intern and Resident Wellbeing in 2020.[5] Recommendations and their associated resources include:

- addressing organizational culture
- developing leadership skills
- addressing conflict in the workplace
- dismantling power dynamics
- establishing a house officer training program oversight committee
- promoting and allowing for health and wellbeing
- addressing barriers to access
- taking a holistic approach to wellbeing
- aligning supporting policies and systems
- limiting financial distress
- enacting flexible scheduling
- implementing maximum duty hours
- redesigning workflows
- enhancing mentorship
- developing quality mentors
- providing constructive performance evaluations

In reflecting on the onslaught of challenges faced during my residency, I'm struck by the resilience it demanded and the growth it facilitated. From battling imposter syndrome to grappling with personal loss and professional setbacks, each obstacle tested my resolve and shaped my journey. Despite the trials, I remained steadfast in my pursuit of knowledge and board certification, drawing strength from the support of mentors and the camaraderie of fellow residents. Now, as I navigate the field with a deeper understanding of its complexities and a commitment to advocate for house officer wellbeing, I carry with me the invaluable lessons learned from overcoming adversity, knowing they have made me a stronger and more compassionate veterinarian.

Adventures in Veterinary Academia

While being in academia has its downsides (lower pay is the big one), I wished I could let my young colleagues know that there are many more upsides in academia. The first and foremost upside is my coworkers—and I mean all my coworkers—including the vet students, the staff, the veterinary nurses, the interns and residents and my faculty peers. We work as a team, and we are all in a growth mindset.

—Terri DeFrancesco, DVM, DACVIM (Cardiology),
DACVECC
(Professor of Cardiology and Critical Care Medicine)

After more than a decade of postsecondary education and a rigorous residency, I was ready to begin my first job as a veterinary specialist. I'd developed a profound passion for teaching during my internship and residency, so I chose to apply for several different faculty positions at academic institutions across the USA and Canada. I started these applications in the third year of my residency program, putting myself forward for academic job openings at Cornell University, Texas A&M University, and the University of Minnesota, among others.

The process of applying and interviewing for academic jobs is rigorous and intimidating, especially for a third-year resident. Most academic applications require a curriculum vitae (CV) listing the education, training, research, teaching, publications, and committee or volunteer work a person has done, as well as a letter of intent describing teaching, research, and clinical aspirations. Once a candidate's application is accepted, they begin the interview process. This usually includes a two-day visit to the veterinary school, where the applicant meets with members of the candidate selection committee, in addition to others in the Dean's Office and teaching hospital. There are tours, meals, and other informal gatherings, as well as one or two presentations where the candidate is asked to share their teaching philosophy and research aspirations. These interviews allow you to get a sense of the school and the people you'd be working with, as well as helping the selection committee determine your suitability for the role.

I remember interviewing at Cornell University, an Ivy League veterinary school ranked No. 1 in the USA in 2008, the year I completed my residency. Rather than moving around the school to meet others and chat informally, I sat in a room where others came to see me for a full day of interviews. While

DOI: 10.1201/9781003347385-6

everyone was polite and some made an extra effort to ease my nerves, it was immediately clear that I wasn't going to be a successful candidate. Each person who sat down in front of me asked, "What's your plan to develop your research program at Cornell?" Research program? Develop it? At the time, I was a third-year resident who had published a few peer-reviewed articles; I was in no position to be creating a rigorous research program to Ivy League standards. After returning to North Carolina exhausted and somewhat deflated, I learned that an internal candidate at Cornell had also applied for the position. With his PhD in addition to his specialty certification, I felt pretty certain that I'd been interviewed only to make the application process appear fair.

My interviews at the University of Minnesota and Texas A&M went more smoothly, and it was exciting to visit other veterinary schools, see the different designs of their teaching hospitals, and learn about research and teaching opportunities from current faculty members. I began to really picture myself as a faculty member of a veterinary school and grew excited to pursue my passion for teaching while performing clinical and non-clinical research.

In the end, Texas A&M offered me a tenure-track Assistant Professor position. While I pondered my future as a young Canadian faculty member in College Station, I learned of a yearlong position being offered at the Ontario Veterinary College (OVC), University of Guelph. The role was temporary, covering for a longstanding and esteemed faculty member in small animal emergency and critical care who was taking a leave of absence for health reasons. The thought of getting to live north of the border again and work at one of the oldest and most respected veterinary schools in Canada was invigorating. Although the idea of looking for another job (and having to move again) in a year's time felt daunting, I decided to apply. I didn't have to feign my enthusiasm about being one of the few emergency and critical care specialists in Canada at the time, and at one of the best veterinary schools in the world (Box 1). During my very positive job interview, I shared plans to continue research on the biomarker capabilities of electrolyte imbalances in critical patients. I met with other faculty members and staff, most of whom had graduated from or done their residency training at OVC, and I felt immediately at home.

Box 1: Top 10 Universities in the World for Veterinary Science in 2024[1]

1. Royal Veterinary College, University of London, United Kingdom
2. University of California, Davis, USA
3. Cornell University, USA
4. Vetsuisse Faculty, Bern and Zurich, Switzerland
5. Utrecht University, Netherlands
6. University of Pennsylvania, USA
7. Texas A&M University, USA
8. University of Guelph, Canada
9. University of Edinburgh, United Kingdom
10. Colorado State University, USA

To my delight, I was offered the temporary position at the OVC, which I accepted. My heart was being pulled back to Canada. So, just one week after I wrote my board certification exam in Phoenix, I packed up my belongings and drove north across the border to Ontario, where I would begin my academic veterinary career. Because my contract began so soon after my exam, I had to rent the upstairs of a house sight unseen and lived solely with the belongings I could fit in my car until my moving truck arrived weeks later. This meant sleeping on an air mattress until my bed frame and other items made the journey! At this point, I recall asking one of my residency program mentors whether I should delay the beginning of my yearlong contract to allow for some downtime. He smiled and shrugged, reassuring me that most academic jobs started off relatively relaxed, a new faculty member having weeks (or even months) to get settled prior to starting their clinic coverage, the most rigorous part of the job.

You can imagine my surprise when I arrived on the first day of my OVC orientation and was told I'd be working in the clinic the following week! It turned out that my colleague had been covering clinics several weeks consecutively while the other faculty member began her leave. She was exhausted, having been the only advisor and mentor available for the emergency and critical care service, including the two residents and four interns currently in training. Eager for a break, she felt it best that I start my clinic duties right away. So began my brutal transition from resident-in-training to faculty member training residents. If the move from veterinary student to intern felt like a jump, the transition from resident to faculty was a giant leap. I could hardly believe that I was the one whom students, interns, and residents were now coming to with questions about managing cases or concerns about speaking with clients.

Thankfully I jumped into the role with gusto, wholeheartedly embracing my new responsibilities and utilizing the recent wisdom bestowed upon me while cramming for my exam just months before. I was keen to teach the residents everything (and more!) that I had learned during my own residency program, and I intended to do this with supplemental physiology and board preparation rounds, in addition to the weekly journal clubs that were already scheduled. Unsurprisingly, my new colleague was somewhat perturbed by my efforts to broaden the teaching opportunities for the current residents, given her own exhaustion and burnout. This led to some disgruntled conversations and requests for me to curb my enthusiasm, which at the time I couldn't comprehend but now understand completely.

This was also my firsthand experience of the competition that can occur in veterinary academia. During my residency, I had witnessed surgeons who competed for cases and research grants and resented each other with obvious vehemence, so the concept of competition among faculty wasn't new to me. However, I soon discovered the intensity of competition for research funding, teaching awards, annual review accolades, top student evaluations, and committee roles in academia. Assessments in academia don't stop once you graduate; they continue through yearly reviews, promotion and tenure evaluations, and student feedback. And let me tell you—these processes are both grueling and humbling.

Promotion and tenure (often referred to as "P&T") is an essential aspect of academic life, requiring faculty to demonstrate excellence in teaching, research, and service. This comprehensive evaluation ensures that faculty members are not only contributing to their respective fields through innovative research, but are also effective educators and active participants in academic and community service. The process typically involves a thorough review of the faculty member's accomplishments, including peer-reviewed publications, successful grant applications, and positive student evaluations. It also assesses contributions to departmental and university committees, mentorship of students and junior faculty, and engagement in professional organizations. Promotion and tenure provides a sense of job security and recognition of a faculty member's hard work and dedication.

While I was initially hired on a one-year contract, after nine months the previous professor officially stepped down from her role and a tenure-track position opened. I applied for and gratefully accepted the role of Assistant Professor, which included an approximate breakdown of 50% clinic responsibilities, 30% research duties, and 20% teaching and administrative work. For most individuals, an application for tenure and promotion from Assistant to Associate or Associate to Full Professor occurs within three to five years. So, four years after I was initially hired, I began the arduous task of preparing my promotion and tenure portfolio with the intention of applying for promotion to Associate Professor. This physically and mentally exhausting process takes months and involves not only accumulating all the previous years' tasks and accomplishments, but also writing portfolios related to teaching, research, and administrative duties, in addition to obtaining letters of reference from faculty members at other institutions. As arduous as it sounds, I was grateful for the opportunity to reflect on and showcase the "fruits of my labor" since my beginning at OVC.

There are also non-tenure-track roles with varied responsibilities, such as administration, student teaching (in clinics, classrooms, and labs), and mentoring graduate students, interns, and residents. These faculty members play a critical role in bridging the gap between theoretical knowledge and practical skills by providing hands-on training in veterinary medicine. They are deeply involved in supervising students during clinical rotations, overseeing case management, and offering guidance on diagnostic and therapeutic decisions. Additionally, they may take on administrative duties such as managing clinical services, while also mentoring interns and residents in their research projects and clinical practice. Despite typically lacking the job security and advancement opportunities of tenure-track positions, non-tenure-track roles can offer a dynamic and fulfilling environment for those dedicated to teaching and direct patient care, contributing significantly to the quality of veterinary education and the development of future veterinarians.

Working in academia offers numerous advantages, including access to cutting-edge technologies and specialized treatments. More than 15 years ago when I chose an academic job over a role in a specialty practice, procedures like subcutaneous ureteral bypass (SUB) surgery and hemodialysis were almost exclusively offered at veterinary teaching hospitals. Moreover, the collaborative environment within academic institutions provides ample opportunities for professional growth and development, with colleagues often sharing knowledge and expertise across disciplines. Faculty members also have the privilege of implementing evidence-based practices, ensuring that they deliver the highest standard of care to their patients while contributing to advancements in veterinary medicine.

However, the benefits of academic life come with unique challenges, notably a lower salary compared to private practice, which can be a deterrent for some individuals (Box 2). Additionally, the demands of academia extend beyond clinical duties, requiring faculty members to juggle teaching, research, and administrative responsibilities, often leading to an imbalance between work and personal life. It often felt to me that the work as a faculty member was "never-ending"; there was always another paper to write, research grant to apply for, study to design, elective rotation to create, or student to mentor. Also, academia is an environment that continuously fosters scrutiny. Whether it be from peer reviewers for a submitted research paper, students during their course evaluations, or the department chair with annual assessments, it's a non-stop cycle of feedback that can leave faculty members feeling perpetually under the microscope. For more on the critical shortage of veterinary specialists and how this shortage disproportionately impacts academia—where attracting and retaining specialists is increasingly difficult—refer to Chapter 12, where I explore the growing demand for specialists and its far-reaching consequences across the profession.

Box 2: Did You Know?

According to a survey of veterinary surgery specialists in 2015, those working in private practice had a higher median income ($206,000 USD) compared to those in academia ($124,000),[2] a trend that persists across most specialties in veterinary medicine.

I poignantly remember my first time receiving student evaluations for my lectures on fluid therapy and CPR. I let out a sigh of relief as I saw that my scores were "very good" to "excellent," but then felt immediately deflated as I read through the comments and saw critiques of my tone of voice and some of the phrases I used. The 80-some positive reviews were immediately abolished by the one or two negative comments that I received. Similarly, when I received my first annual faculty review and was given an assessment of "good" rather than "very good" or "excellent," I felt like I'd been punched in the stomach. After what seemed like an excruciating year covering half of the clinic schedule, mentoring residents, taking on a new graduate student, and successfully applying for research funding, a "good" was perceived as a "meh" and a clear indication to me that I should be doing more.

Navigating the promotion and tenure process in academia, especially in the face of large clinical service responsibilities, also presents its fair share of challenges. Balancing the demands of clinical work with scholarly pursuits often leaves little time for traditional research endeavors, such as publishing in prestigious journals or securing external funding. While the importance of diverse scholarly activities beyond research is increasingly recognized in academic veterinary medicine, existing evaluation criteria may not fully capture the value of clinical service engagement. Based on examples in other healthcare professions, it's clear that we need to rethink how we assess and reward scholarly contributions in veterinary medicine. Providing mentorship, fostering a culture that values various forms of scholarship, and developing tailored assessment methods are key steps toward ensuring that faculty efforts in clinical, diagnostic, and scholarly domains are appropriately acknowledged and incentivized. This shift not only enhances patient care and career satisfaction, but also elevates institutional standing and advances the broader veterinary profession.

Despite these downsides, many veterinarians, myself included, find fulfillment in academia's intellectually stimulating environment and the opportunity to make a meaningful impact on both students and the broader field of veterinary medicine. The satisfaction derived from mentoring the next generation of veterinarians and witnessing their professional development is unparalleled. While the trials of academia are undeniable, in my humble opinion, the rewards of shaping the future of veterinary medicine far outweigh them.

6

A Departure from Academic Life

Many of us had to fight hard to even get into vet school. We had to make our whole lives about achieving the goal of becoming a veterinarian for many years, so once we have achieved that goal, it's hard to remember who we were before all of that stress and hard work. It's like it (severe competition, overworking, stress, exhaustion, selflessness, etc.) becomes a part of our soul and mindset that I feel many of us can't separate ourselves from even after we have graduated.

—Christine Nawas, BScH, DVM
(Small Animal Associate Veterinarian)

To say that people were shocked when I announced that I was leaving my Assistant Professor job would be an understatement. Some even expressed indignation, certain that I was making a big mistake. They knew how much I loved and was succeeding in my role in academia, and they simply couldn't comprehend how I would be fulfilled doing anything else. You can imagine their confusion when they learned I was abandoning academic work entirely to pursue freelance work!

In 2013, when I made my decision to resign, I'd published more than 25 manuscripts, helped supervise nine graduate students, mentored seven emergency and critical care residents, overseen four summer veterinary students, and successfully submitted my application for promotion and tenure. All of this in the less than five years that I had served as a faculty member. There was no doubt that I loved my work and was proficient at it. Yet, for reasons I couldn't put my finger on, it didn't feel sustainable. At the time, I didn't recognize it, but, in hindsight, I was already experiencing the early signs of burnout—an issue that has plagued many in our profession. I explore this in more depth in Chapter 27, where I unpack the symptoms, causes, and lasting impacts of burnout in veterinary medicine, drawing from both personal experiences and broader industry insights.

The reality was that outside of work, I was struggling. I felt out of place in Ontario, the most populated province in Canada. Nearly everyone I worked with at the veterinary school was born there, most having completed their veterinary school, internship, or residency (or all three!) in Ontario. My col-

DOI: 10.1201/9781003347385-7

leagues had nearby family and established friendships and felt entirely "at home." This meant that making social plans was often challenging, as people were inevitably busy with old friends or family on weekends. I recall planning "ladies' nights" for the female faculty members and having some really enjoyable conversations with colleagues over cocktails and a meal. But I was the only person who planned those events, and they were few and far between.

As I neared my midlife, I also grappled with not having my own chosen family. I'd always envisioned getting married and having children. Yet despite signing up for Match.com and other dating websites (this was before dating apps!) I'd had little to no success in meeting a compatible partner. After several failed relationships that never felt quite right, I started to worry that my "person" was not living in southern Ontario.

Similar to the East and West Coasts of the United States being vastly different in both geography and general vibe, so too was the difference between Ontario and Alberta, the province where I grew up. Ontario, with its population of more than 14.2 million residents, is filled with natural bodies of water, including some of the largest lakes in North America. Alberta is populated by 4.3 million people and virtually land-locked (Box 1).[1] When I dabbled in sprint triathlons in Ontario, I quickly stopped doing races because I was utterly terrified of swimming in open water. Southern Ontario is also known for its "rat race" mentality, heavily focused on work, status, and material belongings, and I was astounded by the competition I experienced, both personally and professionally. This was in stark contrast to the more laidback Alberta, where life felt simpler, the people seemed friendlier, and there was less pressure to keep up with the Joneses.

Box 1: Did You Know?

Alberta is one of the prairie provinces in western Canada and has approximately 500 lakes,[2] in comparison to Ontario's more than 250,000.[3]

In addition to the sense that I somehow didn't belong in Ontario, I began to experience a plethora of health problems. I developed gastrointestinal symptoms consistent with irritable bowel syndrome (IBS), which were confirmed with an endoscopic procedure that ruled out Crohn's or Celiac disease. I struggled with chronic insomnia that led to exhaustion and crankiness, which no doubt stemmed from late nights working and time spent on-call. I had symptoms of depression, including feelings of severe sadness, restlessness, and irritability. I felt persistently anxious and preoccupied with worries about what the future held for my work and general happiness. On Sunday evenings, prior to starting a week in the clinic, my worry culminated in anxiety attacks when my heart would race, my breathing would quicken, and I'd be up most of the night unable to sleep (Box 2).

> **Box 2: Did You Know?**
>
> Anxiety attacks occur in response to a perceived stressor or threat and often follow a period of persistent worrying. Symptoms vary in severity from mild to severe and include nervousness, irritability, increased heart rate, rapid breathing, trembling, sweating, a sense of impending danger, difficulty concentrating, or sleep disturbances.[4]

At first, I told myself that these symptoms were normal and experienced by most people with stressful jobs or demanding careers. But when I shared my problems with my naturopathic doctor and, later, my family physician, they expressed concern. My naturopathic doctor suggested that I try to scale back work and take better care of myself. I scoffed at the idea that work could be the source of my problems, but I agreed that a healthier diet, probiotics, and vitamins were worth trying. I committed to exercising more to manage my stress and found myself running, swimming, or attending group fitness classes nearly seven days a week. When coworkers and friends saw me outside of work (and not wearing scrubs), they gently shared their concerns about my weight. I had always been slim with an athletic build, but my intense aerobic exercise coupled with ill health had led to marked loss of body and muscle mass.

After a year of adding tinctures, adrenal restoring herbs, and other non-medicinal concoctions to my daily regimen, most of my symptoms continued. I'd recently been through a breakup and the relationship had been considerably unhealthy. I'd somehow convinced myself that any relationship at this stage in my life was better than no relationship, so I allowed the verbal and emotional abuse to persist. Afterward, I couldn't fathom how I'd stayed with an abusive partner for so many months, instead of standing up for myself and demanding the treatment that I deserved. I questioned my life decisions and my capacity for being in a healthy relationship; ultimately, my self-esteem plummeted and my depression worsened. I'd never been prescribed an antidepressant before, but I obliged when my physician suggested it. I also briefly sought counseling, but never fully disclosed the extent of my troubles. My anxiety and depression symptoms improved with the medication, but my feelings of isolation and uncertainty persisted.

At this point my naturopathic doctor's pleas for me to consider stepping away from work were growing louder and more urgent. But thoughts of leaving my colleague alone as the only faculty member for our specialty, putting a strain on service coverage, resident mentoring, and student teaching, only led to more anxiety. I finally met with the university's human resources (HR) department to discuss whether I would qualify for some sort of medical leave. I doubted that this was a path I would choose and wasn't convinced that my situation would even qualify me for a leave, but I felt the need to consider all options. I was grasping for alternatives to resignation that would leave the least amount of fallout. The HR representative, with whom I met for more than an hour, urged me not to resign, assuring me that my mental and physical symptoms combined with the concerns of my healthcare team would qualify me for a medical leave or short-term disability. But after months of considering this option, I felt that it would be the least tenable for my team.

And so I did what many veterinarians in our profession have done when their work situation feels unsustainable. I turned in my resignation. I told people that I felt the need to be closer to family and friends in the province where I'd grown up and that I'd be pursuing freelance work as an emergency and critical care specialist and public speaker. Both were true, but I didn't reveal the true extent of my health concerns. In fact, I'd made my decision based on the recommendations of my healthcare team, my ongoing mental and physical health struggles, and my desire to do what I believed would be best for my colleagues moving forward. This meant giving six months' notice so that my position could be filled prior to me leaving at the end of 2013.

Once the decision was made, I felt relief, trepidation, and excitement. I've always been someone who has thrived on change and new beginnings, so I set my sights on what I was certain would be a successful transition to a fulfilled and balanced life. I listed my home in Guelph that I had purchased just three years before, sold most of my new furniture, and gave away my old furniture to residents or interns in need. Then I packed up the rest of my belongings and flew across the country in time to spend Christmas with my parents and new dog, which is where I stayed for the next six months.

By this time, I had gratefully adopted another Standard Poodle named Faith, who had come into my life during the final year of my residency, had moved with me to Ontario, and would accompany me back home to Alberta. She was another one of my parents' dogs who had been purchased by a breeder and handler in New Orleans as a puppy. Sadly, when Hurricane Katrina struck Louisiana in 2005, the home of Faith's owner was destroyed, and she was forced to relocate to Florida. Months later, she resigned herself to the fact that she needed to focus on rebuilding her life and could not afford to show or care for Faith. So my parents eagerly offered to take Faith back, after which they promptly had someone drive her more than 600 miles to me in North Carolina. My parents insisted that I needed a new dog to keep me company after the loss of Ronnie and they assured me it would only be "temporary." At first, I was furious with my parents for "forcing" a dog on me when I felt I had nowhere near recovered from the loss of my last dog. However, it didn't take long for Faith to win over my heart, despite being terribly fearful, ridiculously hyper, and occasionally growling at strangers. With a tincture of time (and a lot of socialization), Faith became my "heart dog" and relentless companion.

In the first half of 2014, I became immersed in setting myself up for free-lance work. I hired a web designer to build a website highlighting my skills and experience as a specialist, speaker, researcher, and writer. I borrowed books from the library on business and networking, and I used their wisdom

Figure 6.1
Faith and Marie at the Ontario Veterinary School when she was a faculty member at the University of Guelph.

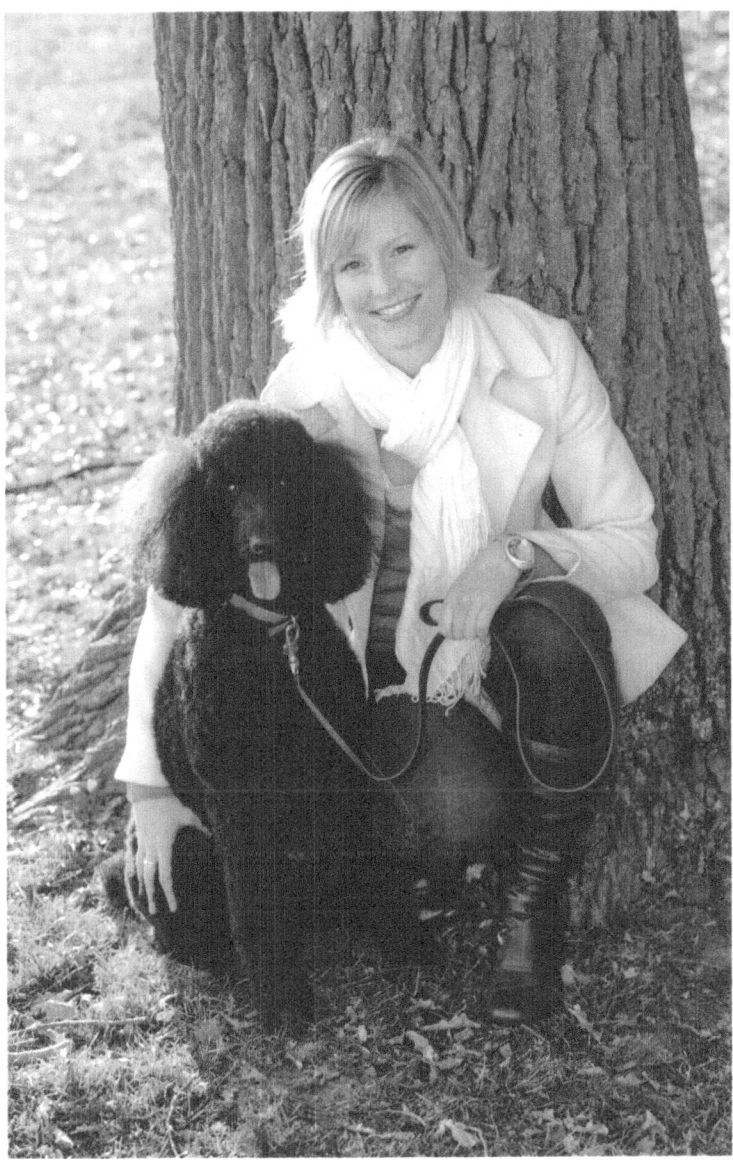

to reach out to most people I knew, sharing my recent career change and asking for advice, connections, or opportunities. I researched corporate veterinary-related organizations and sent letters of intent to Elanco, Hills, IDEXX, and Pfizer (now Zoetis). Because I remained passionate about continuing to provide education and training to veterinarians and technicians, I hired a consultant to help me create a business plan for offering in-clinic consulting, lectures, and training for veterinary practices in western Canada. I even applied for a part-time position as an instructor at the local animal health technology school where veterinary technicians were trained. Continuously putting myself out there was exhausting, and, initially, the lack of opportunities that materialized left me feeling a strong sense of remorse.

Thankfully I eventually got some breaks. I was invited to be an assistant editor for the Journal of Veterinary Emergency and Critical Care, responsible for facilitating the peer-review process. My passion for writing and editing served me well, although it was a very small role that offered no financial compensation at the time. I continued to volunteer for the newly established VetCOT (the Veterinary Committee on Trauma), and I spearheaded the creation of a large trauma database for dogs and cats (Box 3). I was also contacted by a publisher who had received a proposal for a textbook on transfusion medicine and blood banking, one of my areas of expertise, and was asked if I would consider co-editing. Not surprisingly, I jumped at the chance.

Box 3: Did You Know?

The Veterinary Committee on Trauma database was begun in 2014 and is a collection of dog and cat case information submitted by Veterinary Trauma Center leads and their staff. As of August 2022, the database had more than 55,000 cases and more than 20 associated research publications.[5]

Taking advantage of my newfound flexibility to travel, I gathered the names and emails of the state and provincial veterinary medical organizations and conferences and sent more than 100 emails asking organizers if they were looking for a speaker with my expertise. At the time I wasn't well known and had been a veterinarian for only a decade, so the responses, when I did receive them, expressed mediocre enthusiasm at best. Nevertheless, I continued my efforts to reach out to anyone I could think of, asserting that I was ready for hire as a locum emergency and critical care specialist, speaker, or consultant.

Eventually, I decided that Calgary would be the better place for me to root myself as a freelance specialist. At the time, the city of more than 1.2 million people was a hub for air travel in western Canada, and home to the University of Calgary Faculty of Veterinary Medicine, VCA Canada headquarters, and two large veterinary specialty hospitals. It felt like a no-brainer for me to live near these potential employers with easy flights out as other opportunities arose. After contacting the specialty veterinary hospital's practice managers, I was offered Friday through Sunday shifts at one of the hospitals to offset the Monday through Thursday coverage of the full-time emergency and critical

Figure 6.2
Faith and Marie after leaving her faculty position to do freelance work.

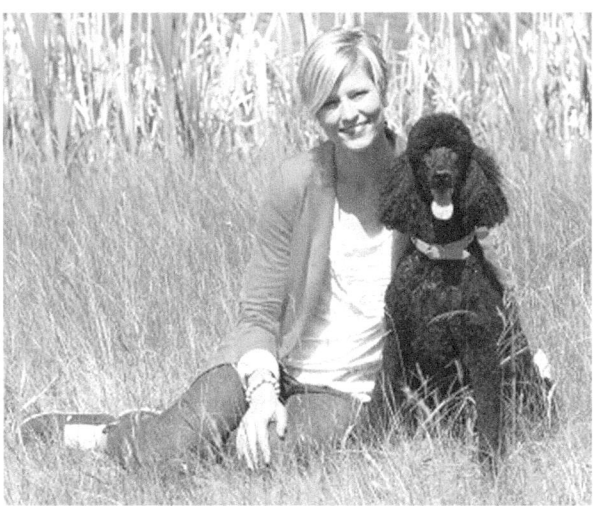

care specialist. I was excited to get back into clinical practice—and to generate income again! So, with a few belongings and Faith in tow, I drove three hours south and stayed at my cousin's house while I sussed out the city. I wasn't sure where these opportunities would lead, but I felt confident that I'd made the right decision in pursuing a fresh start.

7

Transforming Overwhelm into Opportunity

Wish there was more on mental health and self-care. Especially self-care and the mental drain this profession can take. Everything from emotional blackmail of clients to dealing with our own guilt. I was told once, you can't care more than the client does. That was somehow supposed to make things all better!?!

—Stephanie Dodds, DVM
(General Practitioner and Practice Owner)

After moving to Calgary, I threw myself into my new business, despite having virtually zero experience being an entrepreneur. I had my new website, some business cards, and the determination to send emails to anyone who would read them, but getting work, especially paid work, wasn't easy for me. Keep in mind that this was 2014 and the current shortage of veterinarians and specialists wasn't present then (Box 1). In fact, the American Veterinary Medical Association Workforce Study released a report highlighting a 13% excess of veterinarians that was predicted, at the time, to continue through 2025.[1]

Box 1: Did You Know?

In 2013, *The New York Times* published an article titled "High Debt and Falling Demand Trap New Vets," which highlighted concerns regarding the number of veterinarians graduating in the United States with student debts exceeding $300k amidst a bleak job market that limited many new grad veterinarians to part-time employment.[2]

Looking back, there was a simultaneous lull in demand for specialists. Friends of mine who'd finished their residency programs after me were finding that the number of roles available in both specialty and academic practice were few and far between. Many of them were having to "sell themselves" to practices to create demand for their services. Emergency and critical care was experiencing growing pains as one of the fastest expanding specialties in terms of the number of new boarded diplomates (Box 2). But there was in-

DOI: 10.1201/9781003347385-8

creasing division within the specialty college: a split between those gravitating more toward emergency medicine and surgery and others who favored the critical or intensive care medicine aspects. It's difficult to market your specialty services to others when it's not completely clear what that specialty does!

Box 2: Did You Know?

In 2008, there were 263 specialists who were board certified in veterinary emergency and critical care medicine. That number more than doubled to 590 specialists in 2016 and, by 2021, it totaled 834 specialists.[3]

Additionally, many owners and managers of specialty practices claimed to function "just fine" with coverage of the so-called core specialties (i.e., internal medicine and surgery). They simply couldn't fathom what a specialist in emergency and critical care could offer. This led to a plethora of threads on our specialty email list related to "selling" our skills, since so much of what we do day to day is cognitive, not procedural. In other words, we spend a lot of time caring for patients in-hospital by managing pain, tweaking intravenous fluids, adjusting medications, and monitoring vital signs. By contrast, our surgery and internal medicine specialty colleagues perform fracture repairs or endoscopic procedures that generate tangible income.

At the time, Calgary had two specialty hospitals, one with a relatively new emergency and critical care specialist who was attempting to grow the service and the other whose leadership were uninterested in creating such a service. I was working Friday, Saturday, and Sunday shifts at the former hospital, but this schedule wasn't desirable long term. Unfortunately, there were no locum (temporary coverage) positions open for emergency and critical care specialists in Canada or the United States at the time. Most hospitals were just getting their feet wet in terms of hiring critical care specialists and none were so established that they were seeking relief coverage.

The limited employment I was able to obtain in clinical practice led me to seek other work that I enjoyed. I kept following up with organizations and conferences that offered continuing education so that I could nurture my passion for teaching by lecturing to veterinarians and technicians. My favorite topics included trauma, fluid therapy, transfusion medicine, blood banking, electrolyte disturbances, shock, and respiratory distress. I spoke at the annual conferences of the Ontario, Alberta, and Canadian Veterinary Medical Associations that year and, for the following year, I lined up speaking engagements in the greater Toronto area, Indiana, Connecticut, Saskatchewan, and Las Vegas. But these events paid only modest stipends and were few and far between, so I needed to work on securing income elsewhere.

I began reaching out to veterinary schools and practices to offer my services as a trainer and educator in their emergency departments. The emergency and critical care specialist at Western College of Veterinary Medicine had recently left her role, and I ended up with a two-week locum to provide teaching and training there and another at North Carolina State University. But the work it took to network and find these opportunities, never mind the exhaustive process of getting a license and arranging travel for these locum stints, left me feeling frustrated and overwhelmed. My answer to this was, of course, to work harder.

Predictably, I fell into a familiar pattern of workaholism, anxiety, and overwhelm. I had few friends in Calgary, so it was easy to dedicate all my spare time to finding more locum, consulting, or speaking opportunities. The cost of living in Calgary was exorbitant; I was forced to rent a small studio or one-bedroom apartment where I'd work hunched over my laptop at my breakfast bar or relocate to local coffee shops. I'd spend hours agonizing over website edits, researching different speaking opportunities, tweaking emails to veterinary practices and organizations, listening to podcast episodes related to online marketing and social media, and learning about thought leadership and business development. I believed that if I could simply work harder, or perfect what I was offering, then I'd find the opportunities I needed and make ends meet. This relentless pursuit of perfectionism, something I later realized was more harmful than helpful, is a recurring theme in my career. In Chapter 22, I dive deeper into the complexities of perfectionism in the veterinary profession, exploring how it intersects with imposter syndrome and its profound impact on mental health and wellbeing.

In doing so, I threw my personal and professional boundaries to the wind, allowing my mental health and wellbeing to dwindle further. I worked incessantly, everywhere I could plug in my laptop and access Wi-Fi. I was also co-editing the textbook on veterinary transfusion medicine and blood banking, which meant dedicating hours at a time and months on end to researching articles, soliciting authors, and writing or editing chapters. It was undeniably interesting and important work, but it was all-consuming and, worst of all, unpaid. And while we'd end up with a published textbook to sell to veterinary teams across the world, the money generated from the royalties of textbook sales are in the hundreds (not thousands) of dollars per year—hardly sufficient income.

The relentless work hours, combined with the undesirable clinic shifts I was working during the weekends, led to familiar exhaustion. I noticed my depressive symptoms starting to flare up again, including feelings of hopelessness, helplessness, and pessimism regarding the veterinary profession, my specialty, and, worst of all, my decision to leave a stable academic job that I loved. I started to experience insomnia again, exacerbated by the occasional swing shifts I was working. My irritable bowel syndrome worsened and I felt constantly sad and cranky. Despite working out routinely and even joining a competitive women's basketball team, my self-esteem plummeted, and I found I no longer enjoyed these activities.

It felt like nothing was in my control. After a drastic move across the country to make a lasting, positive change in my life, I was right back where I started, on the hamster wheel of perfectionism, workaholism, and depression. Yet again, I couldn't see a sustainable way forward in veterinary medicine and began to question whether I was cut out for self-employment. Research telling me that entrepreneurs experience depression at rates higher than most employed individuals was no consolation (Box 3).

Box 3: Did You Know?

A nationwide survey of nearly 500 Canadian entrepreneurs found that 62% felt depressed at least once per week and nearly half (46%) believed their mental health problems interfered with their ability to work. Mental health concerns were more often reported among females, those with business in the growth or early stages, and those with fewer employees or lower revenue.[4]

In the face of these feelings, I did what many veterinarians who are struggling do. I pushed my concerns aside, put my head down, and continued to work, forging ahead on my path to self-destruction. Inevitably my decision to blindly persevere came back to me at tenfold karmic speed. I was rushing around Calgary running errands after speaking in Florida, striving to get as much done as possible before leaving to speak at a conference in Indianapolis. I had a podiatrist appointment to deal with chronic pain I was experiencing while running and was late after squeezing in an unimportant (but seemingly urgent) car repair. As I was cruising, flustered and late, down a busy street, I was T-boned by another car making an illegal left turn. The impact on the driver's side pushed my car out of the intersection, leaving me in a state of total shock. As sirens blared, my first thought was "now I'm definitely not making my podiatrist appointment" and my second was "how will I get to the airport for my speaking gig?" I was able to get myself out of the car despite horrific pain in my left shoulder, wrist, and thumb, and paramedics confirmed that I'd likely suffered a sprain. I extricated my purse and backpack with my undamaged (thank goodness) laptop inside and called my cousin to pick me up. Once home, I burst into tears, the reality of dealing with my injuries and impending travel hitting. I had no idea who to call or what the next logical step was.

The pain in my upper body was getting worse by the minute so I called my brother to take me to the ER, where a physician prescribed anti-inflammatories, icing, and a splint for my sprained wrist and thumb. I also had a suspected brachial plexus injury from the pull of the seatbelt across my left shoulder, which would resolve itself with pain relievers and time. The physician cautioned that I'd probably experienced a mild concussion and whiplash, counseling me on the symptoms to watch for; all difficult or impossible for a person who lives alone (as smart as Standard Poodles are, Faith was unable to identify concerning features of a severe concussion and dial 911).

Back home, I took Faith for a quick walk with my good arm and considered how I was to get through the next few days (and potentially weeks) without two healthy hands for typing or a car for driving. I contacted the conference organizer and we decided to wait and see what the next few days would bring before adjusting the plan. I had some looming due dates for articles, so I asked for extensions on those. I contacted my insurance company to arrange for a temporary rental car. Then I went to bed, hoping that this was all just a horrible nightmare that I would wake up from the next day.

Sadly, the next morning brought not relief, but a raging headache, excruciating neck pain, and persistent numbness and tingling in my left arm. I knew right away that the day would be a write-off in terms of getting any meaningful amount of work done. Instead, I contemplated everything that had led me to this point. I replayed the events of the previous day, the needless rushing around, the shock of the accident. Then I rewound further to my decision to move to Calgary and take up freelance work. Finally, I reran my decision to leave the Ontario Veterinary College, where I was well paid, doing work that I loved, and achieving more than I'd thought possible when I pursued my veterinary degree.

It seemed unfathomable that these decisions had led me to the place I found myself now: disoriented, dejected, and disillusioned. Suddenly I realized that this car accident, which had physically halted my life, was a sign from the universe telling me to stop and reassess. Why did I find myself in the perpetual daily grind of perfectionism, workaholism, and ill health when I wanted nothing more than to live a well-balanced, happy life? And what on earth did I need to do to get to that place before the next car accident put me in the hospital (or worse)?

8

From Crisis to Compassion

Clinical medicine is as much about the people as it is about the pets. You'll have a more fulfilling career if you can find joy in working with people and have a heart for service.

—Jessica Pritchard, VMD, MS, DACVIM (SAIM)
(Veterinary School Professor and Veterinarian)

My car accident served as a metaphorical wake-up call to make sustained changes in my life. In the fall of 2014, right around the time of my accident, the news broke that Dr. Sophia Yin, a renowned veterinarian and pioneer in animal behavior and low stress handling, had died by suicide. Dr. Yin authored *The Small Animal Veterinary Nerdbook*—a handbook I'd routinely referred to throughout my fourth year of veterinary school. Her suicide shook me to the core, as it did the veterinary community as a whole. The grief that followed led to difficult questions about the role the profession may have played in her untimely death.[1] Dr. Yin's passing was a stark reminder of the mental health challenges many veterinarians experience. Her premature death raised important questions about suicide and the stigma surrounding mental health in veterinary medicine. I delve deeper into these critical issues in Chapters 25 and 29, where I examine the impact of suicide within our community and discuss the urgent need for open conversations and proactive measures to support our colleagues.

While I hadn't had thoughts of suicide myself, I knew that I needed to do more to take care of my mental health. My thoughts of hopelessness and helplessness, in addition to my anxiety, sadness, and irritability, were impacting my daily decisions and functioning. I wasn't sleeping well and I felt perpetually exhausted. I no longer enjoyed or made time for activities that I used to look forward to. Most troublingly, I was really starting to dislike the contradictory person I had become: working incessantly while wanting more balance; feeling resentful while not setting boundaries; striving for perfection while paralyzed by procrastination; and generally feeling frustrated with not being able to make lasting positive changes in my life.

Given that I'd achieved most of what I set out in my life to do, the latter feeling was especially difficult for me to comprehend. How was it possible

DOI: 10.1201/9781003347385-9

that I could experience every kind of career success yet be unable to figure out how to manage my own wellbeing? My accident and the forced break that followed gave me the impetus and time to consider the question carefully. I began to evaluate my patterns of workaholism, perfectionism, and absence of work-life balance, and I decided to dive deeply into therapy. My childhood best friend had been seeing a psychologist and having what she referred to as "life-changing epiphanies." This psychologist focused on reprogramming beliefs formed during early childhood experiences that ultimately inform our future thoughts, feelings, and behaviors. These so-called limiting beliefs are perceived as truth; they pertain to how the world works, as well as how inter-actions with others unfold. And the worst part about these limiting beliefs is that they can prevent a person from achieving their most important goals and desires. Using cognitive behavioral therapy, in combination with Emotional Freedom Technique (EFT) (Box 1), I spent dozens of hours in therapy iden-tifying my limiting beliefs, focusing on the feelings and sensations that arise with them in my body and tapping my body with my fingertips to reprogram the belief.

Box 1: Did You Know?

Emotional Freedom Technique (EFT), also known as tapping or psycho-logical acupressure, is an alternative therapy believed to alleviate physi-cal pain and emotional distress by tapping on specific meridian points on the body. Developed by Gary Craig, EFT aims to restore balance to the body's energy system, addressing disruptions that are thought to un-derlie negative emotions and pain. Although ongoing research is being conducted, EFT has been utilized to treat conditions such as anxiety and post-traumatic stress disorder, with proponents suggesting that it accesses the body's energy and signals the brain to reduce stress and restore equilibrium.[2]

Almost immediately I began to see benefits in my everyday thought processes and actions based on this reprogramming. Beliefs such as "I'm not good enough," "I am wrong," and "I don't belong" had once prompted me to work harder to prove myself, strive for perfection to hide my flaws, or isolate myself from others when I felt ashamed. Now I could see these false convictions for what they were and could reexamine the unhealthy behaviors and patterns that sprung from them. Whereas before I felt helpless to control my thought tendencies or reactions, I now felt empowered by a newfound understanding of my disposition and inclinations.

It was on the advice of my psychologist that I also completed a mindful-ness-based stress reduction (MBSR) program. Jon Kabat-Zinn, bestselling author and creator of the Center for Mindfulness in Medicine, Healthcare, and Society at the University of Massachusetts Medical School, created the curriculum for the eight-week program and described it comprehensively in his book *Full Catastrophe Living*. The program, developed in 1979, remains to this day one of the most scientifically researched approaches to mindfulness (Box 2). Serendipitously, Mindfulness Institute.ca was offering an eight-week MBSR program in Edmonton, specifically tailored for professionals. It offered training on mindfulness, cognitive behavior, and self-regulation skills, thereby helping participants mobilize their inner resources to facilitate learning, growth, and healing. Enhanced self-care and positive shifts in attitudes, behaviors, and relationships were proclaimed benefits. I signed up on the spot.

Box 2: Did You Know?

A large review of research studies published in the *Journal of Alternative and Complementary Medicine* in 2009 demonstrated that mindfulness-based stress reduction (MBSR) in healthy individuals reduces stress and enhances spirituality. MBSR also showed benefits in reducing ruminative thinking and anxiety, while increasing empathy and self-compassion.[3]

The program included weekly 2.5 hour in-person sessions and a daily personal practice. Our facilitator was a psychiatrist and Assistant Clinical Professor at the University of Alberta with a clinical focus on helping those with a background of early life or combat-related trauma. During our first in-person session, I was introduced to approximately 20 other helping professionals, including physicians, nurses, psychologists, teachers, social workers, and one lawyer. I was the only veterinarian in attendance, which seemed fascinating to others in the group. We were given a booklet that included brief descriptions and research pertaining to mindfulness, reflections for the week, and instructions for our daily personal practice. I listened intently as our facilitator introduced us to the foundations of a mindfulness practice: non-judging, patience, beginner's mind, trust, non-striving, acceptance, and letting go (none of which were in the repertoire of my approach to life), and, afterward, we sat in meditation for 20 minutes—what felt like an excruciating eternity to me at the time.

In the weeks that followed, I learned more about mindfulness techniques, including using breath work to anchor the mind in the present moment, as well as yoga, which aimed to bring awareness to the mind, body, and breath. I learned that daily activities such as washing the dishes, driving the car, and walking my dog could be performed mindfully whereby attention was given to the body's sensations while going through typically mindless motions. We even spent a session talking about the benefits of mindful eating and spent more than ten minutes (I'm not exaggerating) holding a raisin and tuning into the look, smell, touch, *sound* (who knew that raisins made noise!), and, finally, taste of the small piece of dried fruit.

Some of the personal practices were particularly challenging, namely the 45-minute body scan. Practiced lying down or sitting up, a body scan can be done self-directed or by listening to a voice recording that prompts the person to direct their attention to the different parts of the body. Inevitably I would fall asleep (especially while practicing laying down) and my inability to stay awake, let alone stay tuned in to the voice, left me feeling frustrated. But I soon learned that this was entirely normal and all part of the process. Each time I noticed my mind wandering, bringing it back to the task at hand was the goal and what would ultimately strengthen the mental muscle of mindfulness.

At the end of the eight-week program, the changes to my focus, self-awareness, and emotional regulation were palpable. Not only was I able to sit through a 45 or even 60-minute meditation without fidgeting or falling asleep, but I could also participate in a similar length yoga class without my mind wandering (for long), while noticing my breath and remaining in postures, even when they felt intolerable. And what was most surprising and exciting to me was how this present-minded awareness and acceptance of my circumstance translated to my personal and professional life. During stressful work situations I was able to stay composed; when my presentation wouldn't project properly at a conference, I could notice the sensations in my body (heart pounding, breath quickening, face burning), recognize my reactive thoughts (I can't believe it! Why is this happening?), and allow the feelings of frustration, fear, or anger to pass by. My preconditioned reactions turned into thoughtful responses, and I saw the positive impact this had on my relationships at work and at home. I continued my daily meditation and deepened my yoga practice after the program ended, becoming a staunch proponent of mindfulness whenever I was given the chance to share.

Then, approximately six months after my accident, I received just over $20,000 CAD from the insurance company in reparation for the damage to my car and to my life. I used more than half of it to purchase a used car and, with the money left over, I vowed to do something *as a gift to myself.* A concept I wouldn't have considered before my therapy.

So, when I learned about a month-long 200-hour yoga teaching training program, I attended the information session with zero hesitation. Sure, I wasn't the most avid of yoga practitioners (I practiced once or twice per week), and I had no intention of becoming a yoga teacher. But I also knew the benefits of yoga as a mindfulness practice and was drawn to the idea of deepening my understanding of and aptitude for the ancient discipline. At the information session, each of the three people who would be leading the training shared their own journeys to becoming yoga teachers. One had stepped away from corporate work years ago to open the studio. Another had spent nearly her entire life learning the ancient philosophies of yoga and was especially devoted to yoga nidra, a meditative practice. I was particularly drawn to the third teacher, who was also an orthopedic surgeon and professor at the University of Calgary. She spoke of how her yoga practice had transformed her clinical and teaching work. I immediately related and her enthusiasm and compassion inspired me to submit my application for the training later that evening.

My yoga teacher training began a few months after, with nine-hour days Monday through Friday, plus two Saturday training sessions a month. To this day, the training was one of the best and most transformative experiences of my life. Not only did I gain a better understanding of yoga philosophy, anatomy and physiology, Sanskrit, postures and alignment, sequencing, and teaching, I garnered a deep appreciation for the practice and its benefits. I learned how my experience on the yoga mat, as a teacher or a student, translated to my behaviors off the mat in my everyday life. For example, during uncomfortable postures, I wanted to shift and adjust to move away from the undesirable sensation—just as I felt compelled to avoid or turn away from experiences in my life that brought discomfort or duress. Over time, I learned to sit with these experiences, become aware of everything that was arising with them, and respond thoughtfully and intentionally when the time felt right.

During the first month of yoga teacher training, I spent lunch hours and weekends reading some of the many books that were recommended to me by others in my class. Some of these were in preparation for a 40-hour introduction to meditation teaching training that I'd also signed up for. They included *The Untethered Soul* by Michael Singer, *Man's Search for Meaning* by Viktor Frankl, and *Secrets of Meditation* by Davidji. I highlighted these books and took notes, just as I had nearly a decade before when I took my board certification exam, only this time I was doing it with the goal of growing as a human being, rather than passing a test.

After I completed the training, I began to see the changes in my life that I'd been hoping for when I first left my academic job. I noticed my perfectionistic tendencies and made concerted efforts to reprogram the beliefs that perpetuated them. I was aware of my proneness to workaholism and focused on establishing boundaries, saying no, and being more intentional about the projects that I was taking on. My communication became responsive and compassionate rather than reactive and combative, and this led to positive transformations within my work and personal relationships. Self-care became a priority for me, especially at times when I would notably slip into my previous patterns. My sleep quality and quantity were better, and my stress was well managed with the strategies I had put in place.

These positive changes were recognized by my friends and peers, leading me to ponder what my life and career might have been like if I'd had some of these strategies in place decades before. I knew in my heart that it was important for me to share these tools with others, and, when at first, I questioned my capabilities and credentials, I spoke with my psychologist about my reservations. She reminded me of my years spent performing research, writing peer-reviewed articles, and speaking on emergency and critical care, and she questioned why the same fervor couldn't also be applied to educating my colleagues on personal and professional wellbeing.

And so I began to dive deeper into the mental health and wellbeing of veterinary and human healthcare professionals. I traveled to the United States to go to the National Wellness Conference and attended the Veterinary Wellness and Social Work Summit, where I completed my compassion fatigue certificate training. I completed the first Mental Health First Aid Training offered by the Alberta Veterinary Medical Association and followed it with Applied Suicide Intervention Skills Training at the Centre for Suicide Prevention. I read dozens of books related to self-care, self-help, self-awareness, self-compassion, emotional intelligence, perfectionism, boundaries, and mindfulness. I studied the published literature extensively to better understand the mental health and wellbeing of veterinarians, veterinary students, and other healthcare professionals. Basically, I devoured everything I could to better my skills and knowledge.

Then, after a decade speaking at conferences on veterinary emergency and critical care, I started to submit topics pertaining to the wellbeing of veterinary professionals. Shortly after, I organized and facilitated my first veterinary wellness workshop and retreat, a combination of lectures, workshops, and experiential practice of wellbeing and mindfulness activities (i.e., yoga, meditation, time in nature). Since then, I've spoken at conferences worldwide and have offered online continuing education programs on concepts of self-care, boundaries, mindfulness, burnout prevention, mental health, and workplace wellbeing. While I can't say that I've mastered my own health and wellbeing, I can now share my personal journey and evidence-based knowledge with others so that they might be inspired to take actionable steps toward sustainable change in their own lives.

PART TWO

What I Learned about Veterinary
Medicine along the Way

9

The Road to Becoming a Veterinarian

Getting into vet school, all the way through from age seven to your application, all you're told is how hard it is and how competitive it is. And you still try. Even my chemistry teacher, when I was asking for predicted grades, suggested that I pick another course. And there's the rejection—you get so much rejection.

—Anonymous

When I mention that I'm a veterinarian, people often express surprise, exclaiming, "I've heard it's harder to get into veterinary school than medical school." Having mingled and studied alongside more pre-med than pre-vet students during my undergrad at the University of Alberta, I don't necessarily buy into this notion. Out of the handful of my friends who aimed for medical school, none of them ultimately made it. Reflecting on my high school graduating class, which boasted nearly 400 students, I can recall one other person who pursued veterinary studies, but I don't know any classmates who became physicians. Now, I don't claim to have kept tabs on everyone's career paths, but the point stands: becoming a medical doctor isn't a walk in the park either.

My journey to veterinary school unfolded relatively smoothly, securing admission on my first attempt after two years in the pre-vet program, fulfilling all prerequisite courses. But this isn't the typical experience. Veterinary schools across the United States and Canada report acceptance rates ranging from 10% to 15%.[1,2] To put that into perspective, for every student admitted, 7 to 10 applicants face rejection. Moreover, the volume of applications in the United States is steadily increasing each year (Box 1).[2] The scenario is somewhat different in the United Kingdom, where roughly 2,400 students vie for 1,200 spots in the Bachelor of Veterinary Medicine (BVetMed) program annually, yielding applicants a 50% chance of acceptance.[3] I've spoken with veterinarians who endured three or four application cycles before finally securing admission. Many of them pursued bachelor's or master's degrees beforehand. Some opted to delay their applications until after completing their degrees, while others pursued their education while awaiting acceptance to their preferred institution. Some veterinary schools, including the Western College of Veterinary Medicine (WCVM), have a maximum number of ap-

DOI: 10.1201/9781003347385-11

plication attempts—for WCVM it's three interviews.[4] Others cite no limit to the number of times a student can apply.

Box 1: Did You Know?

In 2019, the number of applicants to veterinary medical colleges in the United States increased by 19% compared to the previous year. This remarkable surge built upon a steady annual growth rate of about 6%–7% over the preceding several years.[2]

Not everyone who applies to veterinary school, even repeatedly, is accepted. During my time as Assistant Professor at the Ontario Veterinary College, I encountered a student working as a summer assistant in the ICU. She displayed exceptional brightness and diligence, consistently posing insightful questions about cases and demonstrating strong clinical skills. I assumed this competent, mature young woman was a veterinary student, but I later discovered she was an undergraduate. When she approached me for a letter of reference for her veterinary school application, I readily agreed. Her extensive animal experience, including volunteering at farms and clinics, research positions in two laboratories, and international exposure to exotic and zoo animals, made her application remarkably well rounded. Yet despite multiple applications and interviews, she was never accepted into veterinary school. She later completed a PhD in epidemiology, which delves into understanding disease patterns and their determinants. Since then, she has pursued a career outside of veterinary medicine and I still regard her as a missed opportunity for the profession.

The process of applying for and getting accepted into veterinary school is challenging for many students. They must complete prerequisite classes that are heavily weighted in the sciences (Box 2) and some schools require a bachelor's degree. Other schools demand that students also write the Medical College Admission Test (MCAT), a standardized multiple-choice exam designed to assess critical thinking, problem-solving, and knowledge of medical concepts and principles. Most veterinary schools require transcripts of high school and undergraduate grades, a written essay describing why the student is choosing a career in veterinary medicine, and letters of reference from at least two veterinarians who have first-hand knowledge about the applicant's experience and aptitude. Veterinary and animal experience in the form of clinical practice, research, animal shelters, animal rehabilitation, public health, livestock care, animal breeding, equestrian activities, or animal-related hobbies are also required, with time requirements ranging from unspecified to more than 150 hours (Box 3). Additional criteria pertain to mental aptitude, motivation, maturity, leadership, social awareness, and communication, as well as knowledge and understanding of the veterinary profession.[4,5]

Box 2: Prerequisite Classes for Admission to the Western College of Veterinary Medicine[4]

6 credits in biology, chemistry, English, math, or stats
3 credits in organic chemistry, physics, biochemistry, genetics, introductory microbiology
21 credits in elective courses

Box 3: Did You Know?

The University of California Davis College of Veterinary Medicine, typically one of the top-ranked veterinary schools worldwide, claims that its admitted applicants have an average of 1,475 hours of quality "hands-on" experience in the veterinary profession.[6]

Because most veterinary schools receive more than double the number of applications to seats, a screening process is used to pare down the applicant pool to a more manageable number. This process commonly includes an average grade cutoff, sometimes supplemented by MCAT scores. While some schools base admissions solely on grades, others require applicants to undergo interviews. When I applied to WCVM, interviews were a prerequisite for all applicants surpassing the grade cutoff. A panel, usually made up of a local veterinarian and two current faculty members, conducted these interviews to get a well-rounded sense of the candidate. However, many veterinary schools have since adopted Multiple Mini-Interviews (MMIs), which involve several stations, each presenting a different scenario or question for candidates to address within a specified time frame.

As a faculty member at the Ontario Veterinary College, I participated in administering MMIs. Paired with a student volunteer, we evaluated applicants' proficiency in various scenarios relevant to veterinary medicine using a structured scoring system. These scores were compiled to determine each applicant's overall score, a critical factor in the admission process. The MMI stations covered a wide range of veterinary topics, including animal welfare, ethics, communication skills, problem-solving, and teamwork. Additionally, candidates were evaluated on their motivation for studying veterinary medicine and relevant experiences.

You might assume that prospective veterinarians could cast a wide net by applying to multiple schools, increasing their chances of acceptance. Unfortunately, this isn't the case for many students who are confined to applying to their designated school by geography and tuition agreements. For instance, living in Alberta meant I was eligible for one of the 20 seats allocated to Albertan residents out of the 70 available seats at the WCVM. A similar allocation was made for residents of Saskatchewan, with the remaining seats distributed among students from Manitoba, British Columbia, Yukon, and the Northwest Territories. This distribution was based on an interprovincial agreement, where provinces subsidized the tuition of students in the program, expecting them to return to practice in their home province. While students had the option to apply for a few Non-interprovincial agreement seats, these non-subsidized seats came with a hefty tuition price tag, over 3.5 times higher than subsidized seats.

A similar scenario exists in the United States, where state governments provide funding to their own state or regional veterinary schools to subsidize tuition for a set number of seats. At North Carolina State University, where I completed my residency, approximately 80% of seats are reserved for in-state residents, leaving the remaining seats for out-of-state applicants.[7] This allocation heavily influences American students' decisions on where to apply for veterinary school, particularly considering the significantly higher tuition costs for out-of-state students. Consequently, this setup restricts the flexibility in applying to different schools, and, in some years, over 150 students may compete for just 20 seats within a program.

Some students, unable to secure admission to veterinary school in their province or state of residence, or even as an out-of-state or non-interprovincial agreement applicant, opt to apply to veterinary schools in other countries. One notable example is the Ross University School of Veterinary Medicine, founded in 1982 by entrepreneur Robert Ross. Ross aimed to provide an alternative option for students seeking training as veterinarians after establishing the Ross University School of Medicine in 1978. As the first privately funded veterinary school in the Caribbean, Ross University, along with two other subsequent Caribbean schools, offers an alternative route to aspiring veterinarians from Canada and the United States. Despite tuition costs exceeding $200k USD, these Caribbean schools admit classes of students three times per year and offer a condensed curriculum without summer breaks, allowing students to complete their Doctor of Veterinary Medicine (DVM) requirements in 3.25 years, shorter than the typical four-year duration of most DVM programs.

During my time in veterinary school, we had two students from Alberta who joined our class after their first year at Ross University, after two of our class's students dropped out. This was a rare occurrence, as most Ross University students complete their non-clinical years in the Caribbean before transferring to an affiliated school in the United States to finish their clinical training. As a resident at North Carolina State University, we often had "Rossies" join us as fourth-year veterinary students throughout the year due to their staggered admissions at Ross University. Having experienced winter temperatures below -30°C (-22°F) during my veterinary school years in Saskatoon, the idea of attending veterinary school in the Caribbean was appealing to say the least! In 2010, I visited Ross University (located in St.

Kitts) to deliver a guest lecture for the students and I got to see its beautiful oceanside campus. The breathtaking setting was captivating, but probably quite distracting too!

It was not until 2011 that Ross University earned accreditation from the American Veterinary Medical Association (AVMA). This accreditation allowed students completing their studies there to take the North American Veterinary Licensing Examination (NAVLE), necessary for obtaining a license to practice veterinary medicine in the United States and Canada. Since then, other veterinary schools worldwide have also achieved AVMA accreditation to admit American and Canadian students who wish to return promptly to their home countries to practice. These schools, located in Ireland, Scotland, Australia, France, Mexico, New Zealand, Korea, and the West Indies,[8] charge annual tuition rates similar to those for out-of-state or non-interprovincial agreement students—typically three to ten times the regular tuition fees— along with additional costs for travel and living expenses. Many of these schools have less competitive admissions processes and accept students throughout the year.

Despite progress in how applicants are assessed, the admissions process for veterinary school remains imperfect, with many qualified individuals turned away due to their MCAT scores or undergraduate grades. The high demand for veterinarians in Canada and the United States has spurred the establishment of privately funded schools worldwide, admitting veterinary students at less competitive rates but with the drawback of higher tuition fees and living expenses. If the demand for veterinarians continues to outstrip the supply, it's likely that these schools will persevere in accepting, training, and graduating more veterinarians.

10

Veterinary Education's Debt Crisis

> The financial reward from my position as a practice owner is not propor-
> tionate to the time and effort given on a daily basis. The large debt accrued
> for my education, which was supposed to be an "investment in my future,"
> now looms over me. I don't mind working hard to achieve a goal. But the
> reward should be proportionate to the effort made.
>
> —Lisha Whitaker, DVM, MS
> (Small Animal Practice Co-Owner)

It's not uncommon for clients to assume that veterinarians are wealthy, due in part to the fees they pay for their pets' care. I've heard stories from countless colleagues who, despite being deeply in debt from veterinary school, are subject to jokes from clients about funding their next vacation or paying for their new car. One colleague shared with me that after presenting the client with an estimate for a complicated surgery on their dog, the client laughed and said, "Guess I'm paying for your new summer house now!" My colleague didn't have the heart to tell the client that she was barely making ends meet. In fact, after ten years of practice, she still owed more than $150,000 in student loans and hadn't taken a vacation in years because she couldn't afford it. The irony of these remarks was stinging.

This misperception exists because many clients don't realize that the fees they pay largely go toward the high cost of running a veterinary clinic—salaries, equipment, medications, supplies, and rent—rather than directly into the veterinarian's pocket. The costs of maintaining a pharmacy, radiology suite, dental office, wellness clinic, and laboratory under one veterinary practice's roof are immense. So, while they think their veterinarian is paying off a luxury vacation or fancy new car, their veterinarian is, in fact, often struggling under the weight of their student debt or the pressures of financing a new practice.

Despite two years of undergraduate university education, four years of veterinary school living away from home, and four years of internship and residency training in the United States, I started my first job as an Assistant Professor at the Ontario Veterinary College with zero student debt. To say that I'm incredibly lucky is an understatement. In comparison, a colleague of mine who is also a board-certified emergency and critical care specialist

DOI: 10.1201/9781003347385-12

completed all her training in the United States. She attended Tufts University as an in-state resident, meaning her annual tuition was $5,000 USD less than her out-of-state classmates. She graduated with $168,000 USD in student loans, which she was able to defer for one year before transitioning to income-based repayment. During her internship and residency training, her income was approximately $30,000 USD per year, not enough to support herself and her husband, who was in graduate school at the time, let alone begin paying back her loan. She worked additional locum shifts outside of her grueling specialty training and, when her residency was complete, her debt load was almost $200,000 USD.

The educational debt of veterinarians has been rising steadily for the last 35 years, and, until recently, it has been outpacing increases in starting salaries. Between 1989 and 2007, starting salaries as a veterinarian in private practice increased at a rate of 4.6% per year, outpaced about 60% by the increase in educational debt, which was approximately 7.4% per year. The subsequent debt at graduation increased from 1.1 times the starting salary in 1989 to 2.0 times the starting salary in 2007.[1] In 2020, the American Veterinary Medical Association's summary of the Economic State of the Veterinary Profession reported that educational debt was increasing at a rate 4.5 times faster than the comparable increase in income.[2]

These numbers have been in accordance with the rising cost of veterinary education, whereby, between 1999 and 2017, resident tuition at US veterinary schools increased by an average of 205%.[3] This led to the average student debt among graduating US veterinarians rising from $56,824 in 2001 to an astounding $157,146 USD in 2020, an increase of about $5,280 or 5.6% per year. If you exclude the <14% of US veterinary students who were able to graduate without student debt during that time, the average debt in 2001 was $67,198 and $188,853 USD in 2020.[4] In 2022, newly graduated US veterinarians faced varying debt burdens, with 38% carrying $200,000 or more in debt, including 13% with debts exceeding $300,000 USD. Conversely, 18% had no educational debt, while 10% held debts below $100,000 USD, reflecting the diverse financial situations among recent veterinary graduates.[5]

The numbers are less stomach-turning here in Canada, but equally concerning. Canadian veterinarians who graduated in 2022 had an average of $53,744 CAD in student debt. This varied depending on the school, the highest amount of debt among those attending the Atlantic Veterinary College in Prince Edward Island ($94,642 CAD), and the lowest among those attending Faculté de médecine vétérinaire in Montreal ($26,667 CAD).[6] One veterinarian I spoke to graduating from the Ontario Veterinary College in 2015 had approximately $55,000 CAD in student debt, a lower number attributed to an educational investment fund her parents had set up and a partner who was earning an income. After purchasing a practice three years after graduation, she needed to pay for a locum to cover the four months she was taking for maternity leave. That year she could pay herself only a meager $30,000 CAD salary from the practice. After owning her practice for approximately five years, she's only just starting to make close to the average associate salary in Ontario.

Research has identified different variables associated with an increased likelihood of graduating with student debt among US veterinarians, one of which is race. In 2022, Black or African American graduates carried the highest mean debt from earning their veterinary degree at $188,820 USD, followed closely by Hispanic or Latino graduates at $183,596 USD, while white graduates had an average debt of $146,213 USD, and Asian graduates had the lowest mean debt at $107,399 USD.[5] Another study investigated student debt among graduating US veterinarians between 2001 and 2020 and found that the university attended was associated with the amount of debt accumulated. In fact, attending Tuskegee University, recognized as the most diverse of all veterinary schools in the United States (it has educated more than 70% of the nation's Black veterinarians), was associated with an increased likelihood of student debt. On the flip side, veterinarians who attended Auburn University (just a 30-minute drive from Tuskegee University), University of California-Davis, University of Georgia, North Carolina State University, University of Pennsylvania, University of Tennessee, Texas A&M University, and Tufts University had a decreased chance of debt upon graduation.[7] These findings, based on 20 years of data, also revealed that having children was associated with higher debt levels—a relationship observed in both female and male veterinarians, though it appeared to disproportionately affect women in 2020 (Box 1).[7]

Box 1: Did You Know?

Following adjustments for cost of living, per capita income, and total education expenses in 2020, female veterinarians with children were three times more prone to have student debt compared to those without children; however, for men the presence of children did not show a similar correlation with DVM debt.[7]

Another variable associated with lower student debt among US veterinarians graduating in 2020 is the percentage of tuition paid by parents or other family members. Analysis reveals that the likelihood of graduating with DVM debt decreased by 2% for every percentage of tuition paid by these sources. Alternatively, for each percentage of tuition paid by educational loans, the likelihood of graduating with debt increased by 14%. The total cost of attending veterinary school is also a factor in student debt at graduation, whereby for a 10% increase in the cost of attendance the likelihood of graduating with student debt increases by 170%.[7]

Not all factors that one would intuitively associate with student debt were found in these research studies. In fact, age, major life events that impact finances, needing to repeat courses in veterinary school, obtaining a dual degree, or being financially responsible for animals during veterinary school were not associated with the likelihood of graduating with student debt.[7]

The cost of obtaining a veterinary degree is on the rise in most parts of the world, due to higher operating costs and lower government subsidies. However, differences in tuition costs remain depending on the country or region and whether the student is considered a resident or nonresident. For example, average annual tuition costs among US veterinary students are $35,000 USD for those attending school in-state versus an average of $50,000 USD for those attending an out-of-state school. In comparison, veterinary students' annual tuition in Canada averages $13,000 CAD, in Australia it averages $11,000 AUD, and in the United Kingdom £9,000 GBP. And if a North American student were to pursue veterinary school internationally in the Caribbean or Ireland, for example, the annual tuition cost would be $23,000–$34,000 plus living expenses ranging from $15,000–$50,000 USD per year.[8,9]

The rising cost of veterinary medical education has been accompanied, until recently, by a slower paced increase in starting salaries. The average starting salary for a Canadian veterinarian graduating in 2022 and not completing an internship or residency was $107,000 CAD, compared to those doing post-DVM training, who made an average of $42,500 CAD.[6] Comparatively, veterinarians graduating in 2022 in the United States were earning $111,000 USD,[5] those in the United Kingdom in 2021 were earning £35,500,[10] and those graduating in 2023 in Australia were earning up to $134,000 AUD.[11]

The slower rise in salaries compared to the increased cost of tuition has historically created a higher debt-to-income ratio among veterinarians worse than that of other professions. For example, in 2016 the average student loan debt for a graduating physician in the United States was $180,000; with their $200,000 average starting income, their debt-to-income ratio was 90%. Comparative numbers for a graduating veterinarian in the United States in 2016 included a student loan debt of $160,000, income of $85,000, and debt-to-income ratio of 188%. Debt-to-income ratios in other professions in 2016 included 164% for dentists, 150% for optometrists, and 141% for pharmacists.[12] Thankfully, the trend of increasing debt-to-income ratio lessened in 2022 among veterinarians for the first time since 2005 (Box 2).

Box 2: Did You Know?

The debt-to-income ratio for new veterinarians in the United States dropped to 132% in 2022 owing to a small decrease in educational debt coupled with rising starting salaries.[5]

The historically high debt-to-income ratio among graduating veterinarians has created a huge financial burden that has major potential consequences for those carrying large amounts of student debt. I know many veterinarians who expect to be paying off their student loans until they're near retirement age and whose loans have delayed or reduced their ability to purchase a home or save for retirement. Research investigating the wellbeing of veterinarians in the United States has demonstrated that student debt and other financial pressures are major contributors to psychological distress and low wellbeing, especially among new graduate veterinarians.[13] Interestingly, a recent study demonstrated that American veterinarians who hired a financial planner were less likely to experience serious psychological distress and more likely to pay off student debt faster than those who did not hire a financial planner.[14]

Concerns about the crippling student debt among veterinarians in comparison to their moderate salaries are worrisome not only for the wellbeing of currently practicing veterinarians, but for the future of the profession. Research analyzing new veterinary graduates in the United States between 2001 and 2021 found that the amount of debt incurred during veterinary school was associated with the choice of career path after graduation. In other words, veterinarians graduating with higher debt levels sought higher paying jobs in the private sector or clinical training that might lead to higher paying jobs. Notably, jobs in the public sector, a field in critical need, were chosen by veterinarians with an average of nearly $25,000 USD less in debt.[14] I've seen this decision play out among colleagues of mine who have completed their specialist training programs and opted for higher paying private practice jobs rather than lower paying jobs in academia. A close friend and resident-mate of mine told me that she would not interview for academic jobs after finishing her residency because her student loans were too high. The efflux of veterinarians and veterinary specialists from public sector jobs into private practice for more competitive salaries is contributing to the widespread increase in job openings in academia.

New veterinarians embarking on careers at corporate-owned practices or group consolidators also have notably higher mean debt ($157,810 USD) compared to those joining private or independently owned hospitals or clinics ($147,472 USD) in 2022. The theory is that they are being drawn to corporate-owned or group consolidators due to a higher mean starting salary of $124,686 USD compared to $105,637 at independent practices, in addition to more generous benefits and signing bonuses (Box 3). Additionally, corporate-owned practices were more likely to provide moving allowances, with 48% offering an average of $6,180 USD, while only 23% of independently owned practices extended a moving allowance averaging $3,626 USD.[15]

Box 3: Did You Know?

Signing bonuses averaging $27,181 USD were offered to new graduate veterinarians by corporate-owned practices or group consolidators in 2022, compared to 42% of independently owned practices offering a signing bonus averaging $10,678 USD.[15]

Unless steps are taken to mitigate the financial burden of veterinary education, decisions about whether to pursue veterinary school or accept jobs in lower-paying sectors such as academia and government will likely hinge on an individual's financial circumstances or the level of support available to them during their training. This has ramifications for diversity and inclusion within veterinary medicine and will likely continue to impact the mental wellbeing of veterinarians after graduation as they strive to pay off their student loans. And while there are some veterinarians who were, like me, lucky enough to graduate without crippling student debt, the salaries paid to most veterinarians today still pale in comparison to those in other medical professions with similar education. I think it's safe to say that most practicing veterinarians are not as rich as the public perceives them to be.

The Hidden Curriculum in Veterinary School

> I remember almost getting into a car accident driving home in the middle of the night (briefly falling asleep at the wheel), after being called in to help monitor anesthesia for an emergency surgery. I remember thinking that I had gained absolutely nothing education-wise from going back to the school in the middle of the night, but could have lost my life. But these were the expectations of students.
>
> —Nicole Stone, DVM (Small Animal Veterinarian)

For many students the white coat ceremony marks their official entrance into veterinary medical training, a moment as scary as it is exciting. The ceremony has become an annual tradition in many veterinary schools around the world, including mine years after I graduated. It signifies the transition into veterinary medicine, embodying the shift into the professional expectations and rules of the field. Students receive a white coat, symbolizing professionalism and empathy in the practice of medicine. This symbolic gesture underscores the care, trust, and professionalism that pet owners expect from their veterinarian, while also reminding students of the importance of balancing excellence in science with humanistic patient care (Box 1).

Box 1: Did You Know?

The inaugural white coat ceremony, initiated by the Arnold P. Gold Foundation, took place at the Columbia University College of Physicians and Surgeons in 1993. Since then, this tradition has proliferated across various disciplines, including medicine, dentistry, pharmacy, osteopathy, and veterinary medicine, being adopted by numerous academic institutions worldwide.

In veterinary medicine, professionalism encompasses the skills, judgments, and behaviors that are expected from a trained veterinarian. Professionalism is taught within three facets of the curriculum: (1) the formal curriculum that represents what a school has planned to teach; (2) the in-

DOI: 10.1201/9781003347385-13

formal curriculum, which is the delivery of the formal curriculum; and (3) the hidden curriculum that is experienced by the students. In the context of veterinary medicine, the formal curriculum includes the classes and course outlines for each year; the informal curriculum is what is taught during each class lecture or laboratory; and the hidden curriculum includes everything in between. Specifically, the hidden curriculum is the information implicitly conveyed by schools, teachers, and peers regarding the different facets and values of the profession.

One might assume that the hidden curriculum would serve to reinforce the concepts and standards taught within the formal and informal curricula, and, in many circumstances, it does. However, the experience that most veterinary students have, especially when they reach their clinical year of training, is that the hidden curriculum often conflicts with the principles and values espoused during their preclinical years. And when faced with this mismatch, students inherently default to the information provided by the hidden curriculum.

I've lost count of the number of times that I, and many of my peers in veterinary school, faced the conundrum of practicing what was being "preached" versus what we were witnessing firsthand from our instructors, professors, and peers. Beginning in the first weeks of veterinary school, binge-drinking and partying were emphasized as the norm for Friday and Saturday nights. Yet studying and getting good grades were also prioritized, often in conflict with the social pressure to attend parties and extracurricular activities. The pressure to get good grades without passing up social opportunities also resulted in students cheating—whether by finding out what was going to be on the exam from senior students or by obtaining copies of exams from previous years. Despite these practices being against our schools' honor code, many of my classmates described them as normal and something "everyone" was doing to pass their exams (Box 2).

Box 2: Did You Know?

An honor code establishes ethical standards within an academic community, relying on trust that individuals will uphold honorable behavior. It typically involves a pledge by students to maintain academic integrity, refrain from cheating or dishonesty, and adhere to ethical conduct. The College of William & Mary introduced one of the earliest examples of such a code in the early 18th century.[1]

As someone who had spent many years in a companion animal clinic, I was already privy to the realities of general practice. Nonetheless, the hidden curriculum became painfully apparent during my fourth year of veterinary school. Most veterinary schools, including mine, have a teaching hospital run by the clinical faculty, most of whom are board-certified specialist veterinarians. Students soon learn the "rules" that will help them to survive during final-year clinical rotations and, ultimately, as a practicing veterinarian. Some of these rules that we learned early on included: (1) don't expect to have a life during certain clinical rotations, especially those with on-call responsibilities; (2) questions are appropriate only without a pet owner present and should in no way indicate that you don't well understand the fundamental concepts; and (3) emotional reactions are frowned upon, especially during or after euthanasia procedures.

Most clinical rotations began early, ended late, and often included on-call responsibilities. There were times when these rotations led students (myself included) to feel more like "cheap labor" as opposed to veterinarians-in-training. In fact, the teaching and learning part of the day often felt like an after-thought or "bonus." Most of the clinical rotations had formal rounds in the morning and/or afternoon, which included structured teaching around relevant cases. However, outside of those opportunities, the slog of admitting patients, completing treatments, performing procedures, and communicating with clients left little time in between for thoughtful conversation or integrated learning.

Additionally, questions weren't always welcomed during busy clinical rotations and were sometimes even received with mockery. During certain rotations there was a history of clinicians rolling their eyes or, worse, laughing at the students' queries, intimidating us into keeping quiet. While many faculty members admittedly have no formal training as teachers, these behaviors conflict with the learning environment and professional conduct expected within a teaching hospital. In short, while the formal curriculum might endorse an environment open to insightful questions and thoughtful conversation, the hidden curriculum suggests the student "should know that already" or that there simply is not time for such conversations.

On the other hand, there are times when teaching and learning are prioritized above the responsibility to ensure that animal pain and suffering is relieved. For example, I can remember witnessing a situation in a teaching hospital whereby a blocked cat was admitted to the emergency room. It's not uncommon for male cats to present with a urinary tract blockage, due to their inherently narrow urethra and a tendency toward urethral inflammation or spasm, especially during periods of stress. In this instance, the cat's owner had recently lost his job and didn't have the funds to pay for the unblocking procedure. As such, he consented to euthanasia. Before going ahead with this, the well-intentioned faculty member asked every student on the rotation to palpate the cat's bladder to feel the abnormal size and firmness and know how to diagnose this condition in subsequent situations. As you can imagine, the cat was severely distressed and uncomfortable. To say that I too felt "uncomfortable" at prolonging the cat's suffering to allow students a learning opportunity would be an understatement. In this circumstance, student learning took precedence over the oath to first and foremost relieve patient suffering.

I still remember my four-week internal medicine rotation during which the students took turns admitting emergency cases to the hospital. This was my favorite part because the cases were challenging, fast paced, and the most interesting, in my opinion. One of the cases I admitted was a large mixed-breed dog that had collapsed at home. He was in shock when he arrived, with rapid breathing, a high heart rate, and an arrhythmia (abnormal heart rhythm). After performing emergency blood work and taking x-rays of his abdomen and chest, we determined that he had a large mass in his belly that was bleeding and that the presumed cancer had spread to form nodules in his lungs. His prognosis was grave, and his owners made the decision to euthanize him.

Having spent hours with his family learning about his otherwise long and healthy life, and after witnessing the sadness that culminated in both his owners breaking down in tears, I found myself also sobbing in the wake of the acute grief around me. I stayed for the euthanasia and arrived late to our end-of-day rounds, my face puffy and my eyes red. And at the end of my clinical rotation when I received my grade, I received the feedback that I was "too emotional" and needed to learn to "hide my feelings" during emotionally charged situations. I still recall the shock I felt at this, having always believed that my empathy and vulnerability allowed me to more effectively connect with my clients and peers.

Research reveals similar sentiments among students who recognize a disconnect between the values and ideals that are espoused by the institution compared to the realities of everyday life in the clinic. In fact, a study following students graduating from the BVetMed (DVM equivalent) program in 2015 at the Royal Veterinary College, University of London, investigated aspects of professionalism that were identified as important or in conflict based on the hidden curriculum. Perhaps unsurprisingly, technical, then communication skills were weighted as being most important in establishing a high level of professionalism as a veterinarian. These were reiterated by the weighting they had on student evaluations, whereby technical skills in performing techniques such as blood draws or surgeries were heavily scrutinized, as were client communication skills such as history-taking, correspondence, and follow-up.[2]

Many veterinary students can attest to the fact that the grades received during clinical rotations often feel arbitrary or artificial. Technical skills are emphasized above all else, yet not all clinical rotations allow for those technical skills to be demonstrated. Second to technical skills is aptitude during client communications, yet many students call or conduct interviews with clients without an assessing faculty member present. How, then, is their client communication to be assessed accurately, and does that put the same importance on this skill as those clinical skills that are more closely monitored and scrutinized? I remember having difficulty assessing grades for the fourth year students on my own ICU rotations when I was a faculty member. Some weeks in

ICU were quieter than others and did not give students opportunities to demonstrate their tasks. We always tried to offer simulations of procedures, but, even then, it was challenging to feel objective in our assessments. Likewise, I had to be mindful not to overemphasize the technical assessments on the evaluation, given the importance of other professional skills such as punctuality, teamwork, and collegiality.

Additional sources of tension pertaining to the professional role arise in the context of compassion and empathy toward animals and owners; lifestyle ethics, including work-life balance; and autonomy and responsibility for the cases being managed. As I experienced during my fourth-year internal medicine rotation, the compassion and empathy that had been endorsed during my pre-clinical training seemed to go out the window the moment I was doing "real life" clinical work. The clinicians I worked with seemed hardened to their emotions and were, in my opinion, sometimes cold and disconnected from the experiences of their clients. When it came to having any sort of a life outside of clinical work, it was difficult to reckon the desire to maintain good habits such as daily exercise and sufficient sleep with the expectation to eat, sleep, and breathe veterinary medicine.

Doing clinical rotations in a 24-hour veterinary teaching hospital seemed to convey unrealistic expectations for what those entering general practice would ultimately experience. Not only did the unrelenting work hours and extensive on-call responsibilities feel inconsistent with most general practice jobs, but students also perceived the faculty specialists to over-identify with the profession and not exhibit a life outside of work. Likewise, students felt that the environment of the veterinary teaching hospital did not provide learning situations that could be translated to clinical practice. Most veterinary teaching hospitals are tertiary referral centers, meaning that they are receiving cases from veterinarians, some of whom are themselves specialists, who received the case from another general practice veterinarian. The fact that veterinary teaching hospitals have access to the latest and greatest tools and technologies, while attending to patients that are either covered by insurance or owned by families with expendable income, creates a sense of "unrealistic circumstances" that do not apply to a veterinarian in general practice.

During my time as a faculty member, I noticed how clinical faculty and their grading methods can either reinforce or shift the hidden curriculum. For example, I saw some faculty openly criticize referring veterinarians in front of students and other team members. While this behavior wasn't common, it was concerning because of how it might shape students' professional development. When I later returned to my veterinary school as a locum in the ICU, I felt the need to step in during rounds, reminding everyone to stay professional and avoid making judgments without the full story. This really highlighted for me the importance of consistently modeling ethical behavior in clinical settings.

Some aspects of the hidden curriculum are less within an individual's control and more a result of the traditions and systems in place (Box 3). For example, the predominance of white women in veterinary medicine, coupled with mostly white men in leadership roles, perpetuates the racial and gender biases that preclude minority students from applying to veterinary school or female veterinarians from pursuing leadership roles. It was also my experience during veterinary school that my male classmates were presumed to be interested in large or mixed animal practice (as opposed to companion animal practice). When large animal demonstrations were performed during laboratories or clinical rotations, a male student was almost always selected to participate. While a consequence of unconscious bias, these behaviors contradicted the formal and informal curricula taught to all veterinary students, regardless of gender.

Box 3: Did You Know?

Popular medical television shows provide rich examples of the hidden curriculum. One study analyzed one season each of *ER*, *Grey's Anatomy*, and *Scrubs*, and identified prevalent themes of the hidden curriculum, including the hierarchical nature of medicine, challenges during transitional stages, patient dehumanization, faking or overstating capabilities, unprofessionalism, loss of idealism, and difficulties with work-life balance.[3]

The hidden curriculum can ultimately influence how veterinarians perceive and cope with mistakes in real-life practice. If the prevailing culture within veterinary school emphasizes perfectionism and places a stigma on errors, veterinarians may be less inclined to disclose or learn from their mistakes, fearing repercussions or judgment from colleagues. Conversely, in learning environments that promote open communication about failures and a growth mindset, veterinarians will be more likely to view mistakes as opportunities for reflection, learning, and improvement. I've spent time in both environments and can attest to the vast differences within the team in terms of communicating and coping in the aftermath of medical errors. For a deeper exploration of how perfectionism and the handling of medical errors impact veterinary professionals, refer to Chapters 22 and 23. Without a doubt, a supportive and psychologically safe workplace culture is essential for facilitating constructive responses to mistakes and promoting professional growth among veterinary teams.

The hidden curriculum's strong influence highlights the need for a focused effort to align the values and principles promoted within the veterinary profession. While classroom teaching and professional conduct guidelines may stress integrity, compassion, and ethical practice, the hidden curriculum can sometimes encourage behaviors and beliefs that go against these ideals. As veterinarians and students navigate the challenges of their training and work environments, they need to be aware of, and question, the norms and expectations they encounter. By actively working to reshape the hidden curriculum to better reflect the profession's core values, veterinarians can cultivate a culture that emphasizes wellbeing, ethical integrity, and compassionate care for both animals and people. In the end, by recognizing and addressing the hidden curriculum's impact, the veterinary profession can move toward a more inclusive, supportive, and ethically grounded future.

12

Meeting the Demand for Veterinary Specialists

Tell me I'm not the only one who's heard a client exclaim that her friend/
sister/coworker/whoever thinks "it's just hilarious that I bring my cat to
the (insert specialty here)." Like, it's just so crazy you could be a specialist
for cats!

—Erin Anderson, VMD, MSc, DACVIM (Cardiology)
(Veterinary Cardiologist)

When people think of veterinarians, they tend to envision the general practice veterinarian their family has been seeing for years; the vet who owns the
practice up the road and is open on weekdays and Saturdays for routine appointments and spay / neuter surgeries. So, when I tell people that I'm an
emergency and critical care specialist for dogs and cats, most of them look at
me with bewilderment, saying, "I didn't know there was such a thing." While
four years of veterinary school provides a solid baseline of skills and knowledge needed to provide preventative and urgent care for animals, some cases
require more complex management or procedures that only specialists with
advanced training can provide. Still, many pet owners make only rare trips to
their general practice veterinarian, never mind being referred to a specialist
for potentially thousands of dollars in veterinary care.

I grew up with veterinarian parents, yet even I didn't realize until my third
year of veterinary school that veterinary specialties existed. I vividly remember sitting in a small animal medicine and surgery class and learning about
the management of cranial cruciate ligament ruptures, the most common orthopedic injury in dogs. This condition is like a torn anterior cruciate ligament
(ACL) in people, and there are two main surgical procedures recommended
if exercise restriction and anti-inflammatory medications aren't successful in
managing the condition. In class, the first technique described was a lateral
suture technique, whereby a "new" ligament composed of strong suture material is implanted outside the knee joint to stabilize it. The other technique described was a tibial plateau leveling osteotomy (TPLO), a more complex procedure requiring equipment such as a bone saw and an orthopedic plate. The
surgery involves cutting the tibia (i.e., the shin bone) and rotating the bone so
that the femur (i.e., the thigh bone) cannot slide backwards. This stabilizes the
joint and eliminates the need for a cranial cruciate ligament altogether. This

DOI: 10.1201/9781003347385-14

procedure was first described in 1993, so by the time I was in my third year of veterinary school, it had only been known for ten years. Given its novelty and the equipment and expertise involved, I learned that referral to a veterinary surgeon specialist was usually required.

My mom was an excellent surgeon and did many complex surgeries herself, and the rare cases that she referred to the veterinary school were simply not on my radar. But hearing my veterinary school professors (all specialists themselves) share information about complex cases sent from GP veterinarians to specialists, I began to wonder what these people did and how I might become one. Up to this point, I hadn't considered anything other than working at my mom's clinic after veterinary school. The idea that a veterinarian could pursue advanced training to garner skills beyond those that I had grown up witnessing was news to me!

The American Veterinary Medical Association (AVMA) recognizes veterinary specialties in North America that have been approved by the American Board of Veterinary Specialties (ABVS), an organization whose mission is to encourage "the development of recognized veterinary specialty organizations promoting advanced levels of competency in well-defined areas of study or practice categories to provide the public with exceptional veterinary service." In 2022, more than 16,500 veterinarians achieved Diplomate (specialist) status in one or more areas of specialization.[1] To obtain Diplomate status, veterinarians must complete rigorous post-veterinary school clinical training and fulfill various other educational requirements, such as performing a research project, publishing a scientific article, and passing an exam. Some areas of specialization include anesthesia, behavior, cardiology, clinical pharmacology, dentistry, dermatology, diagnostic imaging and radiology, emergency and critical care, internal medicine, neurology, nutrition, oncology, pathology, radiation oncology, sports medicine and rehabilitation, surgery, theriogenology, and toxicology (Box 1).

Box 1: Did You Know?

The American Veterinary Medical Association recognizes Veterinary Specialties™ within their respective Veterinary Specialty Organizations™, which include the following:
American Board of Veterinary Practitioners

- Shelter medicine
- Reptile and amphibian
- Exotic companion animal
- Canine and feline
- Equine
- Food Animal
- Dairy

- Swine health management
- Avian
- Beef cattle
- Feline

American Board of Veterinary Toxicology
American College of Animal Welfare
American College of Laboratory Animal Medicine
American College of Poultry Veterinarians
American College of Theriogenologists
American College of Veterinary Anesthesia and Analgesia
American College of Veterinary Behaviorists
American College of Veterinary Clinical Pharmacology
American College of Veterinary Dermatology
American College of Veterinary Internal Medicine

- Cardiology
- Small animal internal medicine
- Large animal internal medicine
- Neurology
- Oncology
- Nutrition

American College of Veterinary Microbiologists

- Virology
- Immunology
- Bacteriology/Mycology
- Parasitology

American College of Veterinary Nephrology-Urology
American College of Veterinary Ophthalmologists
American College of Veterinary Pathologists

- Anatomic pathology
- Clinical pathology

American College of Veterinary Preventive Medicine

- Epidemiology

American College of Veterinary Radiology

- Radiation oncology
- Equine diagnostic imaging

American College of Veterinary Sports Medicine and Rehabilitation

- Canine
- Equine

American College of Veterinary Surgeons

- Small animal surgery
- Large animal surgery

American College of Zoological Medicine
American College of Veterinary Emergency & Critical Care
American Veterinary Dental College

- Equine dental

The process for specialization goes something like this: (1) graduate from veterinary school to obtain a Doctor of Veterinary Medicine (DVM) or equivalent degree (the University of Pennsylvania refers to their veterinary degree as a Veterinariae Medicinae Doctoris (VMD); (2) complete a year-long internship training program or equivalent clinical practice experience; (3) finish a three or more year residency program; and (4) study for and pass the board certification exam to achieve Diplomate status. If you factor in all this advanced training, most veterinarians complete at least four more years of study, in addition to their veterinary and pre-veterinary school education. Many veterinarians have a bachelor's or master's degree prior to veterinary school, which can culminate in 12-plus years of veterinary-related education to become a specialist.

And if you thought getting accepted into veterinary school was competitive, applying for and matching with internship and residency programs is on a whole other level. Most of the recognized programs are facilitated by the Veterinary Internship and Residency Matching Program (VIRMP), which is sponsored by the American Association of Veterinary Clinicians. VIRMP follows the principles established by the Physicians National Intern and Resident Matching Program whereby the prospective intern or resident selects a program or programs to rank. An application is completed, which includes a letter of intent, transcripts, class ranking, and recommendation letters, and it is submitted through the VIRMP website. The academic institutions or specialty hospitals offering the internship or residency program review the applications and perform the interviews. Then applicants and academic institutions or specialty hospitals provide their confidential rankings and VIRMP uses computer software to match the prospective interns and residents with the highest available option on their rank order list. The results are then provided to applicants and academic institutions or specialty hospitals on the same day (often referred to as "Match Day"), which typically takes place in February, a few months in advance of the June or July program start date. Applicants and institutions or hospitals are not allowed to withdraw from the match after they have provided their rankings. Those in violation of this rule are not permitted to participate in VIRMP for three consecutive years after the year of violation.

In 2022, there were 2,094 veterinarians in the match, including 1,019 applying to internships, 538 applying to residencies, and 537 applying to both. The reason a veterinarian might apply for both an internship and residency is to ensure that if they do not match with a residency program, they will have the option to pursue another year of internship training. The overall applicant match rate in 2022 was 54%, with 66% of applicants matching with an internship and 38% of applicants matching with a residency program. Some of the most competitive small animal residency programs in 2022 were cardiology, equine surgery, exotics/wildlife/zoo, large animal surgery, and small animal surgery, all of which had less than 25% of applicants match with a program. The highest number of applicants were to small animal surgery, with 238 applicants applying for 43 programs, 98% of programs matching with a resident, and only 22% of applicants matching with a program.[2]

My specialty program, emergency medicine and critical care, had an applicant match rate of 70% in 2022, with 90 applicants vying for 79 positions and 63 matching. Most of the matches were at academic institutions (39/42 programs filled), whereas several referral practices did not match with an applicant (24/37 programs filled). The discrepancy between applicants and program matches is attributed to unqualified applicants, as well as the tendency for more applicants to apply to academic institutions, potentially due to concerns about a lower passing rate for the certification exam among those in private- or corporate-owned referral practices (Box 2).

Box 2: Did You Know?

In 2018, a study was published revealing that the first-time pass rate between 2010 and 2015 for residents of the American College of Veterinary Emergency and Critical Care (ACVECC) was 77% for residents trained in academic programs compared to 47% for residents trained in private or corporate referral practice.[3] This statistic raised concerns that a disparity exists among training programs at the time, making some non-academic training programs seem less desirable.

There is no doubt that the demand for specialists is growing as more and more pet owners become aware of the advanced techniques that are available for animals. According to the American Veterinary Medical Association, between 2007 and 2017 the number of specialists in the United States increased by almost 50%, whereas the overall veterinarian population grew by less than one-third. In 2021, specialists comprised approximately 12% of the estimated US veterinary population (approximately 14,500 specialists among 124,000 veterinarians).[4] However, job openings for specialists are growing exponentially, suggesting that residency program openings cannot keep up with pet owner demands in practice. The deepening human-animal bond that leads owners to treat their pets as family members is putting pressure on veterinary specialists to provide cutting-edge care. While 20 years ago it might have seemed outlandish to provide mechanical ventilation for a dog with pneumonia or perform hemodialysis for a cat with kidney failure, as described in Chapter 13, both techniques are now commonplace in the specialty of emergency and critical care.

In 2018, there were 693 ACVECC Diplomates, a dramatic increase over ten years from 263 in 2008, the year that I achieved board certification. And at the end of 2020, the number of emergency and critical care specialists had risen again to 832.[4] Yet despite the dramatic rise in the number of specialists, the demand, as evidenced by the number of job openings, far exceeds the supply, as indicated by the number of residency programs. A report released in 2022 titled "Pet Healthcare in the US: Are There Enough Veterinary Specialists? Is There Adequate Training Capacity?" confirmed that the number of emergency and critical care specialist job openings at hospitals owned by five large veterinary corporate entities in October 2021 was 182, whereas the number of new emergency and critical care specialists estimated to enter the job market in 2022 was 78. This means that the number of job openings per new emergency and critical care specialist in 2022 was 2.3. The numbers are even worse for specialties such as small animal surgery and small animal internal medicine for which the job openings per new specialist at those companies alone were 2.8 and 4.1, respectively.[5]

Dramatic steps are being taken to try to fill the vacant veterinary specialty positions across Canada and the United States. Recruiters regularly approach residents during their first or second year of training and many of the large veterinary corporations that own specialty hospitals throughout Canada and the United States are sponsoring residency programs. This involves providing funding to a school to cover a resident's salary, benefits, and other agreed-upon expenses in exchange for the resident working for their sponsoring company for a predetermined time (usually 3 to 5 years) after their training program is completed. The frequency of sponsored residency programs is on the rise and is even being offered by academic institutions struggling to fill vacant specialty positions within their faculty and by industry partners hoping to increase the number of board-certified specialists. While the incidence of residency sponsorship was rare when I completed my program, it has become commonplace and will likely grow as more academic programs are approached with offers to fund additional residency candidates. The US Army also funds residencies for Army Veterinary Corps officers on active duty, whereby residents are paid by the federal government, receive salary and benefits based on rank, and complete service obligations determined by the length of their training program.

Unfortunately, increasing the number of internship and residency programs will not be sufficient to meet the demand for specialists, especially if the number of applicants to these programs does not grow concurrently. Every year it seems that more and more ACVECC residency programs have open spots without a matched resident. Simply not enough qualified veterinarians are applying to these programs. One of the reasons why veterinarians opt out of advanced training programs is because the salary has traditionally been a fraction of what they would make as a general practitioner or non-specialist veterinary working in emergency practice. This has prevented veterinarians from underprivileged backgrounds, without family financial support, or with massive student loans from considering advanced training. In response to the need for more program applicants, the salary for many internship and residency programs has increased to meet at least a living wage, if not to offer an income comparable to what a newly graduated veterinarian would make in general practice.[6] Whether this recent change leads to an increase in applications in the coming years remains to be seen.

The increasing demand for board-certified veterinarians raises uncertainty about whether sponsored residency training programs and improved salaries can adequately address the growing need for these specialists. This shortage is already having a negative impact on veterinary medicine in various regions of Canada and the United States. I frequently read posts in a Facebook group for veterinary specialists who are moms about the scarcity of specialists and how it is impacting practice. Stories about surgeon specialist shortages, for example, are leading to extended wait times for emergency surgery referrals. Consequently, general practitioners in certain geographical regions are increasingly feeling pressure to perform surgeries beyond the scope of their routine practice, attempting complex procedures like gallbladder surgeries, lung lobe resections, or adrenal gland removals. These challenges have prompted lengthy and emotional discussions without the group regarding the ethical dilemma of turning away such cases and the moral stress this creates, in turn, for referring veterinarians. The urgent requirement for additional specialists to alleviate the mounting caseload is glaringly evident. Although the toll stemming from the disparity between the supply and the demand for veterinary specialists has yet to be quantified, it's clear that this situation is impacting the wellbeing of all veterinarians, particularly as pet owners seek advanced veterinary care.

13

Stories from the Veterinary ICU

I really like getting patients who come in the door half dead and being able to fix them and send them home to their families. But I'm very much in the "just because we can doesn't mean we should" camp of critical care. I find it ethically challenging when people want to pursue futile care but palliative care or euthanasia is likely in everyone's (pet, client, team) best interest.

—Janine Calabro, DVM, DACVECC (Medical Director)

As an emergency and critical care specialist, it's not uncommon for pet owners to tell me that they would do anything and everything to save the life of their furry family member. Yet many people are genuinely surprised to learn that intensive care is available for dogs, cats, and other species, just as it would be for a human. A relatively new veterinary specialty, Intensive or Critical Care Medicine began in 1989 when the American College of Veterinary Emergency and Critical Care was recognized by the American Veterinary Medical Association, and it has grown exponentially since. When I began veterinary school in 2000, there were only a handful of Critical Care Specialists working across Canada, and today these specialists can be found in nearly every major city throughout the country.

Most large veterinary emergency and referral hospitals in urban centers have their own intensive care unit (ICU), typically located centrally. This space is comprised of specifically manufactured cages that allow for 360-degree access to the patient, as well as oxygen cages, mechanical ventilators, dialysis machines, plasma thawing devices, a manual defibrillator, fluid and syringe pumps, as well as devices that monitor heart rate, ECG/EKG, blood pressure, oxygen saturation, carbon dioxide, blood flow, and more. Having visited human ICUs, I can attest to the fact that veterinary ICUs possess the same life-saving equipment and monitoring devices. The main difference is that human ICUs contain beds filled with people whereas veterinary ICUs contain cages usually filled with dogs and cats. Aside from that, the beeps and bustle of the ICU are startlingly similar.

Also like human medicine, veterinary ICUs house the sickest patients in the hospital, belonging to different services and specialties. The most common are patients with bleeding disorders requiring blood transfusions; endo-

DOI: 10.1201/9781003347385-15

crine disorders requiring electrolyte and insulin administration; respiratory disorders requiring oxygen supplementation, intubation, or ventilator support; neurologic disorders requiring constant monitoring for seizure activity or brain swelling; toxin ingestions that need therapeutic plasma exchange for toxin removal; infectious diseases that require isolation and intensive care; and various forms of organ dysfunction such as liver, pancreas, and kidney disease or failure. There are many serious medical conditions that require intensive care such as immune-mediated diseases, complicated diabetes mellitus, epilepsy, and cancer. A myriad of surgical patients can also require intensive care, including those hospitalized for an intestinal foreign body, stomach torsion, ruptured spleen, or trauma.

Animals hospitalized in the ICU often have at least one intravenous (IV) catheter, including a "long line" or PIC (percutaneous IV catheter) placed for blood sampling and fluid or blood product administration. It's not uncommon for veterinary ICU patients to also have a second IV catheter, nasal oxygen cannula or feeding tube, and an assortment of cords attached to a multiparameter monitoring device. More recently, telemetry has become commonplace in veterinary ICUs, limiting the many cords traversing between patients and devices. Accompanying these devices is the steady sound of beeps, alarms, and other noises that alert the veterinary team to any abnormalities.

It's often said among veterinary ICU teams that the "pump-to-patient ratio" is an accurate indicator of the severity of illness of critically ill patients. Intensive care medicine is often a juggling act of various fluid, electrolyte, blood product, and drug infusions that require half a dozen or more fluid and syringe pumps for administration. Inevitably, the more dire a patient's status is, the more pumps they will need. To say that these are high-stakes cases is an understatement. The costs of managing critically ill dogs and cats can easily lead to bills exceeding $10,000 USD, which, unless covered by pet health insurance, must be paid by the pet's family upon discharge from the hospital.

Over my last two decades in veterinary ICUs, I've seen a dramatic increase in treatment costs, as well as the emotional and financial lengths that pet owners will go for their furry family members. Whereby cases exceeding $10k used to be shockingly rare, today most ICU veterinarians would not bat an eyelash at providing a pet owner with an estimate exceeding $15k. While inflation and the cost of veterinary care have admittedly risen during the last 20 years, some of this increase can be attributed to the level of sacrifice that owners are prepared to undertake to save their pet. Procedures such as mechanical ventilation for respiratory failure or hemodialysis for renal failure can result in bills exceeding $20k. The cost of intensive care has undoubtedly driven many owners (including veterinarians like me!) to purchase pet health insurance and is what contributes to the high cost of premiums for certain insurance plans.

I can vividly recall the first patient I managed whose bill exceeded $10k. It was during the early 2010s when I was a faculty member at the Ontario

Veterinary College (OVC) and the patient was an elderly large breed dog who had experienced a complication after emergency surgery at a referring veterinary clinic. The dog presented with air in his chest and fluid in his abdomen, secondary to an abdominal surgery that was not performed correctly. He was hospitalized and underwent another two emergency surgeries to correct damage that had occurred during the first surgery and to remove sponges that had been left in the abdomen following that initial emergency surgical procedure. Unfortunately, this dog developed an infection after the second surgery at our hospital and required a third abdominal exploratory surgery. Sadly, his condition continued to decline, and his protein levels dropped significantly, despite several plasma transfusions. Ultimately his owners made the difficult decision to perform euthanasia. His bill was nearly $15k, which, accounting for inflation today, would be more than $20k.

It's important to contrast this case with a similarly expensive case that had a very positive outcome and illustrates the value of team-delivered care within the ICU. More than a year later, a young cat arrived in the ICU at the OVC having ingested toxic lilies. Cats are particularly susceptible to kidney failure when certain species such as the Easter, Japanese, Stargazer, Casablanca, and tiger lilies are ingested.[1] Exposure to the pollen alone (for example, if a cat were to brush past a stamen and lick the pollen off the fur while grooming) has the potential to cause life-threatening kidney damage. This cat was less than a year old and presented to our ICU Service with severe kidney failure that required dialysis therapy.

Because this was before the OVC had acquired a hemodialysis machine, the cat underwent peritoneal dialysis therapy, whereby a fenestrated drain is placed into the belly of the patient and specifically formulated fluid is instilled into the abdomen to remove toxins and electrolytes from the bloodstream by pulling them into the belly from where they are drained. This process repeats itself every few hours for days (or weeks), essentially functioning to prevent toxin buildup in the body until the kidneys can recover. With the help of the critical care team who placed the peritoneal drain, PIC line, and feeding tube, as well as the ICU veterinary nursing team who provided the hourly care, after two weeks and dozens of rounds of peritoneal dialysis, the cat went home. A clear differentiator in this case is that this cat's family had purchased pet health insurance that covered the entire bill minus their $1,000 deductible. This case highlights the positive outcomes that can happen while under the care of a dedicated ICU team if the owner has the financial means or insurance coverage to pay for the care.

A few years after this cat's successful recovery with hemodialysis, the OVC acquired a hemodialysis machine and now employs dialysis IV for dogs and cats with kidney damage or failure who require renal replacement therapy (Box 1). They are not alone in their capacity to provide so-called advanced renal therapy for animals. The American Society of Veterinary Nephrology and Urology lists more than 20 hospitals in the United States and more than a dozen throughout the rest of the world that offer renal replacement therapies, including hemodialysis, with even more offering the less technically challenging peritoneal dialysis.[2] Suffice it to say, veterinary medicine is not far behind human medicine when it comes to some of the techniques available to ICU patients, which, incidentally, utilize equipment and machines designed for humans.

Box 1: Did You Know?

Hemodialysis is a treatment used for severe kidney failure in pets, typically performed over 5-7 days, and in some cases for weeks. It helps manage life-threatening complications like fluid overload, electrolyte imbalances, and toxin buildup in the blood. While it doesn't improve kidney function; it provides critical support while the kidneys heal.

The mechanical ventilator (or critical care respirator) is another device that most veterinary ICUs use: it's a machine made for use in humans that has been commonly employed for critically ill animals. Ventilators became widely known to the public during the COVID-19 pandemic when they represented a marker of illness among those infected and hospitalized. It was understood that if you contracted COVID-19 and required ventilation, your illness was markedly more severe than someone who was hospitalized and did not require ventilation. Incidentally, early on during the COVID-19 pandemic when ICU equipment such as high-flow oxygen devices and mechanical ventilators, were in high demand, the low supply among human ICUs resulted in many veterinary ICUs lending their ventilators to their local human hospital for use. This, of course, meant that mechanical ventilation would not be an option for any veterinary patients presenting to the hospital in respiratory failure. This was deemed a necessary sacrifice to save critically ill human patients in need of ventilatory support.

I remember the first patient I sent home during my residency after being mechanically ventilated. He was a middle-aged Miniature Dachshund who presented to me in congestive heart failure. This Dachshund had a previously diagnosed heart murmur suggesting degenerative mitral valve disease, a common condition among small breed dogs that occurs when there is thickening and abnormal closure of one of the heart valves, causing leakage and abnormal buildup of fluid in the circulation. In its severest form, mitral valve disease can lead to heart failure, whereby fluid builds up inside of the lungs cause an increased breathing rate and difficulty getting oxygen into the bloodstream. The Dachshund was in severe distress upon arrival at the hospital and within hours it necessitated that we place a tube in his airway and begin mechanical ventilation. This is usually begun because an animal cannot breathe on their own, such as in patients with brain injury or paralysis who cannot get enough oxygen with other forms of supplementation or is fatigued and essentially too exhausted to breathe unsupported. In this case, the Dachshund was unable to sustain his blood oxygen levels despite supplementation in an oxygen cage, and he became too tired to breathe on his own after a few hours in the hospital.

Thankfully, soon after beginning mechanical ventilation, the Dachshund's oxygen levels stabilized, and, after a few days, he was weaned from the ventilator. This process involves gradually decreasing the sedation required for a patient to tolerate the presence of an endotracheal (breathing) tube in their airway. Light anesthesia is maintained to prevent animals from chewing on the tube while receiving mechanical ventilation, and the goal is for the patient to eventually begin breathing on their own. Once a patient can sustain their oxygen levels with limited ventilator support or oxygen supplementation, reversal medications are given to remove the effects of any reversible sedatives. When the animal is conscious, the breathing tube is removed. While the weaning process can often be a series of attempts and resumptions of mechanical ventilation, in the Dachshund's case he was successfully weaned from mechanical ventilation on the first attempt. And, just a few hours later, he promptly bit me on my nose (a "thank you for saving my life" that I'll never forget!).

The most gut-wrenching and uplifting cases that I can recall in my career to date have been mechanically ventilated. Years ago I cared for a young French Bulldog who had aspirated after her routine spay surgery and developed pneumonia that required ventilation. After more than two weeks of mechanical ventilation, which included consultation with a human critical care specialist (she was the first documented case report to receive a special form of mechanical ventilation previously utilized only in human ICU patients),[3] she was eventually discharged from the ICU. Her owner, one of the most dedicated and kind pet parents I have had the pleasure of interacting with in my career, kept in touch with me throughout her dog's life, messaging me on social media each time her dog celebrated another birthday and, most recently, when she passed away.

Many, if not the majority, of ventilator cases do not have such positive and uplifting outcomes. I can recall another Miniature Dachshund puppy who was admitted in respiratory failure after chewing on an electrical power bar. Not only had the puppy sustained electrical burns to the commissures of her mouth, she developed acute respiratory distress syndrome (ARDS) (Box 2), a common and life-threatening sequelae of electrocution. Despite more than two weeks of mechanical ventilation and intensive care, her condition didn't improve and, with the uncertainty of whether her lungs would recover or sustain permanent scarring and the need for lifelong oxygen support, her owners made the painful decision to euthanize her. This was devastating for everyone involved, including her entire ICU team and her extended family who visited daily.

Box 2: Did You Know?

ARDS is a serious condition where dogs experience sudden breathing failure due to fluid buildup and severe lung inflammation. Sadly, it's a life-threatening problem, and many dogs with ARDS do not survive. Common causes of ARDS include pneumonia, smoke inhalation, near drowning, electrocution, aspiration, serious infection, or systemic inflammation.

The highs and lows of working in the ICU are difficult to capture for those who haven't had the firsthand experience of bringing animals back from the brink of death or euthanizing patients after weeks of hourly treatments and tireless care. Whether nursing animals who are unconscious and ventilated for weeks in the ICU, or conscious and receiving renal replacement therapy, the devotion to patient care by the entire ICU team, including the committed pet parents and their families, is unparalleled by any other specialty. While the shifts can be emotionally taxing and the cases mentally challenging, the high-stakes environment lends itself to some incredible wins among the excruciating losses, which most veterinary ICU team members wouldn't trade for anything.

14

Navigating Euthanasia in Veterinary Medicine

> When someone says "I couldn't become a vet because I love animals too much and wouldn't be able to perform humane euthanasia," I wish they knew that it's hard for us too.
> —Kathryn Sippel, DVM (Small Animal Veterinarian)

I vividly recall my first encounter with euthanasia. It was during my early elementary school years on a Sunday when my mom received a call from a long-time client. They'd made the difficult decision to euthanize their cherished family dog. Although I was unaware of the exact cause, it was evident that he'd been unwell for some time and the family had prepared for this final farewell. Accompanying my mom to the clinic, as I often did on weekends, I waited in the background while she spoke with the dog's owners and returned cradling an endearingly scruffy terrier mix. Too young to comprehend the situation, I obediently held the dog as my mom administered an injection into his vein. The little animal was so frail that he needed more of a tender embrace than restraint. As my mom injected the blue-tinged liquid into his leg, he swiftly grew limp in my arms. Tears streamed down my face as the reality of his passing sank in, transforming the lively companion into a still memory even as I held him.

My childhood experience likely resonates with many of my clients, who, over the years, have faced the emotional challenge of attending their pet's euthanasia. In the past, it was common for pet owners to leave their animals at the veterinary clinic, avoiding those final moments. This changed as families began to choose to be present during the procedure, often conducted in an exam room after the pet was briefly taken elsewhere for catheter placement. Today, veterinary clinics offer comfort rooms, aiming to provide a more soothing environment for euthanasia. Pet owners are frequently given the opportunity to remain with their beloved animals throughout the entire process, from sedation to the administration of euthanasia drug. Moreover, the availability of at-home euthanasia services has grown, allowing families to bid farewell in the familiar surroundings of their home or backyard. These changes in euthanasia practices reflect the strengthening of the human-animal bond, with pets increasingly regarded as cherished family members whose loss is mourned akin to that of a human loved one.

DOI: 10.1201/9781003347385-16

The term "euthanasia" finds its roots in the Greek words "eu," meaning "good," and "Thanatos," representing "death." Over time, due to the emotional weight associated with euthanasia, various euphemisms have emerged to soften the finality of the procedure. These euphemisms, such as "put to sleep" or "put down," attempt to convey the act in a gentler light. Another commonly used phrase is "crossing over the Rainbow Bridge," inspired by a narrative penned by Scottish artist and animal enthusiast Edna Clyne-Rekhy in 1959, following the loss of her beloved dog, Major (Box 1).[1] This narrative, along with similar poems, has provided solace to countless individuals grieving the loss of their pets. Personally, I have also found comfort in the imagery of the Rainbow Bridge, a sentiment I've shared with families since my teenage years, working alongside my mom at her veterinary clinic, and continuing throughout my career.

Box 1: Did You Know?

Edna Clyne-Rekhy was 19 years old and living in Scotland when she wrote a story portraying a serene place, described as "just this side of heaven," where pets are restored to full health, injuries vanish, and they frolic endlessly with companions under perpetual sunshine. She conveyed that the only absence is their cherished human companion, awaited until the day they reunite at the Rainbow Bridge, embarking on their journey into eternity together.[1]

More than 30 years later and 20 years into my career as a veterinarian, I've euthanized hundreds of animals. While most of these compassionate farewells have taken place in the presence of the pet's caregivers, some have occurred within the ICU setting with my team, because either the owner opted not to be present or was unable to attend. Following a euthanasia, it has become almost customary for the pet's owner or family to express, "this must be the hardest part of your job." I often respond by acknowledging the profound difficulty of bidding farewell but also emphasizing that it's one of the privileges of being a veterinarian. As Anne Quain eloquently articulates in her article "The Gift: Ethically Indicated Euthanasia in Companion Animal Practice": "'the gift' refers to the privilege we have as veterinarians to end suffering."[2] While performing such a procedure may appear to be the most challenging aspect of our profession, veterinarians often contend with a multitude of other demanding scenarios. From witnessing animal neglect or abuse to navigating complex moral dilemmas, the true challenges of veterinary practice extend far beyond the act of euthanasia.

While numerous studies on veterinarian stress in regions like North America, Australasia, and the United Kingdom have highlighted euthanasia as a significant factor, recent focus group research in Canada has uncovered a different perspective. Contrary to popular belief, the act of euthanasia itself is not the primary source of distress. Instead, findings from a 2019 study published in *The Veterinary Record* revealed that the most challenging aspect for veterinary team members was engaging in discussions about euthanasia with families. Moreover, the study demonstrated that successfully navigating these discussions and facilitating a "good death" for the animal resulted in an enhanced sense of wellbeing for the veterinary team. A "good death" was characterized by interviewees as one that was "humane," "peaceful," "smooth," and "quick," ultimately bringing an end to the companion animal's suffering.[3]

Navigating euthanasia in veterinary practice is far from straightforward; it's a nuanced terrain with varied experiences. I've encountered instances where I've guided clients seamlessly through the decision-making process, with them by their pet's side throughout the procedure and leaving the clinic tearful but grateful that their beloved companion is no longer suffering. Yet, there have been countless other scenarios that deeply troubled me. Some clients have hesitated to euthanize their pet despite clear indications, while others have insisted on euthanasia despite viable treatment options. These situations create profound moral conflict for us as veterinarians. We're tasked with balancing the principles of beneficence (doing good) and non-maleficence (doing no harm), striving to act in the best interest of the animal while respecting the autonomy of the pet owner. Most of the time, transparent communication fosters understanding, and decisions align smoothly. However, there are moments of dissonance, where the desires of the family diverge significantly from our professional recommendations. These instances underscore the intricate ethical dilemmas inherent in euthanasia discussions, where we strive to navigate with sensitivity and compassion, a commitment to the wellbeing of our patients, and the wishes of our clients.

It is not uncommon for veterinarians and pet owners to have divergent views on the best course of action for an animal. And it's important to recognize that there's no absolute "right" or "wrong" decision when it comes to euthanizing a pet; rather, everyone is making the choice that feels right for them in their unique circumstances. That's why I tend to refrain from answering the common question posed by many pet owners facing this decision: "What would you do if this were your pet?" There are myriad factors influencing an owner's decision, from their personal beliefs and financial situation to their bond with the animal and life circumstances. I choose not to share my personal opinion to avoid adding complexity or inadvertently implying judgment. Instead, I assure pet owners that I'll support whatever decision they make. Whether they opt for further treatment, consent to transition to palliative care, or choose euthanasia, my priority is to provide them with comfort and validation in their decision-making process.

Unfortunately, there are euthanasia scenarios that undeniably weigh heavily on veterinarians; these are typically referred to as convenience or objectionable euthanasia. Ethically indicated euthanasia, as defined by the American Veterinary Medical Association (AVMA) Guidelines for the Euthanasia of Animals, aligns with the animal's welfare and best interests. In stark contrast, convenience euthanasia involves putting down a physically and mentally healthy animal due to the owner's circumstances, such as financial constraints, time limitations, or an inability to care for the animal. On the other hand, objectionable euthanasia is simply euthanasia that a veterinarian disagrees with.

A survey published in *The Veterinary Record* in 2018 revealed that 80% of the nearly 500 surveyed veterinarians in the United States had declined a euthanasia request at some point in their careers, with one-third reporting turning down such requests a few times each year.[4] Another study of nearly 900 North American veterinarians found that 93% had received what they considered to be inappropriate euthanasia requests, of which 40% had never complied and 38% had rarely complied with these requests.[5] These statistics underscore the high frequency of complex ethical dilemmas veterinarians face when confronted with euthanasia requests that challenge their professional and personal convictions.

My first encounter with euthanasia still feels like yesterday, etched permanently into my memory. It's just one of countless moments in my veterinary career where I've grappled with the profound responsibility of guiding families through the decision to say goodbye to their cherished pets. But beyond my own experiences, there's a broader conversation among veterinarians about euthanasia—one that explores our attitudes, perspectives, and the complex ethical terrain we navigate. Studies, like one conducted in Austria, offer fascinating insights into how factors like gender and years of experience shape our views on euthanasia scenarios. The study published in 2016 surveyed veterinarians to gauge their attitudes toward euthanasia of small animals. Nearly 500 veterinarians provided responses to questions evaluating demographic variables, such as gender, age, and professional experience, to identify correlations with viewpoints on euthanasia. Interestingly, female veterinarians and those with fewer years of experience were more inclined to disagree with convenience euthanasia scenarios. Additionally, more veterinarians working together appeared to alleviate moral stress related to euthanasia, suggesting that collaborative environments may offer crucial support to veterinarians facing such ethical dilemmas.[6]

I've spoken with numerous emergency veterinarians who have refused to euthanize pets that show no apparent signs of illness or injury, especially when there's limited history available about the owner or the animal. On the other hand, I've also heard unsettling stories from emergency vets who've granted similar euthanasia requests, only to discover later that the pet was perfectly healthy and cherished by someone else in the family. Sometimes, these veterinarians are told that the animal has been unwell for an extended period or has behavioral issues that pose a risk to others. However, without access to medical records from the primary care veterinarian, which are often unavailable after regular business hours, the emergency veterinarian is left to weigh the owner's account against the pet's wellbeing. These scenarios undoubtedly weigh heavily on the veterinary team, torn between wanting to trust the owner and ensuring the best outcome for the pet, who may be perfectly healthy and possibly treatable or rehomable.

A study published in 2023 highlights the significant variability in euthanasia protocols among New Zealand veterinarians, with many clinics lacking standard procedures for dogs and cats. Moreover, it reveals a deficiency in training during veterinary school on emotional support for clients (Box 2).[7] These findings are consistent with my own journey, where I learned most of what I know about euthanasia from mentors and coworkers in practice. It's alarming to realize that formal training in euthanasia or end-of-life conversations was absent during my veterinary school years, leaving me to navigate these sensitive situations on the job. Despite veterinary schools today offering some education on communication and case-based learning regarding end-of-life scenarios, as a speaker and advocate for wellbeing I'm frequently asked to address the mental health implications of euthanasia and offer coping strategies. This highlights the urgent need for more comprehensive training in euthanasia and client communication throughout veterinary education and beyond. By prioritizing the emotional aspects of euthanasia in veterinary training, we can better support veterinarians and improve the overall experience for both patients and families.

Box 2: Did You Know?

In a recent survey, over one-third of veterinarians in New Zealand said that they received no training in dealing with emotional clients or managing compassion fatigue and nearly three-quarters learned from experiences or discussions with colleagues after graduation.[7]

When discussing euthanasia of healthy animals, it's crucial to consider the experiences of veterinarians working in shelter environments and those involved in mass depopulation events. A comprehensive review published in the *Journal of the American Veterinary Medical Association* analyzed research papers focusing on the effects of euthanasia on individuals working in animal shelters, veterinary clinics, and research facilities. The findings, primarily based on studies involving shelter workers, revealed that those who perform euthanasia can suffer from traumatic stress reactions that significantly impact their wellbeing.[8] This toll is particularly understandable in the context of euthanizing healthy animals in shelters when adoption isn't possible. However, a separate study in the *Journal of Occupational Health Psychology* in 2014, which surveyed over 500 Australian veterinarians, found that objectionable euthanasia wasn't directly linked to depressed mood or suicide risk. Instead, the frequency of euthanasia overall showed a slight association with depression, suggesting that veterinarians who performed euthanasia more frequently were more likely to experience a depressed mood. Interestingly, those working in low socioeconomic areas, compared to average socioeconomic conditions, also showed a higher likelihood of experiencing depression.[9] This could be attributed to their increased exposure to convenience euthanasia situations, where owners couldn't afford ongoing care, even if the circumstances weren't considered objectionable.

Discussions within veterinary circles often revolve around the idea that performing euthanasia could be a traumatic event for veterinarians, possibly leading to post-traumatic stress disorder (PTSD). While euthanasia situations aiming for a "good death" are common, there are instances perceived as resulting in a "bad death," where animals may exhibit distressing behaviors like vocalization, gasping for air, or jerking movements before passing away. These experiences cause distress not only to the pet owner but also to the person performing the euthanasia. In the Canadian focus group study mentioned earlier, veterinary team members who perceived a euthanasia as resulting in a "bad death" reported negative impacts on the wellbeing of both the client and the veterinary team member. Moreover, some owners experience overwhelming grief upon learning of their pet's passing, leading to emotional labor for the veterinary team, particularly when clients are inconsolable.[3] A study published in the *Australian Veterinary Journal* surveyed over 100 veterinarians in South Australia in 2015, revealing that 40% of respondents agreed or strongly agreed that dealing with grieving clients had adversely affected their mental and physical health.[10]

Scholars and professionals in the field have broadened the discussion by introducing the term "perpetration-induced traumatic stress" (PITS) to describe the emotional impact of mass euthanasia of healthy animals in veterinary medicine. Unlike PTSD, which originated to explain the psychological aftermath of harrowing experiences among war veterans, PITS emerged in 2002. It was observed that American veterans of the Vietnam War who directly participated in or believed they caused human deaths were significantly more prone to PTSD than those who only witnessed such events.[11] This phenomenon has been studied among animal workers, including veterinarians, veterinary technicians or nurses, as well as research and animal shelter staff. Research indicates that 11% of participants report moderate levels of traumatic stress symptoms, with higher levels of euthanasia-related stress linked to a shorter length of time working with animals and elevated concerns about animal death.[12] Moreover, PITS has been associated with distress among animal workers and veterinarians involved in mass depopulation scenarios, such as handling infectious disease outbreaks or addressing border closures that require culling thousands of healthy farm animals destined for the food supply. The act of euthanizing healthy animals in these contexts remains a challenging ethical dilemma, despite the focus on preventing or alleviating suffering. In many of these situations, similar emotional impacts have been noted, such as in the aftermath of animal hoarding situations where euthanizing multiple animals may be necessary to address the welfare of those involved.[13]

Although I haven't experienced working in a shelter environment or encountered many cases involving the euthanasia of apparently healthy animals, I've personally found there's a limit to how many animals I can comfortably euthanize in a single shift. When faced with situations where an animal's life could have been saved with proper treatment, my distress is palpable. One euthanasia particularly haunts me: a puppy left at the doorstep of the emergency clinic where I worked. With limited money available from a small "Good Samaritan Fund," we diagnosed the puppy with parvoviral enteritis, a severe intestinal virus. Initially, I held onto hope that we could nurse him back to health for adoption. However, as his condition worsened and he required more intensive care, it became clear that we needed additional resources beyond what our donated funds could provide. Despite reaching out to local animal shelters and welfare organizations, their capacity to accommodate puppies with the virus was already stretched thin. Ultimately, I had to euthanize this sweet Pitbull mix puppy alone in the isolation room of the hospital, tears streaming down my face. Poignant experiences like this, coupled with witnessing the intense grief of pet owners, remain vivid in my memory. Yet, paradoxically, I believe my capacity to perform euthanasia compassionately is one of my greatest strengths as a veterinarian.

The emotional toll of performing euthanasia can be significant, especially when it involves healthy animals for whom alternative options are not available. This responsibility often leads to traumatic stress reactions that deeply impact the mental wellbeing of veterinary professionals. As we navigate these complex scenarios, it's imperative to advocate for the mental health and support of those involved, recognizing that compassion in veterinary medicine extends not only to the animals, but also to the practitioners who bear these heavy decisions. By addressing the emotional ramifications of euthanasia and promoting robust support systems, we can help alleviate the burden carried by veterinarians and, ultimately, foster a healthier and more compassionate veterinary community.

Ethical Dilemmas and Moral Stress

> You need support to deal with the intense experiences associated with eu-
> thanasia, massive trauma, and moral and ethical decisions and medical
> reasoning that becomes part of everyday life for us in this field.
> —Kathryn Arbic, DVM (Locum Veterinarian)

Decades ago, if someone had told me that veterinarians routinely experience
moral distress, I wouldn't have understood what they meant. The notion that a
veterinarian might know the ethically correct course of action but feel unable
to carry it out was entirely foreign to me. Growing up in my mom's companion animal practice and throughout veterinary school, I rarely encountered
or discussed these kinds of ethical dilemmas. But today, I recognize moral
distress as a major source of psychological strain for veterinarians. Whether
it's suspecting a client of animal abuse or disagreeing with a colleague about
a treatment plan, ethical conflicts are a common—and often painful—part of
veterinary medicine.

As veterinarians, we continually navigate the delicate balance between advocating for the patient's welfare and fulfilling our obligation to the client or
owner. Instances where these interests clash inevitably result in moral stress.
As discussed in the previous chapter, the most common ethical dilemmas occur during euthanasia decision making: when a pet owner requests euthanasia despite viable treatment options being available or, conversely, when the
patient is suffering, yet the client refuses euthanasia. In the intensive care unit
(ICU), the latter scenario is particularly frequent. Often, we grapple with cases
deemed futile, where proposed treatments offer little chance of success or may
result in prolonged suffering or dependency on critical care, such as mechanical ventilation. These situations can provoke profound distress among veterinary technicians and nurses, who feel forced to administer treatments they
perceive as unnecessary and potentially harmful, with minimal likelihood of
a positive outcome. Ultimately, veterinarians find themselves caught in a situation where they are compelled to provide care they believe to be ethically
questionable.

One particular case stands out in my memory as emblematic of creating
moral distress stemming from futile care. At the time, I was working in the

DOI: 10.1201/9781003347385-17

ICU of a large specialty referral hospital. A Yorkshire Terrier was admitted, having previously undergone tracheal stenting due to tracheal collapse. Tracheal collapse is a condition that affects certain breeds like Yorkies and Pomeranians, where the windpipe becomes compressed, hindering breathing. To alleviate this, a tracheal stent, akin to a small cylindrical scaffold typically made of metal or plastic, is inserted into the narrowed section of the trachea. This stent acts as a support to keep the airway open, allowing air to flow more smoothly into the lungs—similar to placing a straw inside a partially compressed hose to keep it open for water to pass through.

While some dogs with tracheal stents go on to live the rest of their life without complication, this particular dog was not so lucky. His disease had progressed, resulting in collapse of his larynx (voice box) and the mainstem bronchi (lower parts of his airways that branch into the lungs). A tracheotomy was performed so that the dog could breathe through an opening in his neck, but that did not fix the collapse of his lower airways. When his breathing effort worsened, despite all of our less invasive options, we had to pass a very long tube through his mouth and down to his lungs, to maintain his oxygen levels and resolve his distress. Unfortunately, multiple attempts to remove the tube so that he could breathe on his own were unsuccessful. It was becoming more and more apparent that the dog would be dependent upon positive pressure ventilation in the ICU indefinitely. Given he wouldn't be able to survive independently, continuing mechanical ventilation for the Yorkie was deemed futile.

Although it took some time for the owners to acknowledge this reality and consent to euthanasia, the impact on the ICU team during his hospitalization was profound. Every member involved in the dog's care—from the animal care attendants and nurses to the client care representatives and specialists—experienced intense moral stress as the dog remained on life support. Questions such as "What's the purpose of this?" and "Aren't we just prolonging the inevitable?" echoed among the team, alongside concerns about the allocation of resources and the inability of the owners to recognize the futility of the situation. As the perceived inevitability weighed on the team, moral stress escalated into distress, evident in conversations filled with anger, frustration, sadness, and confusion (Box 1).

Box 1: Did You Know?

Moral stress refers to the discomfort or unease that individuals experience stemming from an ethical dilemma or a situation where a veterinarian faces a difficult choice between two or more options, each of which has moral implications. *Moral distress* occurs when individuals are aware of the ethical conflict between their values and actions but also feel powerless to act in accordance with their values due to external constraints or pressures. This can lead to emotional suffering, frustration, and a sense of moral compromise.

In the realm of veterinary medicine, moral injury is a consequence of a significantly morally distressing event that manifests as a profound and enduring psychological response when individuals witness a violation of their core moral principles (Box 2). Veterinarians, in particular, may confront moral injury following events like mass euthanasia in disaster situations. I recall a conversation with a longtime friend and dairy veterinarian in British Columbia's Lower Mainland after they grappled with devastating flooding.[1] He recounted the anguish of having to euthanize more than one-third of a client's herd, unable to save them from the rising waters and deep mud. The emotional toll was immense as he witnessed the submerged animals and the grief-stricken farmers, many of whom cried over the loss of their animals. Like many veterinarians in similar circumstances, he buried his emotions to continue working, but the memories of that event haunted him, underscoring the lasting impact of moral injury in our profession.

Box 2: Did You Know?

Moral injury occurs when an individual's fundamental moral beliefs are violated, leading to deep emotional wounds or feelings of betrayal. It often arises in high-stress or traumatic situations, such as disasters or when individuals experience moral distress. It can result in feelings of guilt, shame, and a sense of moral disintegration.

A comprehensive review, spanning over two decades of research on work-related stressors affecting the mental health of veterinarians, underscores ethical dilemmas as a significant source of stress.[2] While there is limited literature on moral stress among veterinarians in situations such as massive depopulation or within the horseracing industry,[3] the majority of available information focuses on moral distress in companion animal practice. A study published in *The Veterinary Record* in 2012 surveyed nearly 60 veterinarians in the United Kingdom (UK), revealing that over half reported encountering one or two ethical dilemmas per week, with a third facing three to five such dilemmas weekly. The survey highlighted three common scenarios: (1) convenience euthanasia of a healthy animal; (2) financial constraints limiting treatment options; and (3) clients insisting on continued treatment despite compromised animal welfare. All scenarios were rated as "highly stressful," with financial limitations being the most distressing. Moreover, over three-quarters of veterinarians felt they had insufficient training in veterinary ethics during their education.[4]

A more recent and extensive study, published in the *Journal of Veterinary Internal Medicine* in 2018, delved into the online survey responses of nearly 900 veterinarians across North America. When asked how frequently they encountered cases where they felt unable to do the "right thing," 49% responded "sometimes," and 13% responded "often." Further inquiry into the distress caused by these situations revealed that half experienced moderate distress, while over one-quarter experienced severe distress. Coping mechanisms employed by respondents included discussing the issue with a partner, friend, or colleague (73%); taking no action (17%); or seeking professional support (12%). The survey also explored perceptions of futility in treatment, with 57% reporting encountering cases where they believed pet owners were requesting futile treatment efforts "sometimes," and 22% reporting "often." When asked if they had ever refused to administer what they deemed futile treatment, the responses were evenly divided, with 51% answering "yes" and 49% "no." Additionally, when questioned about prioritizing the needs of animal owners over those of their patients, 60% responded "yes," while 40% said "no." A follow-up question "Do you feel conflicted about this?" revealed that half responded "sometimes" and one-quarter responded "often."[5]

Animal abuse is another significant source of moral distress for veterinarians. A study published in *The Veterinary Record* in 2022 examined survey responses from over 200 veterinarians, primarily from the UK. The study found that 62% of respondents had encountered or suspected cases of animal abuse in the previous year, with dogs, cats, and rabbits being the most commonly reported species. Neglect emerged as the most prevalent form of abuse, followed by physical abuse such as gunshots, bruising, and fractures.[6] These cases can cause profound distress among veterinarians and their teams, not only because of the suffering witnessed or imagined for the animals, but also due to the lack of clear guidance on how to handle and report such cases to the authorities.

In many jurisdictions, veterinarians are mandated to report instances of suspected or confirmed animal abuse to local authorities. In Alberta, where I currently live, every registered veterinarian must report to a peace officer if they have reasonable grounds to believe that an animal is being or has been abused or neglected. Under the Animal Protection Act, veterinarians are not held professionally accountable for breaching client confidentiality when complying with this directive. However, while the Canadian Veterinary Medical Association has a position statement dating back to February 2018 emphasizing a veterinarian's duty to protect animal health and welfare by reporting any firsthand observations suggestive of abuse or neglect, they also caution that veterinarians "may not be immune from liability from reporting in good faith."[7] In other words, not all jurisdictions provide legal protection to veterinarians when breaching confidentiality to report suspected cases of animal abuse.

The hesitation on the part of veterinarians to report such cases extends beyond concerns about legal repercussions, such as potential litigation or complaints from clients or owners. There is also the inherent challenge of accurately determining whether abuse has occurred. Veterinarians typically rely on their clinical findings, such as physical examinations and X-rays, as well as conversations with the owner to assess the situation. However, conclusively establishing whether an injury was deliberate or accidental is often speculative. Veterinarians must navigate a delicate balance between advocating for the animal's welfare and maintaining their relationship with the client, who may be directly or indirectly involved in the alleged abuse. This ethical dilemma contributes to the moral stress experienced by veterinarians. Additionally, there is apprehension that drawing attention to the abuse or abuser could exacerbate the situation for either the animal or the partner of the abuser, as animal abuse and intimate partner violence are closely linked.[8]

Fortunately, I've encountered very few instances of firsthand animal abuse in my career. However, a few years ago, I cared for a critically ill cat believed to have been abused by the owner's ex-partner. When I learned what had happened and examined the cat's injuries, I was overcome with nausea and sadness. It was difficult to comprehend how someone could inflict such pain on a defenseless animal like this sweet cat. The realization that the perpetrator might still be interacting with other animals—or people—filled me with fear and anger. I felt an immediate moral obligation to ensure the cat's survival and to prevent further harm. Reflecting on my colleagues' position when the abuse was first suspected and they confronted the owner, I could empathize with the difficult task they faced. Despite the discomfort, I recognized that addressing such concerns is not only a legal requirement in my province, but also an ethical responsibility—to protect the animal and any potentially affected individuals.

Undoubtedly, morally stressful situations, now referred to as potentially morally injurious events (PMIEs), profoundly affect the wellbeing of veterinarians. A study in the *European Journal of Psychotraumatology* found that nearly 90% of UK veterinarians surveyed had experienced a PMIE, significantly correlating with symptoms of post-traumatic stress disorder (PTSD).[9] Additionally, the same researchers conducted interviews with a dozen veterinarians, revealing that PMIEs led to considerable psychological distress, including guilt, shame, and reduced confidence.[10] Even veterinary students are not immune to moral stress, as demonstrated by a study in the *Journal of Veterinary Medical Education*, where over 80% reported experiencing moral stress related to animal treatment, with less than half receiving training in coping mechanisms.[11] Recognizing this, a comprehensive analysis published in *BMC Veterinary Research* in 2021 concluded that veterinary curricula should incorporate courses addressing ethical dilemmas and moral stressors.[12]

Over the past five years, a surge of research studies has explored diverse approaches to alleviate moral stress among veterinarians. These methods include implementing ethics rounds,[13,14] hosting discussion groups, and integrating veterinary social workers into practice settings.[11] Notably, North Carolina State University has adapted a human clinical consultation committee model to establish an ethics committee within its veterinary teaching hospital.[15] These initiatives underscore a collective effort to develop and refine strategies aimed at reducing the impact of morally stressful or ethically challenging situations on veterinary team members.

Ultimately, veterinary medicine diverges from human medicine in its lack of a safety net ensuring universal access to necessary treatment for every animal. Unlike healthcare for humans, where systems like insurance often cover costs, veterinary care heavily relies on owners' financial means. Without widespread pet health insurance coverage, most owners bear the full expense of veterinary treatment, leading to disparities in access to care based on financial capability. While some owners may struggle to afford necessary care for their pets, others may opt for additional treatments, potentially resulting in futile care and extension of an animal's suffering. Even if veterinary medicine transitions from its current fee-for-service model or achieves universal pet health insurance coverage, morally stressful situations surrounding pet treatment will likely persist.

Veterinary professionals are often left navigating these morally ambiguous and ethically challenging scenarios, which contribute to the rising levels of psychological distress within the profession. Dealing with situations where financial limitations dictate care—or where owners' decisions lead to prolonged suffering—creates moral stress, compounding the emotional toll of veterinary work. This constant strain can leave veterinary professionals emotionally exhausted, which contributes to burnout, a growing issue within the profession, explored in detail in Chapter 27. Ethical training and institutional support are essential to help veterinarians manage these complex situations. Only through addressing the root causes of moral stress can the profession foster a more compassionate and sustainable environment for both animals and the professionals who care for them.

16

The Paradox of Compassionate Veterinary Care

Although it can be very stressful and demanding and draining at times, it is also in my opinion the most fulfilling and rewarding and noble profession on the planet.

—Gregory Clark, BSc, DVM
(Companion Animal Veterinarian)

When I ask veterinarians what brings them satisfaction in their job versus what causes them stress, the responses are overwhelmingly similar and surprisingly dichotomous. Satisfaction inevitably stems from the ability to help others—pets and their families. This can range from the splendor of bringing animals back from the brink of death to the smallest of saviors such as removing a painful torn toenail. In my 20 years of practicing as a veterinarian, I can recall countless ways in which I've helped animals and their owners—from the first time that I unblocked a cat with a urethral (urinary tract) obstruction to the treatment of numerous animals with wounds, broken bones, acute vomiting or diarrhea (or both!), kidney failure, heart disease, breathing problems, toxin ingestions, and hundreds of other maladies. I can safely say that I've directly or indirectly, through my teaching, mentorship, and teleconsulting, saved or improved the lives of thousands of animals. In doing so, I've also enhanced the lives of thousands of humans who are or were attached to those animals. When I think about the magnitude of this, and the decades I have left in my career to assist more dogs, cats, and clients, I'm filled with an indescribable sense of pride, fulfillment, and joy.

I can still remember the first time I thought to myself "I saved that dog's life!" I was a few weeks into my internship at Washington State University and a one-year-old neutered male Cairn terrier presented to me while I was working an emergency shift. He collapsed when he came in, his mentation was dull, and his pulses were rapid and weak. His breathing was fast and shallow, and his gums were pale. I was concerned that he was bleeding internally, but with no known trauma we weren't sure of the cause. We inserted an intravenous (IV) catheter to administer fluids and, when he was more stable, we performed X-rays (this was before it was common to have an ultrasound machine in the ER to scan the chest and belly for fluid). The X-rays confirmed our

DOI: 10.1201/9781003347385-18

suspicion of fluid around the lungs and in his abdomen, and we subsequently performed a thoracocentesis (chest tap) to remove the fluid and resolve his labored breathing.

It turned out the fluid was blood, so we collected it sterilely using a blood transfusion set so that we could perform an autotransfusion (returning the blood to the dog) later on. Blood tests revealed prolonged clotting times, and we diagnosed what was later confirmed to be anticoagulant rodenticide toxicity. The dog recovered quickly after receiving a plasma transfusion and vitamin K to replenish the depleted clotting factors. His owners were relieved and expressed their gratitude with thank you cards and treats for the entire ICU and ER team. After some careful detective work, they discovered that tenants sharing their vacation home had recently put out rat poison on the property, which they promptly discarded during their next visit.

It's stories like this that most people envision when they think of what veterinarians must love about their jobs. It should be unsurprising, then, that what causes most veterinarians stress, myself included, is an inability to help animals and their families (Box 1). Whether it's because we don't have the answer or diagnosis or we're prevented from performing necessary tests or procedures or in some other way we're hindered from coming to the aid of a patient or client, it literally cuts us to the core. I remember an awful situation that transpired when I was a resident. I was working in the emergency room and a four-month-old male Pitbull was brought in by his owners after being attacked by one of the family's other dogs. His vital signs indicated that he was in shock, so we immediately placed an IV catheter to administer fluids while we completed our exam.

Box 1: Did You Know?

A workforce survey in the United Kingdom found that an overwhelming majority of veterinarians agreed with the statements "veterinary work is stressful" (83%) and "veterinary work is enjoyable" (93%).[1]

His forelimb was obviously broken and he had extensive bite wounds covering his body, some of which needed stitches. He was also covered in scars from what looked like old bite wounds and his fur was caked with dried urine and feces. He was thin and noticeably unkempt, and his injuries and scars led us to suspect that he was being used for dog fighting. We explained to the owners that his leg was broken and would need to be splinted and that his wounds would need to be cleaned and bandaged or sutured closed. When we followed that with the estimated fee for his care the owners were indignant and insisted our recommendations were unnecessary. They asked for antibiotics for the wounds and said they would take him home to heal.

As any veterinarian would be, I was distraught by this situation. I could not fathom sending this puppy home in shock and pain, left to heal on his own. Given his filthy condition, I worried that his wounds would get infected and that he might become septic and die. Or worse, that in his weakened state he would not be able to defend himself from the other dogs and would be attacked again and this time killed. My stomach turned and my eyes welled up as I tried to convince the owners that veterinary care was best for their puppy. They countered with the simple fact that they could not afford the care, which was when I suggested they consider other options such as surrendering the puppy or consenting to euthanasia. Granted, the last thing I wanted to do in this situation was put to sleep an otherwise healthy puppy that I knew we could save, but euthanasia seemed more humane than leaving the puppy to fend for himself at home.

Even after involving my supervising faculty, a kind and compassionate specialist with a calm demeanor and exceptional communication skills, we weren't able to change the owners' minds. We subsequently said that we'd finish treating the puppy's shock, bathe him to wash off the excrement and clean the wounds, splint the leg, and prescribe additional pain relievers and antibiotics for them to take home. We advised that sending the puppy home without X-rays, more extensive wound care, and stronger pain relief was against our medical advice and we had them sign a legal form acknowledging this. After treating the puppy and sending him home, I felt sick thinking of the potential horrible outcomes he might face. After discussing the situation with another faculty member, we decided to contact Animal Control to request they follow up to ensure that the puppy was not suffering at home. As we'd feared, Animal Control officers visited the home and found the puppy lying in a soiled kennel, demonstrating signs of pain. They seized him and brought him back to North Carolina State University, where he was cared for and then fostered while his former owners awaited trial for animal abuse and neglect.

Thankfully, situations like these typically occur only once or twice in a veterinarian's career. While veterinarians working in shelter medicine are more often faced with distressing situations involving neglect, abuse, or mistreatment, in most general practices these situations are uncommon. That said, there are many other stressors that veterinarians experience on a daily or weekly basis that counterbalance the satisfaction they derive from helping their patients and clients (Box 2). A survey completed by nearly 1,800 veterinarians in the United Kingdom (UK) found that the largest contributors to stress were the number of hours worked, making professional mistakes, client expectations, and administrative or clerical tasks. An additional worry, most commonly reported among veterinarians who graduated within the last five years, was managing their own finances. When considering only those veterinarians working in clinical practice, the main stressors were the possibility of client complaints or litigation, unexpected clinical outcomes, and out-of-hours on-call duties. All of these stressors were especially reported among women, younger veterinarians, and those working in small animal practice.[2]

Box 2: Did You Know?

According to a 2005 survey of more than 1,900 New Zealand veterinarians, the main sources of stress were hours worked, client expectations, and unexpected outcomes.[3]

The same survey results of UK veterinarians also determined that the greatest sources of satisfaction were good clinical outcomes, relationships with colleagues, and the intellectual challenge and learning associated with veterinary medicine.[2] Similarly, a survey completed by more than 50 veterinarians working in the University of Veterinary Medicine Vienna found that satisfaction was most derived from helping animals, having an interesting job, interacting with colleagues, and lifelong learning.[4] Likewise, a "reasonable income" and a "good working atmosphere" were most related to satisfaction among more than 1,900 German veterinarians surveyed in 2016, with the former being more important to male veterinarians and the latter being more important to female veterinarians.[5]

A more recent survey of more than 270 veterinarians in Australia asked for responses to the prompt "I derive pleasure in my work as a veterinarian when…". In order of the frequency of responses received, professional expertise (22%), positive outcomes (20%), job characteristics (19%), relationships (16%), recognition (10%), and helping (7%) were most commonly shared.[6] It seems that what all veterinarians want is to utilize and grow their expertise to help animals and their owners. If they can do that with good case outcomes, a reasonable income, positive working relationships, and recognition from others, they can derive satisfaction in their work.

The largest study investigating practice-related stressors among more than 11,000 veterinarians in the United States was conducted in 2014. Veterinarians were given a list and asked to select three factors that they considered most stressful about veterinary medicine. The list included demands of practice; practice management responsibilities; making professional mistakes; client complaints; dealing with personal, staff, or client grief; client expectations of being expert in all veterinary subject areas; animal deaths (from illness or euthanasia); competition with other veterinary practices; ethical challenges; fear of malpractice litigation; educational debt; poor social support; unclear management and work role; lack of participation in decision making; and other. "Demands of practice" was the most commonly selected stressful factor. Among practice owning veterinarians, practice management responsibilities and competition with other practices were additional commonly reported stressors, whereas relief and associate veterinarians more commonly reported professional mistakes, educational debt, unclear management and work role, and lack of participation in decision making as stressful factors.[7]

In their research paper titled "Reviewing a Decade of Change for Veterinarians: Past, Present and Gaps in Researching Stress, Coping and Mental Health Risks," Stetina and Krouzecky illuminate the multifaceted stressors inherent in veterinary medicine. Through an analysis of 30 quantitative and mixed methods studies, they identify a range of stressors, with social stressors emerging as particularly influential.[8] These encompass the intricate human-human interactions intrinsic to veterinary practice, indicating that communication challenges and interpersonal dynamics significantly contribute to stress levels among veterinarians. While many stressors experienced by veterinarians are not unique to the profession, such as those stemming from co-worker relationships or management issues, veterinary medicine stands apart due to its fee-for-service structure. Because pet owners are financially responsible for the care of their furry family members, this creates a distinct set of stressors that veterinary professionals navigate on a daily basis.

What has often struck me as poignant when reflecting on the highs and lows of veterinary practice is the dichotomy between the compassionate work we do as veterinarians and the stress or compassion fatigue we experience in turn. This so-called paradox of compassionate work has been articulated by Canadian sociologists Polachek and Wallace as the reward and cost of practicing veterinary medicine.[9] After interviewing and surveying veterinary care providers, the researchers affirm the complexity of veterinary medicine, whereby making a difference to animals and building relationships with pets and their families result in greater compassion satisfaction. Conversely, barriers to patient care from pet owners and witnessing client grief are associated with greater compassion fatigue. Perhaps most intriguing is the finding that forming relationships with animals is associated with both increased compassion satisfaction and compassion fatigue, which we'll discuss more fully in Chapter 26. It underscores the complexity of working in a profession where that which brings joy also represents one of the greatest sources of sorrow.

If you asked me about my most satisfying moments in veterinary practice, I would recount memories of collaborating with interns, residents, veterinary technicians, and students in caring for patients at the Ontario Veterinary College's ICU. These moments include successfully bringing animals back from the brink, forging connections with the families of my patients during their darkest farewells, and sharing in their moments of greatest joy as they leave the hospital with their beloved companions. Conversely, my most stressful instances in veterinary practice entail gut-wrenching cases that remained in the hospital for weeks without improvement, grueling days punctuated by difficult interactions with clients or team members, and high-stakes situations where families faced uncertain outcomes despite significant financial investments.

Despite the abundance of joyful memories, they often take a back seat to the challenging cases and situations I have encountered. Recognizing the human tendency toward negativity bias, I continue to embrace the rewarding aspects of this profession while acknowledging the inherent tension and strain it can bring. Ultimately, the paradox of compassionate work within veterinary medicine is one of both triumph and turmoil. Veterinarians are uniquely positioned to experience extraordinary satisfaction from the lives they save and the bonds they forge, yet they are also vulnerable to deep emotional fatigue due to the barriers they face and the grief they witness. As we've explored, the very relationships that bring joy and fulfillment can also lead to stress and burnout. This intricate balance underscores the necessity for greater awareness and proactive measures in supporting the wellbeing of veterinary professionals. Compassionate work is both a gift and a challenge, and understanding this duality is the first step toward creating a more sustainable and supportive environment for veterinarians.

Compliments, Complaints, and Client Incivility

We are making health care recommendations that we truly believe are in the best interest of their pets and when they say things like "you're all about the money" or "I thought you cared about pets, but I guess you just care about money" we internalize that. We take it home. We stress about it. And it eats us alive.

—Jennifer Deeks, RVT
(Registered Veterinary Technician)

I remember the first time a client yelled at me. I was in junior high school and working a Saturday shift at my mom's practice. I enjoyed these shifts because they were relatively low-key. We didn't schedule surgeries or major procedures, the shift ended in the early afternoon, and I worked alongside a small team of a veterinarian and veterinary technician. I functioned mainly as a receptionist answering the phone, scheduling appointments, and greeting and checking out clients, while occasionally assisting with patients. On this particular day, we were exceptionally busy and had three "walk-in" urgent appointments, one of which needed to have a minor laceration repair performed. This had led to our regularly scheduled appointments running behind and a client who'd been waiting for nearly 40 minutes was growing increasingly impatient.

At this point in my life (and budding veterinary career), I'd received no formal training in client communication and the only sentiment I recall learning was "the customer is always right." I apologized to the client for the long wait, explaining that we had additional dogs and cats who needed more urgent care and the vet would get to his dog's annual checkup and vaccines as quickly as possible. We moved the client to an exam room where he became increasingly agitated until, after waiting almost an hour, he stormed out of the room, came to the front desk, and told me that the wait was preposterous, we didn't appear to be busy, and that he'd seek his veterinary services elsewhere (I'm paraphrasing here). As you can imagine, this was said loudly, red faced, and in such close proximity that I remember flinching and stepping backward to gather myself. I couldn't think of a reply, leaving him to stride out of the practice and our hospital manager to follow up the next Monday to try to appease and ex-

DOI: 10.1201/9781003347385-19

plain. I don't think I took a breath for the entirety of my interaction with him and was relieved, to say the least, that he never returned to the clinic.

When I've posed the question as to what they feel most challenged by, my colleagues and friends in the veterinary profession almost always respond with one word: clients. They then follow with stories about unrealistic expectations, hurtful accusations, board complaints, negative online reviews, non-compliance, and even lawsuits. The anecdotes that are shared range from humorous and eyeroll-inducing to downright jaw-dropping and could likely fill an entire book (or mini-series) if given the opportunity. But the impact of negative client interactions goes beyond providing memorable stories, as shown by a growing body of recent research examining how client incivility and complaints affect all members of the veterinary team.

A study published in 2021 in *The Veterinary Record* shared responses from 18 veterinarians in the United Kingdom (UK) who conducted telephone interviews detailing their exposure to a range of rude behaviors from clients. These included clients ordering the veterinarian around, talking over the veterinarian, making demeaning comments, accusing the veterinarian of being money motivated, refusing to pay for treatment, and yelling or using a rude tone. These behaviors were attributed to abrasive personalities, financial concerns, and feelings of frustration, worry, helplessness, or grief. Responses to these behaviors ranged from scheduling more or less time to communicate with the client, empathizing with the client's concerns, actively listening to try to understand the client's perspective, using more assertive communication, or asking the client to seek veterinary services elsewhere. Still, the consequences of these uncivil client interactions were numerous and included increased stress, diminished self-confidence, emotional upset, and mental health challenges. Some of the veterinarians who were interviewed even shared a desire to reduce working hours or leave the veterinary profession after repeated incidents of client incivility.[1]

While most veterinarians empathize with pet owners facing high costs or worrying about their pet's outcomes, many express frustration with clients who hold unrealistic expectations. When the open-text responses of more than 1,400 American veterinarians were reviewed to determine the most significant practice-related stressors, unrealistic expectations for treatment ("Client unrealistic expectations / taking their problems out on us") and expectations of availability ("Client expectation of being always available") were two commonly described situations of client-related stress.[2] I regularly witness situations in veterinary practice where clients refuse diagnostic tests, insist on treatment based on assumptions, and then become frustrated—or even file complaint or lawsuits—when their pet's condition doesn't improve. It becomes a no-win situation for the veterinarian—unable to pursue a diagnosis due to client refusal, yet still held to the unreasonable expectation of having all of the answers. And sadly, the incivility of clients is not just felt by veterinarians but, rather, by all members of the veterinary team (Box 1).

Box 1: Did You Know?

An online survey published in *The Veterinary Record* in 2022 gathered more than 250 responses from veterinarians, veterinary nurses, animal care assistants, practice managers, and client care assistants in the United Kingdom. Experiences of client incivility such as being put down, ignored, and yelled, shouted, or sworn at predicted higher levels of burnout and depression or anxiety symptoms among the team members.[3]

When I speak to newly graduated veterinarians or students who are finishing their training, concerns about client complaints and lawsuits are top of mind when they consider the stress of beginning clinical practice. This sentiment is demonstrated in research conducted in the United States evaluating the biggest practice-related stressors. Of the more nearly 12,000 veterinarians surveyed, nearly one-quarter named client complaints and 1 in 10 cited fear of malpractice litigation as the most stressful in veterinary medicine. Indeed, the same survey revealed that 13% of respondents were planning to leave veterinary medicine, with 22% citing client complaints as a reason.[4] While many formal complaints are dismissed or not investigated (Box 2), the consequences can still be dramatic for those receiving them.

Box 2: Did You Know?

Complaints received by the Veterinary Council of New Zealand spanning several decades (1992–2016) were almost entirely related to technical competency (67%) or professional behavior (32%). Two-thirds of complaints were dismissed or not investigated and just 1.5% were upheld due to insufficient technical competency concerns.[5]

The frequency and impact of client complaints are especially notable among veterinarians who are board-certified specialists in internal medicine. Online surveys were completed by nearly 100 veterinary internists in 2017 and revealed that two-thirds had received a client complaint during the previous six months. Cost of care was cited as the most common reason among more than half of the specialists. Nearly all respondents worried about client complaints being made against them with more than one-third worrying "most" or "all of the time." Shockingly, 35% said they had been verbally assaulted by a client and 29% had been threatened with litigation in the previous six months. As a result, nearly three-quarters had changed the way they practice medicine to avoid client complaints and 44% had considered changing their career because of complaints made against them.[6]

The consequences of client complaints stretch beyond feelings of worry or career dissatisfaction, and they impact all members of the veterinary team (Box 3). A focus group study conducted in the UK between July 2020 and March 2021 included veterinarians, registered or student veterinary nurses, and management or leadership team members. The emotional impact of client complaints was all-encompassing as participants described issues with concentration; sleep disorders; lack of personal fulfillment in previously enjoyable activities; impaired clinical confidence; fear in performing clinical work or communicating with clients; and emotional withdrawal from partners, friends, and family members.[7]

Box 3: Did You Know?

An online survey distributed via several Facebook groups involving more than 550 veterinary support team members, including veterinary technicians, veterinary assistants, veterinary receptionists, and kennel staff members, revealed that nearly half felt depressed because of a client complaint made against them and more than half reported that a complaint negatively affected their enjoyment of the job. Approximately 1 in 4 considered changing their career because of client complaints made against them.[8]

Without a doubt there are incidents when a pet owner's dissatisfaction is warranted. Veterinarians are not perfect, and they make mistakes, as we'll discuss in Chapter 23. However, more and more veterinarians are finding that clients' expectations are increasingly unrealistic—expecting immediate answers without diagnostic testing and without incurring any cost. And when situations do not unfold in this way, the response from clients is swift and can be downright mean. I've lost count of the number of veterinarians I know (myself included) who've been screamed at by an owner in front of a waiting room full of other clients, sworn at over the phone, accused of something incomprehensible, threatened with negative reviews or sidewalk picketing, or confronted with board complaints or lawsuits. And, very often, these occur amidst uncontrollable adverse events such as a drug reaction or a foreseeable complication when an owner was non-compliant or did not follow medical advice.

A colleague of mine shared a story about an older feline patient of hers with chronic kidney disease and an undiagnosed intestinal ailment that was likely inflammatory bowel disease or cancer. The cat had irritated skin in the area where the fur was clipped for intravenous catheter placement, and the owner was irate with the veterinarian when she saw this. The skin healed with topical treatment and an e-collar to prevent licking, but the owner didn't follow up with the recommended diagnostic and treatment options for the kidney and gastrointestinal disease. As such, the cat was euthanized after she declined at home.

The circumstances that unfolded around this cat's hospitalization and following discharge are almost unbelievable. The client called the police to say that her cat was being held hostage at the hospital; filed a cruelty complaint against the veterinarian with humane law enforcement; filed a complaint against the veterinarian and hospital with the Office of Consumer Protection at the state's Attorney General's Office; filed a veterinary licensing board complaint against the veterinarian; and filed a bar complaint against the attorney assigned to defend the veterinarian via her Professional Liability Insurance Trust (i.e., malpractice insurance). And if that wasn't enough, three years later the client sued the veterinarian, the hospital, and the state government jointly for $10 million in damages. Not surprisingly, all of the complaints and lawsuits were dismissed, but the distress this caused for the veterinarian involved, for nearly four years after the death of the cat, is incontestable.

Situations of client non-compliance or refusal of care that result in unfavorable outcomes for pets are numerous and distressing for the veterinary team in many ways. Veterinarians have chosen the profession primarily to help animals and their owners. Part of the Veterinarian's Oath is "I will strive to … relieve animal suffering," which is often hindered by clients who don't follow the veterinarian's instructions or recommendations. While these situations can stem from miscommunication by the veterinarian or misunderstanding by the client, it's ultimately the veterinarian who is held responsible when the animal suffers. As an emergency and critical care specialist, I spend a lot of time helping clients and their pets on an emergent basis. The situations are never planned, the required care is costly, and the outcomes are rarely guaranteed.

Sadly, numerous times in two decades of practice I've had owners refuse treatment for their pet. Most often this is for financial reasons, but sometimes this stems from a disregard for medical advice or treatment recommendations. When a patient is discharged from the hospital against a veterinarian's recommendation, it is regarded as a discharge AMA (against medical advice). While this is documented in the medical record to ensure that the veterinarian's recommendations and client's refusal are noted, many times it results in hurtful accusations, veterinary medical board complaints, negative online reviews, and lawsuits from clients when the pet does poorly at home. Discharging patients when we know they will suffer without medical care is already distressing for the veterinary team involved and to then be accused by the owner of being uncaring, or unwilling to provide care at a reasonable cost, adds proverbial salt to the wound.

The situation can be compounded when the veterinary team attempts to ensure a patient receives care by offering an owner who is unwilling or unable to pay to surrender their pet to the hospital. In 2022, an emergency and specialty referral hospital in Maine admitted a German Shepherd puppy who had ingested a wooden kabob skewer. The skewer had punctured the puppy's intestine, and he was demonstrating signs of infection and shock, requiring emergency surgery to save his life. The owners were given an estimated cost for his care ($10,000) and were asked to leave half of the estimate as a deposit prior to surgery. Payment options included a credit application, which was not pursued by the owners. When the dog's condition became dire and the need for surgery was imminent, the clients had still not consented to surgery nor paid their deposit. The option was then given to the owners to surrender their puppy, so that someone who could cover the cost of care could then adopt him afterward. The owners signed legal documents turning the ownership and care of their puppy over to the practice. Subsequently they launched a media campaign that included social media posts and news stories claiming the practice refused to give them their dog back when they came up with the money for surgery.

Initially, the veterinary practice refused to comment to preserve client–veterinarian confidentiality, but was then faced with a public backlash that included threats to "burn down the hospital" and "kill [their] staff and their families." They ultimately released a statement describing the details of the puppy's critical condition at presentation, conversations with the clients, and attempts to obtain consent and the deposit for surgery, as well as clarification that the owners had at no point contacted the hospital with the funds to cover their puppy's bill. In the meantime, the incessant threats by the public and attempts to jam the practice's phone lines so that emergency calls were unable to get through had taken a tremendous emotional toll on the entire veterinary team.[9]

I wish I could say that this situation was a one-time occurrence, but in truth, harassment via social and mass media campaigns led by angry clients are impacting veterinarians more commonly worldwide. A friend of mine practicing locally as an emergency veterinarian experienced a similar situation just a few years ago, when the owner of a Pitbull and a member of a prominent Pitbull rescue group launched an online campaign against her and her hospital. She was harassed, bullied, and threatened online until she removed her social media profile. The practice received hundreds of phone calls every hour from all over the world in an attempt to shut down business to the practice and prevent emergency calls from getting through. The police and veterinary governing body were aware of the situation, but little could be done given that most of the people inciting the phone and online attacks were outside of the country. To this day my friend experiences tremendous anxiety at the thought of this worse-case scenario turned all-too-common occurrence in veterinary medicine.

I would be remiss to speak about clients in veterinary medicine without highlighting some of the positive experiences that I've had. Indeed, one of the aspects of general practice I missed most when I became a critical care specialist was the ongoing relationship I had with clients who would return year after year for their pets' annual exams and vaccines. There's something special about the relationship built with many of these clients—individuals who become cherished friends whose visits are eagerly anticipated on a yearly (or more frequent) basis. My mom practiced veterinary medicine in her clinic for more than four decades during which she saw two-, three-, and even four-generations of families come through her waiting room. She cherished many of those relationships, which were the highlight of her career as a veterinarian and practice owner and which led her to delay retirement for many years.

Even though I see most of my clients only once during their pet's emergency visit or stay in the intensive care unit, I often experience tremendous gratitude from clients who are both elated and relieved for the care they have received. Very often, one euthanasia procedure or routine surgery in the emergency room is followed by a box of chocolates, a plate of fresh baked goodies, or a handwritten note. I have a large collection of cards (and more often nowadays, screenshots of emails) saved from those moments in practice, which I turn to when faced with another client's uncivil behavior. Most of my clients are respectful of my time and expertise, express a true desire to understand and follow my recommendations, trust my diagnostic and treatment plan, and acknowledge the challenges that are inherent in our veterinary work. Despite the negativity bias that leads me to focus on the bad client who spoils the proverbial bunch, I strive to offer each of my clients the benefit of the doubt, knowing that all of us have shown up as lesser versions of ourselves during stressful or challenging situations. Because at the end of the day, clients and veterinarian teams both want the same thing: for animals to be helped in the most efficacious, easiest, and cost-effective way.

18

Examining Toxicity in Veterinary Practices

> Toxicity is prevalent in our field. Creating positive culture among staff is
> attainable, but if toxicity is coming from "above" me, my hands are often
> tied other than being a kind and supportive leader among the toxic ones.
> —Connie Lovello, CVPM
> (Certified Veterinary Practice Manager)

I've walked into veterinary practices where the tension was palpable and the toxicity was apparent from the moment I stepped through the door. During a locum in one hospital, eye-rolling, gossiping, back-stabbing, and other malicious behaviors were so rampant that it felt like a competition in making other team members miserable. Daytime vet techs would leave undesirable tasks for the overnight techs, the lead tech would hoard information so that nobody else knew what was going on, and the patient binder was filled with nasty comments about things the previous shift team had not done (or not done well enough!). These toxic behaviors weren't just demonstrated by vet techs. The specialists on other services would avoid speaking to me and instead send a student or intern to relay that they wanted something changed with their patient, or that they disagreed with a recommendation I'd made. And during rounds, it was normal for residents to ridicule the referring veterinarian or intern for their perceived mishandling of the case prior to transferring it to a specialist's care. As someone who has always prioritized professionalism and compassion for others, these behaviors were shocking and disorienting.

Toxicity within the veterinary field has become a more openly discussed topic in recent years. Once considered isolated to specific workplaces, it's now acknowledged to exist in varying degrees across many veterinary hospitals and practices. A 2014 study, conducted in Canadian companion animal practices, shed light on this issue. The study surveyed nearly 50 veterinary team members, including veterinarians, technicians, and kennel attendants. Participants were asked to rate statements describing a toxic environment on a scale from 1 to 7, covering aspects like poor communication and resistance to change (Box 1). The results revealed a correlation between higher toxicity scores and lower job satisfaction, along with increased burnout symptoms, including emotional exhaustion and cynicism.[1] The study's findings were replicated in 2016 among ten companion animal veterinary practices in the

DOI: 10.1201/9781003347385-20

United States, reaffirming the impact of toxic environments on all members of the veterinary team.[2]

Box 1: Statements Used in a Survey to Assess Toxic Environments among Companion Animal Veterinary Teams[1]

I am sometimes pulled in too many directions.
I am overloaded with responsibilities.
Sometimes there are conflicting messages in the clinic.
I am sometimes overruled by others, even when I am following the clinic protocol.
There are communication breakdowns in our clinic.
There is tension in the clinic.
I am frustrated with my job.
The team is being brought down by someone with a negative attitude.
There is uncertainty in our clinic about why decisions are made.
Some of my coworkers resist change.
Sometimes my credibility with clients is undermined by my coworkers.
My coworkers will not do things if they don't feel it is their job.

A study published in *Frontiers of Veterinary Science* in 2015 conducted focus group interviews of veterinarians and veterinary technicians in Ontario, Canada, aiming to understand the causes of toxicity in veterinary companion animal practices.[3] The researchers identified several toxic attitudes that contribute to a toxic environment, as along with environmental factors that enable these attitudes to emerge and persist (Box 2). During the focus group discussions, participants described scenarios where individuals sought to monopolize tasks or information, leading to frustration and resentment among team members. I've heard of this from a practice leader I once worked with, whose team member responsible for managing all of the hospital's IT problems held exclusive access to passwords and codes. Of course, this is less of an issue if the person is always available (and willing to help) but, in this case, the team member often called out sick and was rude and belittling to anyone who came to him for support.

Box 2: Toxic Attitudes and Contributors to a Toxic Environment Identified by Companion Animal Practice Focus Groups[3]

Toxic Attitudes
Wanting to Be the Go-to Person
Mood Polluters
Personality Issues

That's Not My Job
Lacking Confidence/Skills/Knowledge
Toxic Environment
Changing the Rules
Lack of Leadership
Lack of Consequences
Not Feeling Appreciated
Having Unreasonable Expectations
Conflicting Demands
Coping with Turnover

Participants also highlighted the toxic attitude "That's not my job," which describes individuals refusing tasks such as answering phones, cleaning cages, holding animals, or doing laundry. Interestingly, this sentiment was not limited to veterinarians but also extended to client care representatives and new team members. It was perceived as a control or ego issue that undermined team cohesion. I've worked in ICUs where veterinary technicians refused tasks they believed were the responsibility of kennel attendants, similarly where veterinarians declined to engage with clients or answer questions if they felt another veterinarian should handle the matter, even on their day off. These situations often lead to frustration, as it implies that individuals are prioritizing their own interests over the team's needs.

Similarly, participants identified "mood polluters," who consistently bring down team morale, and individuals with "personality issues," who, despite technical skills, fail to integrate with the team. Focus group participants also shed light on the frustration caused by individuals who lack confidence, skills, or knowledge, which ultimately affects trust and team effectiveness. I've observed and experienced the irritation that arises when a team member constantly second-guesses their actions or struggles to make decisions. This often leads to tasks requiring double-checking and frequent assistance, increasing the workload and reducing overall efficiency—ultimately undermining the purpose of teamwork.

The focus group also identified several facets of a toxic environment, all of which I've sadly experienced. "Changing the rules" is something I've seen in several practices, beginning when I was a veterinary student. I recall a client coming in to ask for medication for her dog's ear infection. We'd not seen her dog in nearly two years, and I told the client she would need to schedule an appointment to bring him in for an exam, enraging the client who demanded to speak to the veterinarian. When I relayed the situation, the veterinarian immediately told the client it was no problem to get the medication without an exam. Despite this going against the practice's policy (and without telling the owner an exception to the rule was being made), the veterinarian sent her home with her ear meds, and I was left feeling confused and devalued.

I've seen this play out in other practices whereby a senior person or specialist on the team will behave inappropriately (e.g., slamming doors, throwing surgical equipment, yelling at team members) and not get reprimanded, whereas a veterinary technician will exhibit the same behavior and get written up immediately. These situations undermine practice policies and create frustration and resentment among team members.

"Lack of consequences" is another factor contributing to a toxic environment. When toxic behaviors go unchecked, they create a hostile atmosphere where unprofessional conduct becomes the norm and motivation to behave appropriately diminishes among team members. Through my experiences working as a locum in different practices, I've seen how failure to hold individuals accountable for their actions can lead to ongoing interpersonal tensions within the team. This issue often stems from a lack of leadership, as in many cases, practice owners and managers are either absent or ineffective at addressing these issues. Many practice owners, veterinarians themselves, lack training in communication and conflict resolution. Similarly, practice managers are often chosen based on their seniority within the veterinary field rather than their leadership skills. This can result in a lack of effective conflict resolution and consequence enforcement within the practice.

Both practice leaders and team members have opportunities to show appreciation for one another. Yet, focus group participants—particularly veterinary technicians—highlight "not feeling appreciated" as a key contributor to a toxic environment. This sentiment often stems from veterinary technicians feeling undervalued, with their education, knowledge, and skills going unrecognized and underutilized. Similarly, veterinary team members and associates may not feel appreciated by their clients or practice owners. Sometimes, this sentiment stems from a simple lack of awareness regarding individual contributions to patient and client care. Unfortunately, other scenarios demonstrate a blatant disregard for the hard work and loyalty demonstrated by veterinarians and other team members. A friend of mine, who worked as an emergency veterinarian at the same practice for nearly a decade, discovered that a newly hired (and recently graduated) emergency veterinarian was being paid a salary over $20,000 higher than hers. Feeling unappreciated and resentful, she approached the owners to request a raise, and ultimately left her role when her request for a salary match was denied.

It becomes clear how various factors contributing to toxicity are interconnected, with many ultimately leading to staff turnover. While some turnover is expected—due to practice growth or parental leave—focus group participants identified "coping with turnover" itself as a contributor to toxicity. The persistent change and the need to build trust and rapport with new team members can cause anxiety and exhaustion; for many, this creates a vicious cycle. Team members leave, whether due to toxicity or not, exacerbating the toxic environment, lowering job satisfaction, and leading to more people quitting.

Additionally, "having unreasonable expectations" was identified by focus group participants as a component of a toxic environment. This involves team members being expected to perform tasks that feel impossible or unrealistic given their skills, abilities, or facility limitations. When consulting with general practitioners, I frequently encounter veterinarians who are managing cases beyond their capabilities. This might occur due to pet owners' reluctance to seek referral to a specialty hospital or because practice owners insist the veterinarian handle cases outside their skill set. Veterinary technicians and nurses are also asked to take on unreasonable tasks, such as monitoring new veterinarians or interns for mistakes or performing the workload of multiple individuals due to staffing shortages. These unrealistic expectations create "conflicting demands," leaving team members unsure of what to prioritize. In small practices, it's not uncommon for one veterinary technician to handle multiple responsibilities simultaneously, such as setting up for surgery, monitoring anesthesia, answering the phone, and admitting and discharging patients. This not only strains individuals, but also undermines patient care.

Interpersonal issues among coworkers are additional contributors to toxicity and workplace stress (Box 3), as identified in studies conducted worldwide. In a 2014 survey published in the *Journal of the American Veterinary Medical Association*, nearly 13% of over 1,400 US veterinarians identified conflict, drama, confrontations, hypercompetitive or unsympathetic colleagues, dysfunctional or hostile work environments, and bullying from team members as primary causes of stress.[4] Similarly, a study published in the *Australian Veterinary Journal* that collected more than 50 survey responses from veterinary professionals working in Australasia in 2021 revealed challenging relationships with colleagues as a prominent theme identified by nearly half of the respondents. Subthemes included interpersonal conflict, mistreatment and bullying, divisiveness between roles (e.g., veterinarians versus veterinary nurses), differing views on patient care, and poor communication.[5] Additionally, a 2020 study published in the *Irish Veterinary Journal* surveyed over 200 Polish veterinarians, with nearly 16% citing conflict with a coworker as a stressor.[6] Even veterinary interns and residents at the University of California Davis Medical Teaching Hospital, surveyed in 2017 and 2018, cited a "lack of collegiality among supervising faculty" as a significant source of stress during their training.[7] These studies underscore the global occurrence of conflict among veterinary professionals.

Box 3: Did You Know?

A study published in *The Veterinary Record* in 2022 shared the results of surveys distributed to UK veterinary professionals to assess their experiences of workplace incivility from clients, coworkers, and senior colleagues. Incivility from different sources had varying effects, with senior colleague incivility predicting turnover intention among veterinarians and job dissatisfaction among veterinary nurses.[8]

Conflict among team members is a prevalent issue in almost every veterinary setting I've encountered. From my early days in practice when I observed tension over mundane tasks like answering the phone during lunch breaks, to witnessing disagreements and even hostility among specialists regarding shift schedules or case management, conflicts seem to be inherent in the veterinary profession. However, concerns about conflict and its impact on stress and workplace culture are not unique to veterinary medicine. According to the American Psychological Association, a significant number of employees (43%) cite "problems with my coworkers" as a major stressor at work, reflecting an increase from previous years.[9] And while many veterinary schools have started incorporating communication training into their curriculum, the focus often remains on resolving conflicts between veterinarians and clients rather than addressing internal conflicts among team members.[10]

Over my decades of experience in many different hospitals and practice settings, I've encountered my fair share of workplace challenges. But I can honestly say that none have been as insidious as workplace bullying. It's a deeply unsettling experience to feel targeted or belittled in a professional setting, where collaboration and respect should be the norm. I recall a time when a senior colleague would constantly undermine my decisions during rounds, eroding my confidence and causing me to dread coming to work. The emotional toll of navigating such toxic dynamics was overwhelming, impacting not only my performance but also my overall wellbeing. Unfortunately, my story isn't unique, as many veterinarians grapple with similar experiences of workplace bullying.

A study published in 2018 aimed to understand how workplace bullying, destructive leadership, and team conflict affected veterinarians in New Zealand, and whether factors like psychological capital and organizational support helped. Researchers surveyed nearly 200 veterinarians and found that about 16% experienced workplace bullying, with higher rates among women and non-managers. Workplace bullying was linked to negative effects like poor physical health, stress, and wanting to quit. Destructive leadership and team conflict also contributed to these problems. However, perceived organizational support helped lessen the impact of workplace bullying on stress and job performance. Overall, the study highlights the importance of addressing workplace bullying and improving organizational support to protect veterinarian wellbeing.[11]

The biannual Merck Animal Health Veterinary Wellbeing Study conducted in 2023 reaffirmed the critical role of a healthy work environment in promoting veterinary wellbeing. The study underscored that factors such as a strong sense of belonging to the team, sufficient time allotted for high-quality patient care, a high degree of trust in the organization, and candid and open communication among team members significantly contribute to overall job satisfaction and lower psychological distress among veterinary professionals.[12] Reflecting on over 20 years of mentoring veterinary technicians and newly graduated veterinarians worldwide, I consistently emphasize the importance of conflict resolution skills. Whether navigating disagreements about treatment approaches or addressing relational conflicts stemming from interpersonal dynamics, effective communication and accountability are paramount.

While the challenges of toxicity in veterinary practices are daunting, they are not insurmountable. Each team member has a vital role to play in fostering a culture of respect and appreciation. By openly addressing toxic behaviors and prioritizing effective communication, we can pave the way for healthier work environments that support the wellbeing of all professionals in veterinary medicine. It is essential for both individuals and leadership within practices and organizations to recognize the impact of their actions and to strive for positive change. When each person prioritizes mutual support, trust, and a commitment to excellence in both patient care and the treatment of one another, the overall experience for pet owners is elevated, ensuring the highest standards of care for their beloved animals. This collaborative effort among veterinary professionals fosters a more compassionate and effective model for animal healthcare, ultimately benefiting all members of the veterinary community.

19

The Burden of On-Call

I didn't realize how anxious it made me until after I changed jobs. Then it was very obvious that my phone ringing immediately made me tense. Took several months of being off call for that response to go away.
—Rebecca E. Linot, DVM (Hospice and Relief Veterinarian)

Being on-call was one of the things I resented most when I was in veterinary practice full-time. My first experience with being on-call was as a student, back when we didn't have cell phones and instead carried a pager. When the pager beeped, we had a number to call and the person who answered told us what was needed. Most of my clinical rotations in veterinary school had some sort of on-call requirement, which was usually shared by the students on the rotation. I can remember being on-call for anesthesia and surgery in case of an out-of-hours emergency procedure, internal medicine for any overnight emergencies, and during my bovine (calving) rotation, when the overnight pages indicated that help was needed to resuscitate dehydrated calves with scours (diarrhea). Some of the on-call responsibilities, such as internal medicine, required staying overnight in the school dormitories located two floors above the teaching hospital. Others allowed students to take their pager home and return to school if necessary—obviously preferable to staying in the communal sleeping quarters.

On-call responsibilities continued during my internship, usually when I was the only veterinarian in the hospital and received pages for any after-hours calls to the emergency service. During my residency (yes, still wearing a pager!) I was on-call during my shifts in the ICU. Unfortunately, this usually meant that after a 12-plus hour shift taking care of the most critically ill patients in the hospital, we knew that we could be paged at any time if the overnight intern, ICU nurse, or another resident had a concern about one of their patients. Very often questions could be answered over the phone, but occasionally I'd have to come back into the hospital, especially if the patient was unstable and needed mechanical ventilation or another treatment that the intern was not trained to provide. I remember some days feeling bone-tired having worked more than 12-hours on "days" and then having to come in overnight for a ventilator case or critical "hit by car." It brought me back to my

DOI: 10.1201/9781003347385-21

60-hour weekend emergency coverage during my internship, where I'd sleep fewer than ten hours and literally feel drunk at the wheel driving home.

During my time as an Assistant Professor at the Ontario Veterinary College (OVC) my on-call responsibilities were at their highest. By then we had cell phones and were expected to be available while on-clinics to answer questions from our emergency interns or ICU residents. Because there was only one other faculty member in small animal emergency and critical care at the time, we shared on-call responsibility approximately 50/50. As the years passed and we both became exhausted by the on-call, we incorporated our most senior (third/final year) resident into the rotation so that they could cover a few weekends and offer us both some reprieve. Despite being lucky to have extraordinarily competent residents who made returning to the hospital rare and during extenuating circumstances, the impact that my on-call responsibilities had on me was significant.

The perceived impacts of on-call duties on veterinarians' job satisfaction, wellbeing, and personal relationships are considerable. They include negative psychological and health consequences, anxiety, inability to relax, sleep and life disruption, and negative relationship effects.[1] I, and other veterinarians I know who have spent time on-call, can personally attest to these factors (Box 1). I remember experiencing severe stress in response to being on-call. This distress was pronounced in situations early on as a veterinarian when I worried I wouldn't have anyone to ask for help if the situation was beyond my capabilities. The physical and mental health effects were also evident, mostly a consequence of sleep deprivation and worry, including muscle soreness or tension, headaches, gastrointestinal upset, and inability to focus. I also experienced severe anxiety that sometimes led to panic while on-call or in anticipation of challenging cases. There's undoubtedly life disruption, given that, when on-call, veterinarians are expected to put on their "professional hat" at any given time and possibly return to the hospital. This precludes certain activities such as social gatherings, substance use, recreational activities, and venturing out of town.

Box 1: Did You Know?

A large survey study conducted in 2017 and published in *Frontiers of Veterinary Science* documented that among almost 2,000 survey responses received from US veterinarians, nearly one-third spent 5–8 nights on-call per month; half reported that their on-call shifts usually included 1–2 consecutive nights; 1 in 10 reported being on-call for more than 30 nights in a row; 3 in 5 reported often or always being on-call over weekends; and 2 in 5 reported often or always being on-call for holidays.[1]

I can remember getting to the end of my five years at OVC and deciding that I couldn't let my on-call responsibilities dictate my entire life. I went from never attending a yoga class, ultimate frisbee practice, or dinner with a friend while on-call to occasionally allowing myself to do this when an experienced resident was on clinics with me. I always communicated when I'd be unreachable, during the occasional hot yoga class for example, and the residents were always very understanding of the need for a "break." Unfortunately, many of my colleagues don't have the luxury of working with another veterinarian, such as an intern or resident, who can troubleshoot the situation and provide initial treatments prior to discussing next steps. This is especially true among rural practitioners, many located several hours drive from the nearest emergency clinic or another on-call veterinarian, who spend much of their time (if not all, if they're a solo practice owner) on-call and available to their regular clientele.

This also pertains to large and farm animal practitioners who typically reside in rural areas and do farm visits or "house calls" for their clients, rather than asking owners or farmers to transport their animals to a veterinary practice. As such, on-call responsibilities are the cause of attrition among many non-urban veterinarians, exacerbating the ongoing shortage of equine and food animal vets who are willing to work in rural areas (Box 2).[2] In speaking with some of my classmates who left mixed and farm animal practice to move to companion animal practice exclusively, not having to spend time on-call was a major reason for the change. Unsurprising, given that more than half of US veterinarians surveyed said that a lack of on-call duties had influenced their acceptance of a job and 60% indicated that on-call duties would have a major role in their acceptance of a future job.[1] A similar sentiment was held among Australian veterinarians in a study published in 2021. Of the nearly 900 current and former veterinarians surveyed, having on-call duties significantly increased the likelihood of leaving clinical practice.[3]

Box 2: Did You Know?

A survey of more than 550 western Canadian veterinarians conducted in 2006 revealed that one of the main factors associated with leaving mixed (companion and large animal) or food animal practice was having too many nights on call.[2]

Based on my experience, some of the dissatisfaction with being on-call stems from concerns about handling cases comfortably and the lack of mentorship early in one's career. This can make on-call situations feel overwhelming and unbearable for new graduates. I remember hearing horror stories from classmates who took jobs at mixed and farm animal practices who were in desperate need of relief, only to be left alone in their first weeks or months of practice (Box 3). This left those new veterinarians feeling ill-equipped and insecure in their abilities, which created resentment and frustration over the broken promise of mentorship during their transition into practice. No wonder those who stayed in their jobs were the veterinarians who felt supported and mentored, thereby gaining confidence in their ability to handle cases on their own (Box 4).

Box 3: Did You Know?

Veterinarians graduating in the United Kingdom in 1998 and 1999 were surveyed during their first two years of practice. Three of five veterinarians were on-call within the first week of their first job and 95% were on-call within the first month. When asked about problems related to their new job, more than half cited being on-call.[4]

Box 4: Did You Know?

A study published in *The Veterinary Record* in 2015 surveyed nearly 400 farm animal veterinarians in the United Kingdom and found that being on-call with an experienced veterinarian in the first job after graduation increased the odds of remaining in farm animal practice.[5]

While many individuals in and outside of the veterinary profession regard time spent on-call as "part of the job," there are undisputable consequences. The negative physical and psychological effects are seen within many industries with out-of-hours responsibilities. These are usually a consequence of working long hours and having to work at night, outside of the body's natural circadian rhythm or sleep patterns. Among general practice human physicians, on-call shifts are associated with anxiety and depression,[6] and physicians consider on-call shifts a major source of stress and job dissatisfaction.[7] Some of this likely stems from the negative impact on sleep and daily routines, but much of it is attributed to inadequate recovery (i.e., leisure) time outside of work.[8] This may be why female veterinarians appear more negatively impacted by on-call responsibilities, given their tendency (in heterosexual relationships) to have more household and childcare responsibilities than men.[9]

Time spent on-call not only poses risks for veterinarian health and well-being, it also poses a risk to personal safety and the care of patients. A study published in *The Veterinary Record* in 2019 investigated the perceptions of veterinarians in the United Kingdom who were working alone while on-call. Many of the vets expressed feeling unsafe when meeting clients alone and in remote locations.[10] Additionally, because on-call shifts can result in sleep deprivation, daytime sleepiness and fatigue can occur impacting sensory-motor and cognitive skills.[11] On-call duties among human physicians increase the risk of work-related injuries and medical errors, and they decrease clinical performance.[12] The latter is typically the result of reduced memory, slower reaction times, hypervigilance, and decreased cognition. When I think back to the mistakes I've made as a veterinarian, the majority occurred because of sleep deprivation secondary to long shifts and being on-call. Given all these effects, and the fact that time off is not commonplace in lieu of time spent on-call (Box 5), it surely comes as no surprise that veterinarians dislike being on-call and that, in turn, it reduces their job satisfaction.

Box 5: Did You Know?

More than 80% of veterinarians in the United States who spend time on-call do not get the day off if called in the previous night.[1]

Much of the research in human medicine that looks at the negative ramifications of on-call duty involves investigating residents. Indeed, motor and cognitive performance are impacted among human medical residents who spend time on-call,[13] and similar concerns are noted among veterinary interns and residents. The results of a survey study of more than 300 interns and residents was published in the *Journal of the American Veterinary Medical Association* in 2022, which found that perceived sleep quality was worse when on-call and the majority felt that fatigue negatively impacted their technical skills, clinical judgment, and ability to empathize.[14] The cognitive effects pertaining to on-call responsibilities were also evident among internal medicine residents studying for their board certification exams. A study published in the *Journal of Veterinary Internal Medicine* in 2022 found that residents were more likely to pass the exam when they did not have on-call responsibilities while studying.[15]

Controversy persists when it comes to how to manage the on-call requirements of veterinarians in internship and residency training programs. More than 20 years ago, the Accreditation Council for Graduate Medical Education established guidelines in human medicine to limit the working hours of physician trainees, aiming to enhance patient safety and the wellbeing of interns and residents. While these guidelines received support, many institutions struggled to adapt, facing challenges in restructuring programs and acquiring necessary staff. Since then, studies on the impact of these duty hour restrictions have shown improved wellbeing for trainees, but at the cost of patient care continuity and an increase in medical errors during patient hand-offs. The effects on resident training vary across programs, with surgical disciplines experiencing more significant challenges. A survey at North

Carolina State University Veterinary Teaching Hospital, staffed by around 100 interns and residents, revealed that a majority reported insufficient time for personal needs and dissatisfaction with their mental and physical wellbeing. While many believed reduced duty hours and on-call would enhance learning, some expressed concerns that the resulting decreased case exposure might negatively impact training.[16]

It's true that to provide 24/7 care for veterinary patients outside of emergency facilities, veterinarians must spend time on-call. This prevents general practices and hospitals from needing to staff trained personnel on evenings, overnight, and weekends when the caseload is low and does not warrant full compensation of veterinarians or team members on the premises. When it comes to financial compensation for time spent on-call, 82% of US veterinarians surveyed received no compensation for merely being on-call; however, more than half were compensated if they were called back into work. Importantly, more than three-quarters of the surveyed veterinarians reported that the money was not worth the inconvenience.[1] So, while the cost savings of paying practitioners only when they need to come in after-hours is commonplace in veterinary medicine, there are clear ramifications for the job satisfaction and longevity of those veterinarians.

The big question remains: what is the solution to having veterinarians spend time on-call? There's no easy answer that doesn't somehow impact the animals, their owners, or other veterinarians in the field. While working as a locum emergency and critical care specialist, I'm typically on-call—both to answer questions pertaining to my own in-hospital (and more complex) cases and to assist interns, residents, and emergency veterinarians who might have questions about incoming critical patients. I've never been compensated for time spent on-call outside of the stipend I'm paid for my shift and an additional supplement if I'm called in. But refusing to be on-call during my locum shifts would undoubtedly increase distress among the in-hospital team, especially if they were tending to a patient they felt needed my expertise.

For general practitioners working in rural settings, the situation is more dire when veterinarians are not available on-call. For many large or farm animal owners in rural communities, no on-call veterinarian simply means no outside-of-hours veterinary care. Or for companion animals and their families in remote areas, not having a veterinarian on-call means driving to the nearest emergency clinic, which could be a distressing hours-long drive (or plane ride) away.

Sharing coverage among independently practicing veterinarians is one solution that mitigates (but doesn't remove) the amount of time spent on-call. This requires that veterinarians work together, communicate, and share caseloads, something that not all veterinarians are committed to. Others advocate for the use of teletriage to alleviate the number of calls fielded by on-call veterinarians during a shift. This allows veterinarians to reduce the time spent on the phone with their clients and to be called by the teletriage service only when their professional advice or on-site assistance is required. Finally, many are suggesting that veterinarians and other healthcare providers be compensated and scheduled for their on-call shifts as if they were a regular shift, essentially providing 24/7 coverage. While this would seem the best solution, the difficulties lie with finding sufficient veterinarians (including those who are willing to work overnight shifts) to fulfill the 24/7 coverage needs.

The burden of on-call duties highlights a pressing issue within the veterinary profession, as these responsibilities lead to dissatisfaction with mental and physical health among practitioners. While on-call shifts are often viewed as an inevitable aspect of the job, they come with substantial consequences that impact both the wellbeing of veterinarians and the quality of care provided to patients. Obviously, there is no clear solution and likely no end in sight for the on-call requirements of veterinarians. To foster a more sustainable work environment, veterinary professionals must advocate for changes that prioritize mental health and work-life balance, such as shared on-call rotations and improved mentorship programs. Engaging in open dialogues about these challenges is essential for creating a supportive and healthy work culture that ensures veterinarians can deliver the best possible care to their patients while maintaining their own wellbeing. As the landscape of veterinary medicine continues to evolve, it is imperative to rethink on-call practices to prioritize the health and happiness of those who dedicate their lives to caring for animals.

PART THREE

What We Now Understand about Veterinarians

20

Professional Identity

For years all of your effort and energy is put into schooling and getting vet hours, and then vet school +/- internship +/- residency consumes your time. There isn't time or energy for other things. It's hard for that not to become your identity.

—Amanda Brand (Veterinary Assistant)

Over the years, I've come to know many veterinarians, and even veterinary students, who have trouble discerning themselves as individuals outside of the work they do. In fact, a common sentiment of veterinarians is that they don't know who they are outside of their role in veterinary medicine. This feeling is pervasive among veterinarians who are unhappy at work and struggling to determine their next steps. Do they find another job? Leave clinical practice? Or exit the profession altogether? When forced to consider the latter of those options, they're often struck by a sense of "who am I if I'm no longer a veterinarian?" I've seen this play out among vets considering retirement as well. I recall working with a renowned small animal emergency and critical care specialist who proclaimed that she dedicated her life to veterinary medicine and her specialty. When health issues forced her to leave her faculty position, she struggled to fully step out of her role and embrace other activities, even after she completely retired.

My mom had the same experience when she retired after owning her practice for more than 40 years. After selling her clinic, she stayed in the practice for several years, explaining that she was dedicated to the clients whose families had been coming to her for decades. She was also an excellent surgeon and performed complex procedures that most of her newly graduated associates did not feel comfortable doing. My mom was also indebted to her team members. Her office manager had been working with her since just after her clinic's inception, a loyalty unmatched in most other practices. There was no doubt that having spent nearly half a century owning and working in her companion animal clinic left her feeling uncertain and scared of what retired life might look like.

Not only did I envision myself in the veterinary profession from childhood, but my parents also shared this vision for me. Whenever someone asked,

DOI: 10.1201/9781003347385-23

"What do you want to be when you grow up?," my parents would proudly declare, "A veterinarian, of course!" I've heard similar stories from fellow veterinarians. This early reinforcement of our professional identity, while well intentioned, fused "being a veterinarian" into our personalities, making it harder to separate the two. While such parental enthusiasm sometimes led us to explore other career paths for a sense of autonomy and flexibility, for most of us the innate passion for veterinary medicine prevailed.

In my coaching work with mid-career veterinarians, I often encounter sentiments like "I don't have any passions outside of veterinary medicine" or "I have no idea what my non-veterinary interests or hobbies are." Many veterinarians find themselves spending their limited leisure time on animal-related activities such as horseback riding, beekeeping, animal fostering, and dog training, all of which are inherently tied to their profession (Box 1). While some find solace and enjoyment in these activities, others express resentment at "never getting a break" from their veterinary role. It's not uncommon for a casual outing to turn into an "ask-the-veterinarian" discussion, leaving veterinarians feeling constantly tied to their profession even during their downtime.

Box 1: Did You Know?

Research performed by Merck Animal Health and the American Veterinary Medical Association in 2023 demonstrates that veterinarians who engage in non-work-related activities such as spending time with family, reading for pleasure, exercising, spending time on a hobby, or socializing with friends have less serious psychological distress and lower burnout scores.[1]

While veterinarians are undeniably passionate about helping animals and their families, the expectation to field veterinary-related questions anytime and anywhere can feel overwhelming. This scenario is akin to a child psychologist being asked for advice on toddler behavior at a dinner party or a general physician being questioned about a skin condition at a professional sporting event: situations that would seem out of place and inappropriate outside of a clinical setting. Yet, veterinarians frequently find themselves dispensing advice during casual encounters, whether on airplanes, in grocery stores, or at social gatherings (as I've personally experienced). These constant demands reinforce the veterinarian identity and blur the lines between professional and personal life. When others fail to acknowledge veterinarians as individuals with roles beyond their profession—such as parents, friends, or family members—it becomes challenging to establish a healthy work-life separation, a crucial practice for preventing burnout among caregiving professionals.[2]

Another growing concern related to veterinary wellbeing relates to *professional identity*, which refers to the set of values and priorities that guide veterinarians' behaviors in their professional roles. *Identity dissonance* occurs when veterinarians' actions or behaviors conflict with their values or goals, leading to feelings of anxiousness, instability, and a reduced sense of control. For example, one of my closest friends from veterinary school decided to leave the profession because she hated her first job. She was feeling overwhelmed and disheartened in a high-volume companion animal practice, where brief client interactions and rushed medical procedures were the norm. This environment clashed with her "people-person" nature, which was tied to her values of quality patient care and meaningful client relationships. Despite her love for animals, she found herself questioning her career choice. However, after transitioning to a small-volume practice with longer appointment times and a focus on comprehensive care, her wellbeing improved significantly. She was able to spend more time with each patient, engage in meaningful conversations with clients, and practice the type of medicine she had always envisioned. This shift not only rekindled her passion for veterinary medicine but also restored her sense of professional fulfillment and purpose.

In veterinary training, students are often immersed in a culture focused on diagnosing and treating cases at an advanced level, which can create a skewed professional identity for future general practice veterinarians. This training emphasizes a "find it and fix it" approach, where the goal is to provide gold standard care based on clear diagnoses and well-defined treatment plans (Box 2). However, the transition to general practice reveals a stark contrast, as cases frequently lack clear diagnoses, client values may differ, and financial constraints are common. This mismatch between the idealized identity instilled during training and the realities of daily practice can leave newly graduated veterinarians feeling ill-prepared, lacking confidence in navigating the complexities of veterinary medicine due to an "identity-behavior mismatch."

Box 2: Did You Know?

Gold standard care in veterinary medicine refers to the optimal diagnostic and treatment protocols recommended for a given condition, incorporating the latest evidence-based practices and expert consensus. It represents the highest level of quality and effectiveness aimed at achieving the best possible outcomes for the patient and is traditionally emphasized during veterinary training.

In 2018, *The Veterinary Record* published a study titled "Identity, Environment and Mental Wellbeing in the Veterinary Profession," which examined the connection between identity and wellbeing among newly graduated veterinarians in the United Kingdom. Researchers utilized narrative inquiry within a private social media discussion group to explore the identities of 12 participating veterinarians. The study identified two distinct veterinarian identities:

(1) an academic, "diagnosis-focused" identity prioritizing definitive diagnoses and evidence-based treatment, and (2) a broader, "challenge-focused" identity encompassing engagement with clients, the veterinary environment, and business aspects. Veterinarians with the "challenge-focused" identity found satisfaction in addressing common practice challenges, such as helping a client with limited finances or navigating challenging pet parent dynamics, while those with the "diagnosis-focused" identity often experienced frustration in similar scenarios.[3]

Having worked in many different practice settings, I've witnessed the impact of these contextual challenges on the veterinary team and how they play out among veterinarians with different professional identities. Understandably, academic and private or corporate referral hospitals have a largely secondary and tertiary referral caseload, meaning most patients have seen at least one other veterinarian prior to presentation. Because these cases are usually sent to a particular specialty for the treatment of a specific condition (for example, a cat diagnosed with lymphoma is sent to a veterinary oncologist for chemotherapy), the pet's family is relatively well prepared for a financial and emotional investment and wants to provide the best care for their pet. So, it's not surprising that most of the veterinarians I work with in specialty practice have a "diagnosis-focused" identity and become easily frustrated with difficult interpersonal interactions or clients who cannot or do not want to pay for the gold standard of care.

I remember working as a locum in a corporate-owned specialty hospital and caring for a cat with severe heart disease, an abnormal heart rhythm (arrhythmia), and congestive heart failure. The cat was diagnosed months before by the practice's cardiologist and, despite the gold standard treatment recommendations prescribed, the owner was not routinely medicating her cat. She returned to me in the emergency room, her cat demonstrating a worse arrhythmia and recurrence of the congestive heart failure. When I spoke to the cardiologist about the progression of the cat's disease, she expressed frustration at the owner's lack of compliance, stating, "I just don't understand why they're here if they won't properly manage their cat's disease." What she saw as the owner not following gold standard care, I saw as a challenge in uncovering the owner's misunderstandings or hesitations about the treatment of this potentially fatal disease. In other words, what for the cardiologist was a frustrating misalignment with a "diagnosis-focused" identity aligned well with my "challenge-focused" identity. After a long conversation with the cat's owner, who thanked me for explaining the complexities of the cat's disease, she finally understood the importance of consistently giving the medications.

Reflecting on that case, I recall feeling tremendous satisfaction in navigating the complexities of client communication. My experience resonates with findings from research on recently graduated veterinarians in the United Kingdom, where those with a "challenge-focused" identity exhibited more markers of emotional wellbeing compared to their "diagnosis-focused" counterparts.[2] In a related study by the same lead author, poor professional wellbeing among new graduate veterinarians was linked to "identity confusion," where inconsistencies in demonstrating a dominant identity (diagnosis-focused or challenge-focused) in practice were observed. Workplace stressors such as financial limitations, lack of compliance, or veterinarian-client conflict, appeared to make academic priorities—a focus on diagnosis and gold standard treatment—more important in how veterinarians saw themselves. This, in turn, made it more difficult for them to understand their professional identity. Interestingly, some veterinarians viewed clients as adversaries, hindering their diagnosis-focused identity goals. Seeking support during client conflicts sometimes reinforced this perception, further weakening their challenge-focused identity centered on fixing veterinary-specific problems. This tension between maintaining a diagnosis and treatment-centered role while striving for positive client relationships was linked to poorer wellbeing.[4]

Given the evidence that supports the positive relationship between a clearly defined and relational-focused professional identity among veterinarians and their wellbeing, researchers Drs. Armitage-Chan and May from the Royal Veterinary College propose a professional studies curriculum to support the formation of a healthy professional identity among veterinary students. They argue that the decisions of veterinarians must be adaptable to any practice situation, whereby the options might range from gold standard to no treatment offered. This would, of course, depend on the many variables present in veterinary practice, including the values and goals of the client and family, veterinary business, and other team members. Drs. Armitage-Chan and May maintain that context must be included in academic conversations related to case management, such as what equipment is available, what the client's wishes are, and whether financial limitations exist. In essence, an emphasis is placed on context-related decision making, whereby the ideal gold standard approach is balanced with the needs of the client and challenges of the situation.[5]

The veterinary school curriculum has changed dramatically since I graduated and continues to change today. Instead of focusing on teaching professional values and behaviors, it is imperative that curricula are designed to help students shape their professional identities. Being a veterinarian involves more than just being a good diagnostician and successfully treating patients. It also involves complex decision making amidst challenging circumstances. Veterinarians must make decisions that balance the needs of the patient, the clients, themselves, and their practice. These decisions are inherently influenced by challenges in the environment, like financial limitations or feeling stressed and tired from a heavy workload. A better curriculum would involve teaching veterinary students how to think critically and handle complex situations, rather than just focusing on finding one right answer to a problem. We also need to be aware of how the curriculum might unintentionally push veterinarians to see themselves only as clinicians. By changing this approach, we could help veterinarians feel more satisfied with their work and boost their mental wellbeing.

Playing the Veterinary Victim and Martyr

There is no badge of honor anymore for working yourself into the ground/ being at the beck and call of the client without looking after yourself, and your needs. I wish I had figured that out much earlier in my career, but now I really focus on teaching this to my mentees.

—Tracey Young, DVM (Associate Veterinarian)

Many veterinarians have a habit of comparing themselves in terms of "who has it worse?," measuring the hours they worked in a day, months worked without vacation, and years working full-time in veterinary practice to indicate their sacrifice for the profession. I remember the first time I told another veterinarian that I'd worked 60 hours as an emergency intern with less than 10 hours of sleep. They responded with: "That's nothing. I used to cover 24-hours with a 30-minute nap." I was flabbergasted, not anticipating a competition. Since then, I've engaged in numerous discussions with veterinarians compelled to battle for the most consecutive shifts worked without a day off or the number of hours worked without stopping to pee (and the urinary tract or kidney infections that occurred as a result). The compulsion to be seen as a martyr for animals and their caregivers is startlingly common.

WebMD defines martyr complex as a psychological pattern "marked by self-sacrifice and service to others" at a person's own expense.[1] Martyr complex is common among care providers and can lead to burnout if left unchecked, something we're seeing frequently among veterinarians and human healthcare providers. The hallmarks of martyr complex include wanting to "be the hero" and, therefore, seeking out opportunities for sacrifice. I've witnessed this in colleagues and friends who are consistently the first to step up when a shift needs to be covered, or a surrendered patient needs to be adopted. In fact, I've lost track of the number of veterinarians I've spoken to who've either slept overnight in their practice to care for a patient or taken animals to their home to administer fluids and other treatments in their bathroom. While these gestures can seem heartwarming and sincere, they're often to the detriment of the veterinarian's wellbeing. And although veterinarians exhibiting martyr complex patterns might never complain, or even minimize

DOI: 10.1201/9781003347385-24

the positive impact they have on their clients or patients, they unrealistically emphasize that their gestures are simply a testament of "how much they care."

Veterinary medicine has fostered a culture of martyrdom for as long as I can remember. For decades, not turning clients away when overbooked, coming into work on days off despite other commitments, and giving out personal phone numbers while craving work-life separation have not only been encouraged but expected. I think back to when I was growing up and my mom listed our home phone number on the practice business card so she could be reached out of hours for emergencies. Throughout my childhood, it was normal for clients to call with questions and for my mom to return to the clinic after-hours to care for a sick pet. And in my mom's 40-something years of companion animal practice, I don't remember her complaining once. For her, and many other veterinarians, this was simply part of the job.

I speak to many veterinarians who have sacrificed their health, wellbeing, and personal life for their clients, patients, and team members. A colleague of mine who is a critical care specialist and medical director often assigns herself overnight emergency shifts rather than asking the full-time emergency veterinarians to take on additional undesirable hours. She admits it's ingrained in her to take on these tasks without pausing to consider whether she truly needs to be the one doing them—or if, given how overtaxed she already feels, it would be more appropriate to ask someone else. Similarly, I speak to veterinarians who feel mentally and emotionally unable to say no to a client's demand for out-of-hours care, or a team member's request to take months of time off, leaving the team short-staffed and overburdened. I question whether the inability to say no or defer to someone else in these situations stems from a true desire to help, a sense of obligation to the team, or an inherent need to be the hero and sacrifice themselves.

While many veterinarians exhibiting patterns and behaviors consistent with martyr complex never complain, there are those who do while concurrently refusing help. In the words of these veterinarians, "it's just easier" if they do it, they "don't mind," or "someone has to do it," so why not them? Those veterinarians who consistently sacrifice their health and home life for the sake of their patients and clients while suffering out loud are entrenched in victim mentality. They seek out opportunities for sacrifice, just as a veterinarian with martyr complex would, but, rather than wanting to "be the hero" for their clients, patients, and team members, veterinarians with victim mentality express anger and resentment over their perceived inability to say no (Box 1).

Box 1: Defining Martyr Complex and Victim Mentality

Martyr Complex: When a person sacrifices their own needs and wants in order to serve others.
Victim Mentality: When a person believes they have no control over their situation.

The subtle difference between martyr complex and victim mentality among veterinarians is best illustrated by a common example from practice. Imagine that it's 5:45 p.m. and the clinic is supposed to close at 6:00 p.m. A long-time client of the practice has just called to say that they're on their way with their Miniature Poodle, who was just attacked by another dog. They're five minutes from the practice, whereas the emergency clinic will be a 45-minute drive in rush-hour traffic. There are two associate veterinarians still working in the practice and one is thinking: "If I don't stay to see this dog, nobody else will," while the other one is thinking "I'll step up and stay late so that my associate can go home." Both veterinarians are experiencing the same level of exhaustion, having worked the same shift, and both veterinarians have family and obligations outside of work they want to get to. The difference is that the first veterinarian is entrenched in victim mentality and is begrudgingly willing to stay late, whereas the second veterinarian is ingrained in martyr complex and insists on "taking one for the team."

Why might there be some veterinarians who exhibit victim mentality while others tend toward martyr complex? The answer is that different causes likely underpin these differing behavior patterns. Low self-esteem is often linked with both martyr complex and victim mentality, in that a veterinarian might seek out opportunities for sacrifice or perceive they cannot avoid them because it's the only way they feel valued for the work they do. Alternatively, these behaviors might have been modeled by their mentors or leaders, perpetuating the culture of sacrifice inherent in many caregiving professions. When a new graduate joined my mom's practice and was asked to put his personal phone number on the clinic business card, I recall seeing hesitation on his face. But he simply shrugged his shoulders and said "okay" and later told me that he guessed this was what was "expected" as a practicing veterinarian.

While it might seem that working alongside a person with a martyr complex would have its advantages (imagine never having to stay late after a shift again!), the negative consequences outweigh the benefits. A veterinarian can sacrifice themself for the rest of the team for only so long until they experience burnout, to the point where they're no longer able to do their day-to-day duties. Recent studies demonstrate that approximately one-third of veterinarians in the United States and half of other veterinary team members are experiencing burnout, including symptoms of emotional exhaustion and cynicism.[2] Ultimately, the mental and physical symptoms of burnout will become too much for an individual with martyr complex, thereby compromising their ability to work at all.

Likewise, working alongside a veterinarian with victim mentality imposes a strain on the entire team. Veterinarians with victim mentality view themselves as a casualty of their circumstances, claiming they have no control over their life and, ultimately, no responsibility for their decisions or behaviors. I used to work with an internal medicine specialist who would insist on coming in for emergencies when she wasn't on-call, staying hours past the end of her shift to call clients, and continuing to care for her in-hospital patients on her days off, despite having other competent specialists (myself included!) in the hospital to take over patient care. All the while, she stated that she felt stuck in a state of burnout and powerless to limit her workload. I remember feeling frustrated and annoyed in my unsuccessful attempts to relieve her caseload, until coming to terms with the truth: that veterinarians with victim mentality are more attached to their story of being powerless than taking responsibility for setting limits to mitigate their burnout.

Ultimately, veterinarians with victim mentality feel safe and validated amidst their challenging circumstances. As the victim, they are not blamed for their actions ("you had no choice but to come in your day off"), they re- ceive attention from others ("you are always there for your clients"), and they are validated by support from others ("you are so committed to your clients by coming in when you're not on-call"). However, by relinquishing responsi- bility to their demanding clients, special needs patients, and incapable team members, they give up their own control over their decisions and behaviors and ability to change their circumstances.

It's important to also consider that there are circumstances when caregiving professionals are forced into the role of martyr. The COVID-19 pandemic is a perfect example of this, whereby human healthcare workers and veterinarians were considered essential service workers and, therefore, expected to relent- lessly continue in their caregiving roles. In many circumstances, veterinarians expressed a desire to stop working because they had immunocompromised loved ones at home or children who were out of school and needed care; yet, they felt a deep obligation to their team members, clients, and patients to con- tinue their work. They ultimately sacrificed the safety of their vulnerable fam- ily members to continue practicing, in what felt like a no-win situation.

Despite the seriousness of the pandemic, the demands of a long-time client, or the needs of a veterinary team, veterinarians (like anyone else) ultimately have control over their choices and circumstances. For years, I've urged veter- inarians to model healthy behaviors when it comes to setting boundaries with clients, taking time away from work, and stepping up to help team members, so that it isn't at the expense of their mental or physical wellbeing. Modeling martyr complex and perpetuating victim mentality across social media and for members of the veterinary team is sadly contributing to the burnout and poor mental health that is so pervasive in veterinary medicine today (more on that in Chapter 24). Recognizing these tendencies, understanding their root causes, and committing to choose different actions is imperative to enhancing wellbeing in the veterinary profession.

22

The Hidden Struggles of Perfectionism

> My perfectionism leads to anxiety. I have to make serious effort to cut my-
> self a break and to not just shut down. It would be very easy for me to
> simply isolate myself from everything . . . can't make mistakes that way.
> —Danièle Lagacé, DVM (Locum (Relief) Veterinarian)

If you asked a room full of veterinarians how many of them identified as
perfectionists, you would undoubtedly see most hands go up. When I speak
to veterinarians—whether at conferences or in practice—I often hear about
their exceptionally high expectations for themselves: a relentless focus on the
cases that don't go as planned, and a belief that they must always have the
correct answer, make the right judgment calls, and avoid any mistakes. Very
often these sentiments are held concurrently with a fear of criticism when
they aren't perfect—whether from clients, peers, practice owners, or management. Some of these worries are legitimate, in response to former client
complaints, veterinary medical board reprimands, or lawsuits when cases did
not go perfectly. However, many of these beliefs stem from the fact that, as a
veterinarian, they believe they should be infallible and that mistakes are simply not acceptable.

I remember considering myself a perfectionist as a young adult. When I
was asked "What is your biggest weakness?" during my veterinary school interview, I responded "my perfectionism." I didn't possess the self-awareness
that I have now to identify and share my true inadequacies, and I'm sure
that I worried that disclosure of any of my "real" shortcomings might mean
I wouldn't get into veterinary school. Either way, I believed this was the best
way to turn a negative question into a positive response. I mean, who doesn't
love a perfectionist, given their attention to detail, thorough checks and re-
checks, and relentless self-scrutiny? Fast forward decades later and I can see
how this personality trait, and clinging to its benefits, has led to significant
psychological distress for me and many other veterinarians.

According to the *Merriam-Webster's Medical Dictionary*, perfectionism is
"a disposition to regard anything short of perfection as unacceptable."[1] It is
typically accompanied by setting unrealistically demanding goals or expectations and believing that a failure to achieve them equates with being a worth-

DOI: 10.1201/9781003347385-25

less person. Examples of how my perfectionism would show up for me as a veterinary student and eventually as a practicing veterinarian included:

- Aiming for perfect scores on exams, assessments, and reviews.
- Wanting all my classmates, coworkers, and clients to like me.
- Believing there was no room for mistakes in my work as a veterinarian.
- Needing things to be done in a very specific way.
- Avoiding things I wasn't already good at or didn't believe I could excel in.
- Setting unrealistic standards for myself and others.

Many would look at this list and think these strategies would serve me well as a vet student and beyond. Indeed, perfectionism, in its healthy form, drives people to succeed. Veterinarians with "adaptive perfectionism" can set realistic goals and accept small failures, while managing the stress associated with achieving reasonable standards. They are typically driven by the desire to do "good work" but are not distressed when they make a mistake or their goals don't become realized. Individuals with adaptive perfectionism report higher levels of self-efficacy and self-esteem and lower levels of procrastination and inferiority.[2] On the flipside, veterinarians and vet students with maladaptive perfectionism are harshly self-critical, and they are usually driven by the fear of failure or criticism from others. The combination of these features leads those with maladaptive perfectionism to experience significant mental health and wellbeing challenges (Box 1).

Box 1: Mental Health and Wellbeing Consequences of Maladaptive Perfectionism

- Depression
- Anxiety
- Obsessive-compulsive disorder
- Disordered eating
- Psychological distress
- Self-harm
- Problematic substance use
- Suicidal ideation

My perfectionism was undoubtedly driven by fear with an underlying belief that I wasn't a good student or veterinarian. This became evident in my behaviors or actions, which worsened during the early years of my career:

- Spending a lot of time after finishing an exam or writing a case record checking and rechecking everything I had written.

- Not speaking up unless I was 100% certain I had the correct answer.

- Avoiding cases or procedures that I hadn't managed or performed before or believed I would be incapable of doing perfectly.

- Refusing to say "I don't know" in front of others.

- Being very hard on my team members if they were not meeting my exceptionally high standards.

- Becoming distressed or feeling ashamed when I would do or say something imperfectly.

Eventually I came to realize that my maladaptive perfectionism was a problem because I felt persistently anxious and fearful regarding my competency at work; I became depressed when cases did not go as planned; I saw my team members walking on eggshells around me, fearing consequences if they didn't meet my high standards; and I struggled to meet deadlines because my work was never good enough. What had propelled me to success as a pre-vet student had left me feeling distressed and disconnected from helping others. While I had been drawn to veterinary medicine because of my desire to help animals and their families, I was now terrified that my incompetencies would cause harm and I lost sight of the ways in which my patients were benefiting from my care.

The negative consequences of perfectionism are documented among professional students, including those in veterinary school. A study published in *BioMed Central Psychology* in 2020 demonstrated that of the more than 1,700 students in veterinary medicine, human medicine, dentistry, pharmacy, and law surveyed in the United Kingdom, those with perfectionism had lower wellbeing scores, higher depression scores, and more suicide attempts. Interestingly, of the six groups of professional students studied, those in veterinary school had the lowest perfectionism scores.[3]

Another study published the same year in the *Journal of Veterinary Medical Education* surveyed nearly 100 vet students in the southeastern United States assessing perfectionism across three dimensions (Box 2) and comparing the results with their Big 5 Personality Traits (Box 3) and resilience scores. The results showed that students with self-oriented and socially prescribed perfectionism were more likely to demonstrate neuroticism, which had a significantly negative correlation with resilience.[4] In other words, students who set high standards for themselves or feel pressure to meet others' expectations tend toward higher levels of neuroticism, a trait depicting emotional instability. This heightened neuroticism negatively impacts their resilience, making it more difficult for them to bounce back from challenges or setbacks. Ironically, the vet school admissions process that emphasizes high grades and interview scores may select students whose perfectionism could become debilitating later in their career.

Box 2: Three Dimensions of Perfectionism According to the Multidimensional Perfectionism Scale[5]

- Self-oriented: setting unreasonably high standards for oneself and being overly self-critical when unable to meet these expectations.
- Socially prescribed: believing that others have established exceptional expectations that one must meet or surpass.
- Other-oriented: having overly high expectations and standards for the people around oneself.

Box 3: Big 5 Personality Traits[6]

- Agreeableness (compassionate/amicable versus rational/discerning)
- Conscientiousness (organized/diligent versus careless/inattentive)
- Extraversion (energetic/outgoing versus reserved/solitary)
- Neuroticism (uneasy/sensitive versus self-assured/resilient)
- Openness to experience (imaginative/curious versus steady/cautious)

Perfectionism among veterinarians is less well documented but often cited in studies investigating causes of work-related stress. A study published in 2019 in *The Veterinary Record* collated the interview responses of 18 veterinarians in the United Kingdom and found an interwoven theme of perfectionism amidst stressors that included poor work-life balance, challenging interactions with pet owners, and dealing with poor animal welfare.[7] These sentiments coincide with another study published in 2015 in the *Australian Veterinary Journal*, which found that during certain stressful events in practice, veterinarians with perfectionism were more likely to feel distressed. Examples of these events included:

- Working in a situation where the owner could not afford to pay for the recommended treatment.

- Carrying out an owner's wishes that were not in the best interest of the animal.

- Balancing the welfare of the human client with that of the animal.

- Assisting other veterinarians who were believed to be providing incompetent care.

- Performing euthanasia for reasons they did not agree with.

- Suspecting animal abuse.

Among those veterinarians surveyed, perfectionism was consistently associated with poorer wellbeing, including high stress and anxiety, and lower resilience.[8]

I remember a situation early in my career when my perfectionism kicked into gear during a stressful time. I was working an emergency shift as an intern and a middle-aged Terrier Mix was presented for increased drinking and urination over the last several weeks, as well as weight loss despite an increased appetite. We performed blood work and diagnosed diabetes mellitus, a disease that requires twice-daily insulin injections in most dogs. After informing the owners of the diagnosis and recommended treatment, they asked for alternative options. They simply weren't willing to commit to the intensive treatment and follow-up required, and they ultimately requested euthanasia. The outcome devastated me, and I thought about it for weeks after. At the time I was against the decision to euthanize and felt incredible distress, believing I had let down my patient by not better advocating for his ongoing care. My perfectionism got the best of me and I felt anxious every time I replayed my failure to convince the owners to pursue the recommended care.

Looking back on the case now, I can see that my perfectionism exacerbated my distress. Had I accepted that not all owners can manage the intense commitment of twice-daily insulin injections and routine follow-up with their vet, regardless of the costs associated, I would have regarded the situation as a "normal" part of veterinary practice. I would have recalled the fact that not all cases turn out the way we want (or expect) them to, and that not all clients can (or want to) afford "gold standard" or the best available care. Yet I was stuck in a cycle of self-criticism and self-judgment over the way I'd conversed with the owners and my fears about the perceptions of my mentors and peers. I was certain they were questioning my ability to practice "best medicine" and care for my patients the expected standard.

Fear of others' perceptions and triggering stressful events are just a few situations where perfectionism rears its ugly head among veterinarians. Another commonly described trigger among individuals with self-oriented perfectionism is the concurrent experience of imposter syndrome. Otherwise termed "imposter phenomenon" or "imposter experience," this is when individuals question their abilities despite having positive evidence that supports their competence. Veterinarians who experience imposter syndrome fear being exposed as incapable "frauds" and tend to attribute their achievements to external factors such as luck, timing, or circumstance, rather than acknowledging their true capabilities.

I first experienced imposter syndrome when I was accepted to veterinary school at the age of 19. Despite being a high-achieving, successful, and well-rounded student my entire life, I was certain the only reason I got in after just two years of pre-vet study was because both of my parents were veterinarians who had graduated from the same school. I recall thinking the "powers that be" must have let me in out of obligation – not because of my years of practical experience, strong grades, or volunteer work. I was certain they'd either made a mistake (and would revoke my acceptance at any moment) or they felt obligated to admit me given my two alumni parents.

These feelings persisted throughout vet school and led me not to tell anyone (except my very close friends) that my parents were veterinarians. I knew that two of my classmates also had close family members who were veterinarians, yet I felt compelled to keep my own two vet parents a secret. I simply didn't want others to confirm my biggest fear: that I wasn't good enough to be there in the first place. My feelings were only compounded when I wrote (and almost failed) my first anatomy exam. I remember thinking to myself "this is it—they're going to realize that they never should have let me in."

But despite later successes, that wasn't where my imposter syndrome ended. Like so many other veterinarians, early in my career and especially during career transitions, my self-doubt and fear of being found out were amplified. When I arrived at North Carolina State University for my new resident orientation, I met residents in other specialties who had done their veterinary school or undergraduate degrees at Ivy League schools like Cornell, Yale, University of Pennsylvania, and Harvard. I felt nauseated with embarrassment as I contemplated how my Canadian university education paled in comparison and stayed quiet so as not to reveal my perceived underlying incompetence.

My imposter syndrome followed me throughout my residency program, especially during morning rounds, where I feared being called upon and not knowing the answer, and during grand rounds, where I was terrified of presenting my research and not being able to justify my methods or results. The persistent distress only exacerbated my self-doubt and perfectionism. I was sure that to keep everyone fooled, I'd never be able to let any of my imperfections show. A hilarious impossibility given that, as a trainee, I was never expected to have all the answers or do everything competently from the get-go. Yet that was the unreasonable expectation that I imposed on myself.

My situation and inner dialogue are echoed by many veterinarians, especially women and those early in their career. In fact, a study published in 2020 in *The Veterinary Record* found that of 600+ veterinarians located predominantly in the United States, United Kingdom, and New Zealand, more than two-thirds met or exceeded the clinical cut-off score for imposter syndrome. This was assessed using a scoring system that asked respondents to rank the truthfulness of 20 statements, such as:

- When people praise me for something I've accomplished, I'm afraid I won't be able to live up to their expectations of me in the future.

- I'm afraid people important to me may find out that I'm not as capable as they think I am.

- I often worry about not succeeding with a project or examination, even though others around me have considerable confidence that I will do well.

- I often compare my ability to those around me and think they may be more intelligent than I am.

This study found that female veterinarians and those with fewer than five years in practice were more likely to score high on the imposter syndrome scale, with many reporting a negative impact on their professional lives.[9]

The finding that early career veterinarians are more likely to experience imposter syndrome mirrors my own experience and that of other medical professionals whose imposter syndrome peaks during times of significant professional change. My imposter syndrome first came to light in veterinary school and flared during each new phase of my training and career, including my transition into mental health and wellbeing advocacy. Every time I embarked on a new project or attempted to acquire a new skill, I heard the voice inside my head telling me that this will be the moment I am "found out" as the fake who's been fooling everyone.

It makes sense that a newly graduated veterinarian would experience this during their initial transition into clinical practice. The same has been seen among human medicine students and physicians whose overall prevalence of imposter syndrome ranges from 22% to 60%. In a comprehensive review of the studies investigating imposter syndrome among practicing physicians or physicians in training, identifying as female, having low self-esteem, and the institutional culture were linked to increased levels of imposter syndrome. On the flip side, having supportive social networks, receiving acknowledgment for achievements, experiencing positive encouragement, and engaging in personal and group reflections act as safeguards against imposter syndrome. It's important to note that experiencing imposter syndrome is also connected to a higher likelihood of burnout.[10]

As I move into the latter decades of my career, I have a better awareness and recognition of my perfectionism and imposter syndrome, including how they adversely impact my work and relationships. I've learned to see these features not as who I am (i.e., a "perfectionist" or "fraud") but as a coping strategy during times of stress, self-doubt, or perceived scrutiny. I've made a conscious effort to recall the truth of how hard I worked to get to where I am today, what I know and excel at, where I need support or am less proficient, and, most importantly, when to let go of the outcomes and perceptions of others I cannot control. This mindset has helped me focus on the positives I bring to those I am trying to help, rather than the ways I might be deficient or lacking. While I can't say that I'm perfect (pun intended) at maintaining these beliefs, it's become a daily practice that supports my mental health and wellbeing.

Beyond career milestones and professional achievements, addressing imposter syndrome and perfectionism is crucial to building sustainable careers in veterinary medicine. Practicing self-compassion—discussed in depth in

Chapter 39—can be transformative for veterinarians, promoting a response to setbacks that values kindness over self-criticism. Reframing negative self-talk, celebrating small wins, and embracing a growth mindset can help combat the feelings of inadequacy common in a demanding field like veterinary medicine. Additionally, mindfulness practices encourage awareness of one's experiences without judgment, allowing veterinarians to refocus on progress and patient care over an unattainable ideal of perfection. Together, these strategies cultivate compassion and resilience, helping veterinarians navigate professional pressures with greater self-acceptance and emotional wellbeing.

The Human Side of Veterinary Mistakes

> Mistakes happen. They are an unfortunate and inevitable part of life and veterinary medicine. Like it or not, missteps, errors, and embarrassments often shape our personal character and professional values as much—if not more—than our successes.
>
> —Jaime Bast, RVT, CCRP, KPA-CTP
> (Registered Veterinary Technician)

I'm often struck by pet owners who share with me their anger and irritation over another veterinarian's mistake. I once attended a wedding and, upon finding out my occupation, one of the guests launched into a story (or, more accurately, a rant) about how an emergency veterinarian had misdiagnosed his dog as having cancer. He said that the veterinarian "didn't know what she was talking about" and he took his dog home. He then reached out to another veterinarian who diagnosed a stomach infection and his dog made a full recovery. He finished by saying that he was so angered by the initial emergency veterinarian's "incorrect diagnosis" that he called the veterinary clinic and "threatened to sue."

So many thoughts and emotions arise when I recall this story. In that moment, I felt angry and frustrated by the pet owner's lack of empathy and understanding toward the emergency veterinarian. I said something along the lines of, "While veterinarians are incredibly smart and capable people, we're still human—we make mistakes." I also explained that without having examined the dog myself, reviewed its history, or interpreted any test results, I couldn't comment on the cancer diagnosis. In my head, I wondered whether the owner had latched onto the word "cancer" as a possible differential, letting fear drown out the rest of the conversation. Reflecting on that, I felt compassion for him—likely blindsided by the possibility of losing his dog and reacting by fleeing the situation.

As veterinarians, we're presented with animals who cannot tell us their symptoms, how long they've been occurring, or whether there's a familial history of illness is—all pieces of information that are invaluable in helping human healthcare providers make a diagnosis. Instead, we rely on family member's observations, our physical examination, and the results of any tests that

DOI: 10.1201/9781003347385-26

we might perform, ranging from blood work and X-rays to CT scans and MRIs. When an animal first presents, especially for an urgent or emergent illness, we often provide owners with our list of differential diagnoses—the list of possible underlying illnesses that the animal might have. This list is often long, varied, and vague. For example, a geriatric cat might present to me emergently after vomiting 10 times over 24 hours. My list of differential diagnoses could initially include everything from organ disease (e.g., kidney failure), endocrine disease (e.g., hyperthyroidism), infectious disease, and intoxication to cancer. As sad as it sounds, cancer is almost always on the differential list, although it's less likely in younger animals.

In my experience, providing an entire list of differentials to a pet owner can be overwhelming (Box 1); therefore, I tend to stick with my top few. But there are some pet owners who want to know every single possibility before committing to a treatment plan or performing tests that might provide more information. Because veterinary medicine is a fee-for-service industry, we must be upfront with pet owners in terms of the costs associated with our exam, tests, and treatments. And when costs run high or an owner is financially strapped, it can be difficult to make decisions with limited information. This contributes to what can be a very emotionally charged and frustrating situation for everyone involved: the owner who wants what is best for their pet and the veterinarian who is doing their best to provide the owner with enough information to decide on next steps. So, what a pet owner might perceive as a "mistake" could simply be one differential in a long list of possible diagnoses.

Box 1: Did You Know?

In veterinary school, students learn the acronym "VINDICATE" to remind them of all the potential systems that can be affected by disease: Vascular (blood vessels and heart), Infectious, Neoplastic (cancer), Degenerative (age-related), Intoxication or Iatrogenic (human-induced), Congenital, Auto-Immune, Traumatic, and Endocrine (hormonal).

This process is similar in human medicine. If I visit my family physician because I have an unrelenting cough, she might tell me that I have post-viral bronchitis or pneumonia. If she gives me an inhaler to treat bronchitis and I don't get better, then later return to have X-rays performed that diagnose pneumonia, did she make a mistake at my initial visit? No, she simply started with the most likely differential diagnosis and advised treatment based on that. Very often in human and veterinary medicine, response to treatment ends up replacing a diagnostic test—if the animal responds to the treatment, then we know our diagnosis was correct.

Now, does that mean that veterinarians don't make mistakes? Well, the answer to that is a clear no. Of course we do. Why? Because we're human.

And humans make mistakes. Especially when we're still learning, trying new things, or functioning in a state of fatigue. I remember once baking cookies on wax paper thinking it was the same as parchment paper and then could not get the darn cookies off the paper to eat them! Or the first time I put on roll-erblades and promptly plowed into a parked car because I didn't know how to brake. Or when I was so tired that I put an outing with my best friend on the wrong date in my calendar and stood her up on the day we were supposed to meet. We've all been there because, as human beings, we are not infallible

I vividly recall what is still, to date, the most gut-wrenching mistake of my veterinary career; a mistake that led to the death of a patient. I was a third-year emergency and critical care resident at the time, working in a busy intensive care unit (ICU) at North Carolina State University, a renowned veterinary teaching hospital. I remember the events as if they happened yesterday. The ICU was full, I was sleep deprived, and I was facilitating the placement of a nasal feeding tube for a dog named Laci, who was being cared for by an internal medicine resident in the hospital. It was a Friday afternoon, everyone was busy, and it was one of those situations when everything that could go wrong did go wrong.

I asked one of the ICU technicians to place the feeding tube and then take an X-ray so that I could confirm it was placed correctly. One of the things that can go wrong when placing a feeding tube into the nose is that it can go into the trachea (windpipe) instead of the esophagus (throat). The first X-ray showed that the feeding tube was placed correctly in the esophagus, but the end of the tube was kinked. I asked the technician to pull the tube back slightly to allow the end of the tube to flip forward toward the stomach and then repeat the X-ray. Unbeknown to me, the tube was removed completely from Laci's nose and replaced. When I went to review the second X-ray, in haste, I only looked to see that the tube was directed toward the stomach (and that the kink was removed), rather than reviewing the entire X-ray; as such, I missed that the tube was now incorrectly placed in the trachea. It was this mistake that led to Laci getting fed food into her lungs. And it is for this reason that she experienced cardiopulmonary arrest and died overnight.

I can still hear the voice of the board-certified radiologist calling me the following Monday, upon reviewing all the X-rays from the prior week. He wanted to make sure that I knew that the last X-ray taken of Laci showed that the tube was in her airway. My stomach clenched and I felt a wave of nausea wash over me. I thought to myself "I killed Laci." What happened after the error was discovered was agonizing. Laci's owners filed a lawsuit against the university and sued everyone involved in her care (including me), resulting in a distressing situation that went on for years. A complaint was filed with the North Carolina Veterinary Medical Board, which correctly identified that despite following the standard of care in this situation (taking an X-ray to con-firm proper tube placement), I had made an error in interpreting the X-ray.

These events took place more than 15 years ago now and I'm certain that I will never forget them for as long as I live. I recall berating myself for the mistake and telling myself that I didn't deserve to practice veterinary medicine. I remember questioning all the medical decisions that I made for weeks. And I recall being terrified to interpret X-rays for months. But most of all, I remember thinking about how I would feel in that situation if it were my dog in the ICU who died because of a medical error.

Almost a decade later, I learned that my experiences after my mistake were not unique to me (Box 2). A study published in *Anthrozoös* in 2018 shared the results of an online survey detailing the experiences and reactions of spay-neuter veterinarians after serious adverse events that resulted in an unintended complication or death. The results showed that the physical and emotional reactions of veterinarians to adverse events are pronounced, with all respondents experiencing an immediate visceral reaction, including signs of anxiety or stress attributed to the fight-or-flight response. The feelings veterinarians described, in conjunction with their physical experiences, included anxiety, guilt, sadness, and self-doubt, as well as empathy for the clients and others impacted by the events. Some veterinarians processed and moved past these feelings within a day or a week, whereas others were deeply affected for months or years after.[1]

Box 2: Did You Know?

An online survey in 2015 of more than 600 veterinarians revealed that 30% were involved in at least one adverse event. Of those veterinarians, 84% had a short term (≤ 1 week) negative impact on their professional life and 56% had a longer term negative impact on their professional life. Of those veterinarians, 78% also experienced short term (≤ 1 week) negative impacts on their personal life and 51% experienced longer term negative impacts on their personal life.[2]

So many feelings are tied to what happened with Laci, which was both life altering and career changing for me. But I'm grateful that I can look back now and take away some very critical concepts from the situation. First, it's because of my experience that I implore veterinarians and other team members to always disclose medical errors to pet owners. In my situation, despite telling my faculty advisor what happened immediately after the mistake was discovered, Laci's owners were not notified about the error until days after they had lost their beloved family member. I'm certain that this fueled their desire to file a lawsuit. Research shows that, in human medicine, when medical errors are disclosed and involved personnel apologize, family members are much less likely to sue. Contrary to what some might think, ignorance is *not* bliss when it comes to medical errors, because the only person who benefits from not coming clean is the person who made the mistake.

So, while the process of telling a client about an error is extremely difficult, especially if it resulted in an adverse outcome or death, in the end full disclosure is best for everyone. In many cases, it allows the animal to receive the treatment that he or she needs, thereby lessening the medical consequences of the error. It also helps to explain otherwise unanticipated problems that the animal might be exhibiting after the mistake is made. It strengthens the relationship between the veterinarian and pet owner, who will trust that the vet will be honest with them no matter what situation arises. And it reduces the emotional distress for everyone involved and helps bring closure and understanding to an already difficult situation.

Second, I believe that mistakes are how we learn and grow and, in the context of medicine, lead to changes in hospital protocol or policy to help prevent errors from happening again. In human medicine, mistakes such as wrong-site amputation have resulted in the standardization of pre-surgery protocols to verify that the correct surgery is performed on the correct location of the correct patient. Likewise, surgical checklists that include pre- and post-surgery sponge counts arose after surgical patients developed complications from sponges left inside of their abdomen. Questions about allergies posed by your pharmacist also arise from incidents in the 1990s involving fatal penicillin reactions. After my mistake, the North Carolina State University teaching hospital implemented the "Laci Rule," which stipulated that every feeding tube would have its correct placement confirmed with an X-ray interpreted by a board-certified radiologist or radiology resident before any feedings would begin.

Third, my final plea to everyone involved in a mistake affecting an animal or owner is to attempt compassion and forgiveness. To pet owners, it's not possible nor realistic to hold veterinarians and other members of the veterinary team to a higher standard than any other human. Veterinarians will make mistakes and hopefully they will handle them in a way that is honest and transparent. And to veterinarians, if another veterinarian says that they have never made a mistake, they're either lying or they simply have not been practicing long enough to make their first one. If we can be compassionate with ourselves and others, including exercising forgiveness in knowing that we all make mistakes, we can recover from adverse events with more comfort and ease.

As a specialist veterinarian, it's typical for dogs and cats to come to me for more complex care than a general practice vet can provide. And it's not uncommon for me to be faced with cases that have been misdiagnosed, mistreated, or mismanaged. I recall caring for a dog who had emergency surgery for a twisted stomach (gastric dilation volvulus [GDV]) at another clinic and was transferred to me in critical condition. The dog had air around his lungs and was bleeding into his abdomen; both complications from the surgery being performed incorrectly. Normally the stomach is tacked to the side of the body wall after it is de-rotated and, in this case, the veterinarian had attempted a technique to tack the stomach around the last rib. In doing so, he had punctured the diaphragm causing air to build up in the chest and collapse the lungs. During subsequent emergency surgeries at our hospital, sponges were also identified in the abdomen and severe bleeding was noted from the spleen that should have been removed during the first surgery. In short, there were several mistakes made, and, in this case, it seemed to be due to negligence and not simply human error.

Medical errors are described as any action or decision that in hindsight appears incorrect or results in an unanticipated outcome. Negligence occurs when the medical care provided fails to meet the standard of care. In other words, an average or similarly trained veterinarian would be expected to recognize and prevent the error that caused the harm. In the case of the dog with the twisted stomach, I felt that the veterinarian was not trained sufficiently to perform the GDV surgery, and he failed to meet the standard of care by not removing the damaged spleen or counting the sponges. The dog subsequently had two additional surgeries to correct the mistakes of the first veterinarian and ultimately died secondary to complications. I spoke with the veterinarian to advise him of his errors and to recommend that he reach out to the owners to express his apologies and condolences. The owners understandably pursued reprimand of the veterinarian via the provincial veterinary regulatory board. I'm not sure how the grievance was resolved in the end, but it was a devastating situation for everyone involved.

It should be clarified that not all medical errors cause harm, not all adverse outcomes result from medical errors, and not all adverse outcomes resulting from errors are due to negligence—such as in Laci's case. In some circumstances, an adverse outcome can be due to unreasonable pet owner expectations. Veterinary medicine continues to evolve and grow, but we still have so much to discover and understand. Consequently, there are countless situations where an animal may be treated for a disease that has not previously been diagnosed or managed successfully. It is important to recognize that, in these situations, the animal may not recover. Likewise, there can be biological variability among animals; a veterinarian can treat three cats for the same condition but only two of them survive. Just as humans have different responses to chemotherapy and other treatments, so can pets. Finally, there can be complications that are unpredictable or unforeseeable. For example, every time an animal is given a vaccine, there is a risk of reaction, just like when you visit your pharmacist to receive your flu shot. While the reaction is an adverse outcome, there is no one to blame.

A study published in *Frontiers in Veterinary Science* in 2019 titled "Medical Errors Cause Harm in Veterinary Hospitals" was designed to evaluate the type and severity of medical errors reported in three veterinary hospitals using a voluntary incident reporting system. Errors were reported over a three-year period and grouped into different categories (Box 3). Based in retrospective review, incidents were also classified as resulting in a near miss (i.e., error did not reach the patient but could have caused harm if it had), harmless hit (i.e., error reached the patient but did not cause harm), adverse event (i.e., error reached the patient and caused harm), or unsafe condition (i.e., circumstance or condition increased the probability of a patient safety event). During the study period, 560 incidents were reported, the equivalent of about 5 errors per 1,000 patient visits. To put this in perspective, approximately 1 in every 1,000 human primary care visits results in preventable harm. Drug errors were the most common error identified in the veterinary study, followed by communication failures. Errors reached patients without causing harm approximately half of the time, but 15% of all incidents resulted in harm to the patient, including 8% that resulted in permanent disease or death.[3]

Box 3: Did You Know?

A 2019 study categorized medical errors occurring in three veterinary hospitals as:[3]

- Drug (medication administration)
- Iatrogenic (procedures or treatments other than medication)
- System (delays, missed treatments, protocol problems)
- Communication (confusion over orders, incorrect patient)
- Laboratory (lost specimen, mislabeled sample)
- Oversight (missed diagnosis, deviation from standard of care)
- Staff (insufficient staff or training)
- Equipment (inaccessible, broken)

No veterinarian wants to make a mistake that results in the death of someone's beloved pet. What happened to Laci has happened to many other animals and is something all veterinarians strive to avoid. But when it does happen, the important thing is that we learn from it and do all that we can to prevent it from happening again. The information gained from recording and evaluating medical errors helps veterinarians understand the primary causes of mistakes with an aim to develop interventions to improve safety for all patients. By fostering a culture of openness and continuous learning, they can not only honor the memories of those lost but also enhance the overall wellbeing of both the veterinary team and the pets in their care.

Mental Health in the Veterinary Profession

> When choosing this profession, we know to some extent that we will be part of the inevitable ups and downs of every pet's life that comes through our doors, but it's time we start talking more openly about how the difficult aspects of our jobs can have serious negative consequences on our emotional wellbeing and mental health.
>
> —Daniel Aja, DVM (Chief Medical Officer)

People often tell me "I wanted to be a veterinarian, but I could never put an animal to sleep." I've always struggled with how to respond. Are veterinarians seen as uniquely disturbed for being able to perform euthanasia? What many people don't realize is that while most veterinarians don't find routine euthanasia procedures emotionally difficult, many do struggle with their mental health—for reasons that are complex and multifaceted. As someone who has lived with major depression since my early 20s and generalized anxiety since my early 30s, I know firsthand how deeply mental health challenges can affect both personal wellbeing and professional life.

According to the Centers for Disease Control and Prevention, more than 1 in 5 adults live with a mental illness and 1 in 25 adults live with a serious mental illness such as schizophrenia, bipolar disorder, or major depression.[1] In fact, by the age of 40, 1 in 2 adults will have, or have had, some form of a mental illness.[2] This means every person is likely to themselves experience or know of someone who has lived with a mental illness. Yet most individuals wouldn't associate words like "depressed," "anxious," "stressed," or "suicidal" with veterinarians, instead viewing us as calm and compassionate professionals (Box 1). Perhaps this is because we tend to hide our personal feelings underneath the veneer of our professional identity, as explored in previous chapters.

DOI: 10.1201/9781003347385-27

Box 1: Did You Know?

Based on survey findings of more than 600 Americans, the public tends to perceive veterinarians more favorably than physicians. Specifically, terms such as "approachable," "sensitive," "sympathetic," "patient," and "understanding" were more commonly attributed to veterinarians, whereas terms like "proud," "arrogant," and "overconfident" were more commonly assigned to physicians.[3]

Yet research studies completed over the last decade suggest that veterinarians (and vet students) around the world have a less than rosy picture when it comes to their mental wellbeing. Beginning in the first semester of vet school, half to two-thirds of students exhibit symptoms of clinical depression, which are more likely among students reporting high levels of academic or transitional stress. This number exceeds that of human medical students, where less than one-quarter experience depression.[4] Another survey study published in the *Journal of Veterinary Medical Education* in 2017 assessed stress and depression among more than 1,200 vet students across 33 schools in the United States and Canada. Two-thirds of the respondents had symptoms of mild to moderate depression with female vet students exhibiting worse symptoms compared to male vet students. But regardless of gender, stress was strongly correlated with depression, meaning those who experienced high levels of stress were more likely to demonstrate symptoms of depression.[5]

Similar findings are demonstrated among veterinary students in the United Kingdom, Austria, and Germany. A survey completed over a decade ago showed that more than half of vet students in the United Kingdom have experienced mental health problems and that mental distress among those students was higher than the general population.[6] Likewise, more than half of Austrian vet students completing an online survey had moderate depression and anxiety. Other notable findings were that 21% had clinically relevant insomnia symptoms, 79% had high-stress symptoms, 23% had symptoms of alcohol use problems, and 39% had symptoms of disordered eating. Like other studies, female vet students were more likely to exhibit mental health symptoms compared to male vet students.[7] Finally, a study of more than 900 German vet students found that they were 20 times more likely to have depression and four times more likely to report suicidal ideation compared to an age-matched general population in Germany.[8]

Most of the statistics among vet students mirror what is seen among veterinarians in the workforce, who also demonstrate higher than average symptoms of mental illnesses. A questionnaire completed in 2007 by nearly 1,800 veterinarians in the United Kingdom showed that symptoms of anxiety and depression and 12-month prevalence of suicidal thoughts were higher compared to the general population.[9] A decade later, an online survey was distributed to Canadian veterinarians and received more than 1,400 responses. The results demonstrated that, relative to the general population, Canadian vets had higher scores for perceived stress, secondary traumatic stress, anxiety, and depression. Remarkably, their 12-month prevalence for suicidal ideation (26%) was nearly 10 times that of the general population (3%).[10] And another study surveying more than 2,000 Australian veterinarians found that one-third reported poor psychological health, which was more prevalent among female, younger, or less experienced vets.[11]

While these statistics clearly indicate an overall higher risk of mental illness among vet students and veterinarians compared to their comparable cohorts, especially when it comes to women (Box 2), there are many personal and professional variables that determine who is more heavily impacted. An online survey of more than 260 American veterinarians published in 2021 found that early-career (< 5 years of experience) and mid-career (5–19 years of experience) vets reported higher mental health symptom burden compared to late-career (≥ 20 years of experience) vets.[13] In the same year, serious psychological distress was documented in 1 in 10 US veterinarians in another survey and was more common among vets less than 55 years old.[14] These findings suggest that the people who persist in veterinary medicine have found coping mechanisms, so that after 20 years working they have a lower symptom burden. Yet age and career stage are not the only characteristics impacting the likelihood of mental health problems.

Box 2: Did You Know?

According to the *World Health Organization*, overall rates of psychiatric disorder are almost identical for men and women; however, prominent gender differences are found in the patterns of mental illness. These differences occur particularly in the rates of common mood disorders such as depression and anxiety, which are twice as common in women. Conversely, alcohol dependence is more than twice as likely to affect men.[12]

Many other studies have sought to determine which factors might be linked with mental health problems among veterinarians. A recent publication analyzed online surveys completed by more than 70 vets practicing in Australia and found that a difficult work environment is tied to negative outcomes like depression, stress, job dissatisfaction, and wanting to leave the job or profession. Even after considering personal resilience—a person's ability to bounce back from trying circumstances—work conditions still affect job satisfaction and mental wellbeing. The research also found that having breaks from, and some control at work is linked to better mental health. The study suggests that while building resilience is important, improving workplace conditions might be a more practical way to enhance mental health and overall wellbeing.[15]

The positive impact of a healthy workplace on mental health has been demonstrated in a recent survey study published in the *Journal of the American Veterinary Medical Association*, which found that working within a healthy culture resulted in a lower risk of experiencing psychological distress. Four factors that were identified as contributing to a healthy work culture included:

- A strong sense of belonging to a team.

- A high degree of trust in the organization.

- Candid and open communication among team members.

- Sufficient time allotted for each appointment to provide high-quality patient care.

That same study also identified non-work-related activities (Box 3) that were associated with a lower prevalence of psychological distress, making the case for having a life outside of work to foster better mental health. Likewise, a survey study of more than 1,000 female veterinarians in Australia found that women with two or more children had less anxiety and depression than those who had never been pregnant, and women working part-time (less than 35 hours per week) had less anxiety or depression than those who worked full-time.[16] It's possible that having children outside of work forces a person to prioritize family and that working part-time allows more opportunities for non-work activities.

Box 3: Did You Know?

In a random survey study of veterinarians in the United States, those who were less likely to experience psychological distress were more often engaged in healthy non-work activities including spending time with family, exercising, hiking, walking, playing sports, reading for pleasure, spending time on a hobby, sleeping at least eight hours per night, socializing with friends, traveling for pleasure, and volunteering.

When I reflect on my own life, there's no disputing that my family history and life circumstances have shaped the highs and lows of my mental health journey. Mental illnesses have affected my family for generations. My great-grandfather died by suicide, and we have a multigenerational history of bipolar disorder. I also have a cousin with schizophrenia and other family members who have experienced major depression or anxiety. Additionally, my experience with major depressive and panic disorders have often paralleled challenging life events, such as relationship breakups, the deaths of family members or pets, and, more recently, becoming a solo parent during a pandemic. For decades I've been under the care of a psychiatrist or other licensed mental health professional, and I've sought counseling ranging from cognitive behavioral therapy to internal family systems therapy for years. And while work-related stress in the form of long hours or lack of sleep has sometimes been a contributing factor to my poor mental health, there are many times in my life where my mental health has thrived despite my preexisting mental illnesses and occupational stressors.

The presence of preexisting mental illness or psychological distress has been attributed to the mental health problems that veterinarians experience. For years, there was a debate among veterinary mental health experts and advocates regarding whether veterinary medicine was selecting for individuals who were "traumatized" and gravitated toward caring for animals to avoid working with people. Some postulated that this was why so many veterinarians felt distressed by challenges with clients or team members. Ironically, so much of the work that we do as veterinarians is people-facing, and yet most of us identify our love of animals as the main reason we chose veterinary medicine.

This theory was investigated in a study published in the *Journal of Veterinary Medical Education* in 2017, which surveyed veterinary students in all years of training at six schools in the United States and Canada. More than 1,100 students completed the survey, which measured Adverse Childhood Experiences (ACEs) (Box 4), depression, perceived stress, and the age at which they wanted to become a veterinarian. Nearly two-thirds of vet students reported at least one ACE; the most common was living in a household with a person with a mental illness, found among one-third of respondents. Vet students with four or more ACEs had a threefold increase in depression symptoms and higher than average stress compared to vet students with no ACEs. However, there was no relationship between the age at which a student chose to become a veterinarian and exposure to ACEs, and vet students were no more likely to report exposure to ACEs before the age of 18 compared to the general population. These findings refute suggestions that vet students enter the profession with a higher risk for poor mental health secondary to their early childhood experiences.[17]

Box 4: Did You Know?

Adverse Childhood Experiences (ACEs) are traumatic events occurring before the age of 18, such as physical or emotional abuse, neglect, or household dysfunction. Examples include parental substance use, divorce, or incarceration, and these experiences can have lasting impacts on mental and physical health throughout adulthood.[18]

Addressing mental health problems among the LGBTQ+ veterinary community is of particular importance, given that non-heterosexual cis men, non-heterosexual cis women, as well as transgender and nonbinary veterinarians and vet students have a higher lifetime prevalence of suicidal ideation and attempted suicide compared with veterinarians in general. Research published in the *Journal of the American Veterinary Medical Association* compiled online survey responses from LGBTQ+ veterinarians and vet students in the United States and the United Kingdom. Transgender and nonbinary vets and vet students also had a higher prevalence of psychological distress compared to non-heterosexual cis men and women, as well as the general veterinarian population. Additionally, exposure to discriminatory behaviors, including homophobic or transphobic language, was associated with a higher likelihood of psychological distress, depressive episodes, suicidal ideation, and previous suicide attempts.[19] Not unlike the general population, mental health problems and suicidal behavior are more common among sexual minorities in the veterinary profession, particularly transgender and nonbinary vets and vet students.

Another question that remains unanswered, based on the available literature, pertains to the impact that veterinarians' mental health problems have in the workplace. Research published in *Frontiers of Veterinary Science* in 2020 demonstrated a complex relationship between veterinarian mental health and client satisfaction. The study took place over a period of several days during which 60 vets completed psychometric surveys to assess their mental health and, concurrently, clients completed post-appointment satisfaction questionnaires. While one would presume that client satisfaction would increase with better mental health scores among the vets, no such relationship was identified. Instead, vets with poorer mental health scores very often had high client satisfaction scores and those with mental health scores suggesting wellness had lower client satisfaction.[20] So it seems that veterinarians might be as good as animals at hiding their distress.

Not long ago, I delivered a workshop to leaders at a specialty veterinary hospital pertaining to coaching and supporting team members with anxiety. We discussed a situation involving one of their team members, who was very anxious when dealing with certain emergency cases and, as a result, became confrontational and combative. When we broke down her behaviors—which included yelling at vet techs, becoming irritated with or avoiding clients, and at times even voicing frustration toward the patients themselves—it became clear that manifestations of her presumed anxiety were impacting client satisfaction, team functioning, and the quality of care. This experience aligns with the sentiments of 25 veterinarians who shared similar observations at a Canadian veterinary conference in 2016, later published in the *Frontiers of Veterinary Science*. One-on-one interviews with veterinarians about how poor mental health affects the provision of care uncovered five main themes related to its impact in the veterinary workplace:

1. Coworker interactions
2. Client interactions
3. Reduced concentration
4. Difficulty making decisions
5. Reduced quality of patient care

So, while client satisfaction might not directly correlate with veterinarian mental health in other research, clearly vets themselves perceive the impact of poor mental health on veterinary team dynamics, case outcomes, and patient safety.[21]

Undoubtedly, the veterinary profession is grappling with significant mental health challenges, particularly among younger professionals and women. The impact of workplace conditions on mental wellbeing is irrefutable, emphasizing the urgent need for enhanced support structures. A positive workplace culture, characterized by connection and open communication, is a crucial factor in mitigating psychological distress. There's a consensus on the heightened risks faced by LGBTQ+ veterinarians and vet students, underscoring the importance of tailored support for this community. The intricate relationship between mental health and client perceptions, while not fully understood, underscores the necessity of addressing these issues for the overall wellbeing of veterinary teams and the quality of patient care. The key takeaway is clear: prioritizing mental health support and fostering a positive workplace culture are imperative for sustaining a healthy veterinary profession.

25

Recognizing Mental Health Stigma

Vets don't talk about their work stresses outside their own tightly knit vet circles. Some of us don't even confide our struggles to our colleagues. We talk about our cases in detail for hours, but many of us still cringe at opening up about the state of our mental health.

—Anita Link, BVSc. Hons.(Class1)
(Small Animal Veterinarian and Mental Health Advocate)

Veterinarians and vet students may have higher than or equal to average rates of certain mental illnesses and suicidal thoughts, yet many resist seeking help. It's a striking irony: professionals known for their compassion and caregiving often avoid turning to caregivers themselves—mental health providers. But when you consider the nature of the veterinary identity and the pervasive stigma around mental health among healthcare professionals, it becomes more understandable why so many in our field have avoided the very help that was desperately needed.

My own stigma has become apparent to me as I reflect on my up-and-down relationship with counselors and other mental healthcare providers. The first time I spoke to a counselor was during my residency, after Ronnie was euthanized. To say that I was a "complete mess" would be a tremendous understatement. I'm certain that I got less than ten hours of sleep over the three days she was hospitalized in the ICU, one of which I spent lying next to her as she nearly died from septic shock due to aspiration pneumonia. While I was grappling with whether to euthanize her, one of my mentors came into the ICU with a middle-aged woman whose name I can't recall. She was introduced to me as "someone to talk to" and I vaguely remember realizing she was a counselor and that my mentor was worried about my mental health. I shrugged my shoulders and said I was "fine," and I'd think about reaching out if I needed to. I found myself in her office a few weeks later, still grieving, but didn't receive advice or support that I considered helpful. With that, I quickly wrote off counseling as a waste of my time.

Years later, when I was an Assistant Professor at the Ontario Veterinary College, struggling to maintain my mental health amidst my preexisting depression and anxiety, as well as newfound burnout, I debated whether to leave

DOI: 10.1201/9781003347385-28

my faculty job or take a medical leave of absence. I clearly recall a Human Resources (HR) representative recommending the latter option. She explained that the reason for my leave would be confidential and that with a doctor's note I could qualify for weeks to months of paid leave to focus on my mental health. She compared it to a person taking a medical leave for chemotherapy, to recover from surgery, or to tend to another physical health concern. Yet I still couldn't wrap my head around it. I knew that my mental health was poor, and I needed some time away from work to address it head-on, but was taking a medical leave appropriate? I struggled with this for months and ultimately opted to resign rather than take a leave that would create questions (and potentially backlash) upon my return.

Looking back on this now, I fully recognize that it was the stigma around mental illness and medical leave that contributed to my hesitation and ultimately resulted in my resignation. Like many other veterinarians I've spoken to, I believed that others wouldn't understand if I needed to take time off to better my mental health or, worse, they might be angry or punish me when I came back (Box 1). The HR representative argued that the leave was justified and that the cause would be kept confidential. But I couldn't help wondering: won't people assume, guess, or eventually find out? And when they do, will they see me as a lesser colleague, mentor, or professor?

Box 1: Did You Know?

Based on the findings of over 1,300 responses to the *British Veterinary Association Voice of the Veterinary Profession* survey conducted in 2019, approximately 18% of veterinarians reported avoiding medical leave because they felt uncomfortable doing so, with higher rates observed among younger vets, particularly those under 35 (25%), and female vets (21%) compared to their older and male counterparts.

It's concerns like these that permeate the studies completed in the last decade investigating help-seeking behaviors and mental health stigma among veterinarians. In 2010, a review of factors influencing the increased risk of suicide among veterinarians was published in *The Veterinary Record*.[1] Stigma associated with mental illness was identified as a key factor, meaning that vets tended to have a negative attitude or belief toward a person or group of people with a mental health problem, which makes them less likely to disclose or seek help for their mental illness. This tendency has been confirmed among veterinarians around the world, including in a survey conducted in 2014 in the United States.[2] Two questions sought to determine the degree of stigma held among vets related to mental health treatment efficacy and perceptions of public support. The statements were:

- "Treatment can help people with mental illness lead normal lives" (assessing attitudes about mental health treatment effectiveness).

- "People are generally caring and sympathetic to people with mental illness" (assessing attitudes about social support).

Veterinarians were asked whether they strongly agreed, somewhat agreed, were unsure or undecided, somewhat disagreed, or strongly disagreed with each statement. More than 9,500 vets provided answers for both statements and were then assessed to determine which demographic and practice variables were associated with negative attitudes toward each statement. Overall, 3% of surveyed veterinarians had a negative attitude toward treatment effectiveness, meaning they somewhat or strongly disagreed that treatment can help people with mental illness lead normal lives. The odds of this negative stance toward treatment effectiveness were higher for males versus females, solo versus non-solo practitioners, those with evidence of serious psychological distress, and those reporting suicidal ideation after graduating from vet school. More years of practice experience was a significant overall predictor of having a negative attitude toward treatment effectiveness.[2]

Even more surprising was that 47% of surveyed veterinarians had a negative attitude toward social support, meaning they somewhat or strongly disagreed that people are generally caring and sympathetic to people with mental illness. The odds of this negative attitude were higher for females, solo practitioners, those not belonging to a veterinary association, those with evidence of serious psychological distress, those with depression during or after vet school, and those with suicidal ideation since graduating from vet school. Older age was a significant overall predictor of having a negative attitude toward social support.[2]

Similar findings and additional insights were gleaned from a more recent survey of veterinarians in Norway published in *BMC Public Health* in 2022, which found that among the nearly 2,600 responses, half somewhat or strongly agreed that "people are generally caring and sympathetic to persons with mental illness," a sentiment more often held by those <30 years of age. Of the 30% of Norwegian vets who had a mental health problem that qualified for treatment, only half of those with serious thoughts of suicide were seeking help. Those vets seeking help were more likely to be female, work in public administration or academia / research, or have a positive attitude toward the treatment of mental illness by somewhat or strongly agreeing that "treatment can help people with mental illness lead normal lives." Working in production animal practice was a factor associated with less help-seeking among Norwegian veterinarians.[3]

Help-seeking behavior was also recently investigated among veterinarians, vet techs, and vet nurses in Australia and New Zealand and published in a study in *Frontiers in Veterinary Science* in 2022.[4] Average scores related to perceived stigma and barriers to mental healthcare were in the moderate range and the factors more frequently limiting access to mental health support were:

- difficulty getting time off work (58%)
- difficulty scheduling an appointment (57%)
- high cost of treatment (52%)

Additionally, the researchers explored how the normalization of psychopathology within the veterinary profession can hinder help-seeking. When unhealthy behaviors or mental health challenges become widespread, they may be perceived as "part of the job" rather than issues warranting support. In veterinary medicine, the researchers suggested that excessive stress and burnout have become so commonplace that they're seen as normal, despite being harmful and deserving of attention and care. Perhaps unsurprisingly, most of the responding veterinary professionals agreed or strongly agreed that[4]:

- fatigue was inevitable in their occupational role (88%)
- they felt pressure to go in to work despite being sick (73%)
- burnout is considered a normal part of the job (72%)

For decades, individuals with a mental health–related stigma have been less likely to seek mental healthcare—a stigma that is more pervasive among men, those in the military, underrepresented cultural groups, and healthcare professionals. What is especially concerning among veterinarians is that those with psychological distress, a history of mental illness, or suicidal ideation are more likely to exhibit mental health–related stigma or not seek help for other reasons. A recent survey of more than 250 veterinarians in the United States found that 80% of vets were not accessing mental health support and, of those, more than half reported at least mild anxiety or depression symptoms. Factors that were positively associated with accessing mental health support included self-awareness, commitment to others (e.g., family, coworkers), and personal fit. Quality of care, utility of care, accessibility, and attitudes were identified as barriers as shared in the free text responses provided in the survey[5]:

- "Many medical professionals don't meet my standards."
- "Mental health professionals don't understand the challenges of my career."
- "Don't have enough time off."
- "Having the time to do so, along with other family member responsibilities, my needs are rarely first."

- "I don't believe in psycho babble."

- "Concerned it will take me a long time to find the right therapist for me."

Many of the disparaging attitudes toward mental health treatment were identified among late career (≥ 20 years of experience) veterinarians who were less likely to report help-seeking intentions compared to mid-career (5 to 19 years of experience) vets.[5]

I used to believe—or at least hope—that the newer generations of veterinarians would be free from mental health stigma and would readily and routinely seek support for their mental health challenges. Unfortunately, the published studies investigating help-seeking behavior for mental health problems among vet students echo most of the findings among working veterinarians. A recent study surveying vet students in the United States identified several barriers to seeking mental health services, including:[6]

- lack of time to attend appointments

- cost of mental health services

- difficulty scheduling an appointment

- lack of knowledge about available services

- lack of availability of services

- lack of trust in mental health professionals

- concerns about providers' sensitivity to diversity issues

- lack of transportation

- concerns about confidentiality

- concerns that mental healthcare does not work

- stigma about seeking mental health services

Stigma surrounding the use of mental health services persists, as demonstrated by numerous studies highlighting its prevalence among veterinary students worldwide. Australian vet student responses to an anonymous survey published in 2019 in *The Veterinary Record* revealed that female vet students reported most often using instrumental support (i.e., seeking help from others) and emotional support (i.e., seeking comfort from others) as coping strategies. Those vet students who demonstrated self-stigma, the negative beliefs that involve feelings of internalized shame, were less likely to use instrumental support and exhibited greater self-blame. Male vet students were also more likely to exhibit self-stigma, particularly those who relied on humor as a coping strategy.[7] Knowing this, I can't help but think of famous comedians who have spoken openly about their depression, such as Sarah Silverman and Jim

Carey. Astutely, Seymour Fisher once shared the concept that comedians attempt to make others laugh to relieve their own anxiety or depression.[8] The so-called sad clown paradox—the contradictory coexistence of comedy and mental health struggles such as depression— might help explain why some vet students use humor as a coping strategy.

Another study published in the *Australian Veterinary Journal* in 2021 found that vet students in Australia reported significantly higher levels of self-stigma compared to non-veterinary students, and that self-stigma was more common among vet students with depressed symptoms.[9] Additionally, a study surveying more than 570 vet students in the United States determined that they were most willing to seek mental health services for issues related to substance use, traumatic experiences, and anxiety; however, they were less likely to do so for sleep problems, as well as family, friend, or romantic relationship problems.

Interestingly, the concept of "pluralistic ignorance" was confirmed among vet students, whereby they underestimated their peers' willingness to seek mental health services (Box 2). In other words, students falsely believed that others were less likely to seek help, even though survey responses showed otherwise. Through statistical analyses and modeling, the authors concluded that public stigma can indirectly influence a student's willingness to seek mental health services. It does so by first shaping self-stigma, which, in turn, affects attitudes toward professional help—ultimately determining help-seeking behavior. This chain of events illustrates how both societal and internalized perceptions can significantly influence decisions regarding mental healthcare.[10]

Box 2: Did You Know?

Pluralistic ignorance can be seen in a classroom setting where a teacher asks if anyone has questions about the material, but no one raises their hand because they assume that everyone else understands it. Many students may have questions, but they remain silent due to the mistaken belief that they are the only ones who are confused.

To truly understand the extent of mental health stigma among US veterinary students, one only needs to examine the candid responses from those completing a survey. These responses highlight prevalent issues in the veterinary profession such as public and self-stigma, ingrained identity norms, perfectionism, autonomy, and presenteeism.[6]

- "How would I be viewed by my mentors and those I look up to in the profession?"
- "I would feel ashamed that I could not help myself."

- "I feel like most of us just accept that it's going to be hard and think we just have to feel miserable."

- "We are used to being on top and the best at everything."

- "It is a terrible feeling admitting needing help. Not being able to do it alone makes people feel worthless."

- "Students who call in sick just to have one day off are stigmatized as 'slackers' or 'not team players.'"

The reasons why veterinarians and vet students do not seek help for their mental health problems are as complex as the reasons why veterinarians die by suicide, which we will discuss in Chapter 29. They may have had a negative experience with a mental health provider, employee assistance program, or workplace counselor, or perhaps are in an unsupportive practice environment or work for someone with limited compassion or understanding regarding mental health. The fact that many veterinarians exhibiting stigma are practicing without other associates makes me wonder: did they chose to isolate themselves further because of their negative social beliefs, or are those beliefs reinforced by the isolation they experience in solo practice? In my own experience, being a member of a provincial veterinary organization that offers free mental health support and annual mental health first aid training has affirmed my belief that others genuinely care about the wellbeing of veterinary professionals.

I can also understand how negative beliefs toward social support can develop early in a person's career, due to a negative personal experience or lack of support during veterinary training. During my residency, after I euthanized Ronnie, I experienced grief that progressed to symptoms of severe depression. One day I overheard one of my coworkers say to someone: "can't she just get over it already?" I was hurt, confused, and embarrassed. I look back now and recognize that this individual was probably dealing with her own "stuff" that was being triggered by my depressed behavior. But, at the time, her comment led me to view my depressive symptoms as an annoyance and to think twice about speaking openly about my struggles. Thankfully, that encounter hasn't prevented me from continuing to seek support for my mental health today, but I can imagine how others might have responded differently after such an experience.

Circumstances have changed dramatically over the last two decades and may help explain the differences in stigma and help-seeking across age groups or years in practice. Twenty years ago, very few vet schools had dedicated social workers or counseling services. Today, however, mental health support is becoming the norm on veterinary campuses, with full-time social workers and psychologists, as well as time off for counseling appointments embraced more commonly by vet schools worldwide. Kansas State University, for example, has been offering on-site counseling services at its veterinary school for more than 15 years, with a steady increase in the number of students seeking support over that time.[11] My own veterinary school at, the University of Saskatchewan hired a social worker ten years after I graduated to provide support for students and staff. Since then, the social work program at my alma mater has expanded to offer services to clients as well, including emotional support, grief and loss counseling, and referrals to community resources.[12]

The discussion surrounding mental health stigma among veterinarians and vet students underscores the complex challenges inherent in addressing psychological wellbeing within the profession. The reluctance to seek help, reluctance to take medical leave, and enduring stigma highlight the need for continued efforts to foster a culture of support and understanding. While progress has been made in raising awareness and providing access to mental health resources, there's still much work to be done to dismantle misconceptions and promote proactive mental healthcare. Ultimately, it's imperative for individuals within the veterinary community to recognize that seeking support is not a sign of weakness, but rather an essential step toward maintaining personal wellbeing and professional resilience.

Confronting Compassion Fatigue

This work is so much more difficult than they train you for. We all become competent diagnosticians and surgeons—that part they can (mostly) teach. What they don't teach, and they don't tell you, is how much of this work involves human emotions and human communication. I was also never told what emotional toll this work will take and was certainly never taught any strategies for combating the compassion fatigue we will all experience. Our profession can be extremely rewarding, but it also is extremely frustrating and disheartening.

—Beverly Wolney, DVM (Relief Veterinarian)

I can vividly recall the first time I lost the capacity to care about what happened to one of my patients. Working in a veterinary teaching hospital's intensive care unit (ICU) alongside two of my residents, we were slammed with critical cases. A cat was undergoing peritoneal dialysis for an acute kidney injury and the ICU was at capacity, meaning there were already dogs overflowing onto the ICU floor because we didn't have enough kennels or cribs. Additionally, we had a dog undergoing mechanical ventilation for an anesthetic complication. We assumed the dog had aspirated stomach contents while recovering from general anesthesia, because he'd vomited while his tube was being removed from his airway. Despite the best efforts of the anesthesia team to suction any fluid from the back of his throat, he'd developed a severe pneumonia. His condition was dire enough that we ultimately had to replace the tube in his airway and provide respiratory support.

Fast forward to nearly a week after starting mechanical ventilation and his condition was worsening rather than improving. His supplemental oxygen needs were higher, as was the pressure needed to keep his wet and infected lungs inflated. His prognosis was becoming poorer, and we believed it was because he'd developed a secondary infection from having a tube in his airway for so long. We refer to this condition as ventilator-associated pneumonia—when bacteria tracks down the tube from the mouth into the trachea and eventually infects the lungs. To prove our hypothesis, we briefly disconnected him from the ventilator, a risky maneuver for any unstable "vent patient," and collected a fluid sample from his airway for bacterial culture. We submitted

DOI: 10.1201/9781003347385-29

the sample to the bacteriology lab (or so I thought) and began the standard waiting time of three to five days for any potential bacteria to grow.

Three days later, we were nervously doing what we could to support the dog while awaiting the new bacterial culture and antibiotic susceptibility results, and I called the lab to see if they had preliminary findings. I was met with the confused response, "we don't have any new samples from that patient." To say that I was distressed by this information is an understatement. My confusion turned to panic and, soon after, to rage. In a very uncharacteristic way, I hung up the phone in the ICU and loudly huffed: "is everyone here completely incompetent?" The tears prickling my eyes demonstrated the anguish behind my anger, as I feared our mistake in not submitting our dog's sample to the lab three days ago had just cost our patient his life. I felt like a worthless failure of a specialist, clearly not a person who was supposed to be leading the helm amidst the dozens of patients in the ICU. This was compounded by an immediate flashback to my last ventilator patient, who had a similar complication and whose owners had ultimately elected euthanasia after nearly two weeks of hospitalization. All I wanted to do was run away and, in doing so, avoid thinking or caring about any of the patients in need of my help.

Some might read this story and feel taken aback by the extremity of my response. I can understand this because I had the same reaction. Hearing the harshness of my words spoken aloud and seeing the downtrodden looks on my residents' faces instantly told me that what I'd said was not only hurtful, but unfair. We were all working our hardest and, simply put, mistakes happen, especially given the immense pressure that all of us were functioning under. Likewise, others might have been surprised by my callous lack of regard for my patients. It's not every day you hear a veterinarian say how *little* they care about their patients' outcomes. This reaction concerned me the most. I had, to that point, always been a compassionate and empathetic vet, caring deeply about my patients, the families who loved them, and my team members who tirelessly tended to them. Believing that I'd stopped caring about my patients was a sign to me that I was no longer fit for my job.

With hindsight, I know that my behaviors were the result of compassion fatigue. According to Dr. Charles Figley, the first to introduce the term, "Compassion fatigue is a state experienced by those helping people or animals in distress; it is an extreme state of tension and preoccupation with the suffering of those being helped to the degree that it can create a secondary traumatic stress for the helper."[1] Dr. Figley aptly dubbed compassion fatigue "the cost of caring" and defined it as a deep physical, emotional, and spiritual exhaustion that can occur among those who routinely work in an intensive caregiving environment.[2] Vicarious trauma, secondary traumatic stress, and secondary victimization are other terms for compassion fatigue. These depict the caregiver's relationship to the patient, or in veterinary medicine, the client or pet owner, whereby empathy leads the caregiver to "take on" the distress of the affected patient or person. A psychiatrist and researcher in trauma named

Dr. Frank Ochberg has said that, over time, a caregiver's ability to feel and care for others "becomes eroded through overuse of [their] skills of compassion."[3]

Individuals who experience compassion fatigue often report feeling trapped by their work, believing they are not successful, and experiencing hopelessness, worthlessness, disillusionment, or resentment as a result.[4] The American Veterinary Medical Association describes a sense of apathy and isolation being most common among veterinarians experiencing compassion fatigue and lists other physical and mental symptoms that also occur (Box 1).[5] The Professional Quality of Life (ProQOL) Self-Score was developed in the late 1990s to offer individuals an objective way of assessing whether they demonstrate symptoms of compassion fatigue and compassion satisfaction, the pleasure a caregiver derives from being able to do their work well. Compassion fatigue is scored based upon two parts: burnout characterized by exhaustion, frustration, anger, and depression, as well as secondary traumatic stress, which is a negative emotional state fueled by fear and work-related trauma.[6] Work-related trauma can be a combination of either primary trauma, for example, witnessing animal abuse or neglect, or secondary trauma, such as supporting an owner who saw their own pet get hit by a car.

Box 1: Did You Know?

Common signs of compassion fatigue include[5]:

- Apathy
- Chronic physical health problems
- Compulsive behaviors such as overeating or gambling
- Difficulty concentrating
- Excessive complaining about work, manager(s), or coworker(s)
- Inability to derive pleasure from previously enjoyed activities
- Isolation
- Lack of self-care
- Mental and physical exhaustion
- Problem substance use
- Recurring nightmares or flashbacks
- Repressed emotions
- Sadness

While at the time I didn't know what compassion fatigue was, let alone that a score to measure its symptoms existed, I can look back and see that my indifference toward my cases, anger toward my team members, and exhaustion that affected me physically and mentally were indications that the cost of caring had caught up with me. As for many other veterinarians in our profession, the immense compassion that I felt for my patients and clients had taken a serious toll. According to a 2020 study published in the *Journal of the American Veterinary Medical Association* that surveyed more than 1,400 Canadian veterinarians, when compared with the general population, vets had significantly higher average scores for secondary traumatic stress and burnout, the two subscales on the ProQOL that show compassion fatigue. These scores were also significantly higher for female compared to male vets, which also mirrored higher perceived stress scores for female versus male vets.[7]

Other research has examined potential risk factors for compassion fatigue among veterinarians, along with exploring additional variables that could be linked to its onset. One of those studies was published in the *Journal of the American Veterinary Medical Association* investigating more than 5,000 full-time veterinarians working in the United States. Survey results that included ProQOL measurements showed that 50% of the veterinarians had high burnout scores and nearly 60% had high secondary traumatic scores, demonstrating that half of the participating vets were experiencing compassion fatigue. Those who spent at least 75% of their time working with dogs or cats had higher burnout and secondary traumatic stress scores than those who spent < 25% of their time. Likewise, female vets and those with less experience were also more likely to have scores consistent with compassion fatigue.[8]

Those in the veterinary profession often say that the rewards of the work come at a cost. I can attest to this. While there are many situations where cases go well, pets are cured, and animals are reunited with their families, there are also a large number of cases that go unexpectedly wrong, where pets die and clients are heartbroken by the loss of their beloved family member. Researchers at the University of Calgary published a study in *Anxiety Stress Coping* in 2018 demonstrating that client grief predicted higher compassion fatigue scores among Canadian veterinary care providers. The study also found that client-related barriers—challenges that interfered with the veterinary professional's ability to care for the animal—were linked to increased compassion fatigue. This can occur when there is a conflict between what a client wants and what is believed to be in the best interests of the animal, or when a client's financial limitations prevent the team from pursuing best practices. On the flip side, making a difference to animals and building relationships with animals and clients are associated with higher compassion satisfaction scores. The paper is aptly titled "The Paradox of Compassionate Work" and describes the contradictory relationship that a veterinarian and client can experience, which can lead to either compassion satisfaction or fatigue.[9]

More recently, researchers have investigated methods to enhance compassion satisfaction and lower compassion fatigue among veterinarians. A study published in 2023 in the *Journal of the American Veterinary Medical Association* examined the relationship between disclosure, responsiveness, compassion fatigue, anxiety, and depression. The researchers gathered over 200 veterinarians who were members of a private Facebook support group. Their survey results showed that self-disclosure online—sharing personal thoughts or struggles—was linked with lower levels of compassion fatigue, anxiety, and depression, but only when responses from others were emotionally supportive. In other words, mental health outcomes improved when self-disclosure was met with validating, caring, and understanding responses. Importantly, the study highlighted that responsiveness acts as a mediator: self-disclosure alone, without empathetic or compassionate feedback, does not have the same positive effect.[10]

It may seem paradoxical that offering compassion for others in distress can benefit the recipient, while simultaneously harming the provider. Which is why, some experts argue that "compassion fatigue with is a misnomer. They suggest that caregivers do not become fatigued simply from feeling concern for others' suffering. Instead, they propose that "empathy fatigue" is a more accurate term—reflecting the emotional exhaustion, overwhelm, and depletion that result from repeatedly sharing in or absorbing another person's pain. This will better be explained once the different forms of empathy are clarified:

- Cognitive empathy is the ability to identify or be aware of another person's feelings. For example, a veterinarian might speak an owner who appears embarrassed and recognize that the owner feels guilty or ashamed for not being able to afford appropriate care for their pet.

- Emotional empathy is the ability to share or experience those feelings. For example, a veterinarian might speak to an embarrassed owner and feel embarrassed when they recognize that they would also not be able to afford the recommended care.

- Empathic concern is the desire to alleviate another person's suffering or improve their situation. For example, a veterinarian might recognize an owner's embarrassment about their financial limitations and reassure them by explaining that their pet still has a good change of full recovery, even with less expensive care.

Harm occurs when healthcare providers—whether veterinary or human— repeatedly experience emotional empathy by continually absorbing the feelings, emotions, and suffering of others. Over time, this can lead to empathy fatigue, when caregivers feel mentally, emotionally, and physically exhausted and struggle to demonstrate empathy in any form.

In veterinary practice, there is no shortage of situations where both the animal and pet owner suffer, and the veterinary caregiver responds with emotional empathy. When an owner struggles with the decision to treat or euthanize their pet, feels sorrow over a terminal illness, or is overwhelmed with grief as their pet fails to respond to therapy, veterinarians can deeply identify with, and even experience the same feelings. Unfortunately, when this happens repeatedly without healthy coping strategies, it can lead to debilitating consequences.

In exploring the delicate balance between being a compassionate, empathic care provider and maintaining professional wellbeing, it is crucial for veterinarians to consider how to sustain their innate gift of empathy without leading to fatigue. Experts suggest that veterinarians can start by expressing empathic concern, sympathy, and compassion, rather than slipping into emotional empathy. This approach involves focusing on the positive impact that can be made in the situation, such as relieving the animal's suffering or comforting the pet owner. Rather than immersing oneself in the owner's or animal's pain, it's more helpful to sympathize with their situation and imagine a future where their distress is alleviated. Research demonstrates that when empathy is expressed as an "other-related emotion" through empathic concern, it leads to positive feelings, better health, and prosocial motivation - the desire to help others. In contrast, when empathy manifests as "self-related emotion" through emotional empathy, it is linked to negative feelings, stress, poor health, withdrawal, and burnout.[11]

In recent years, it has helped me to remind myself that the traumas of my patients and their families are not my own. During heightened emotional situations with clients, I've found myself mentally repeating phrases like "this is not my tragedy" or "this is not my distress.". This simple mantra has served as a steadfast reminder to separate my client's experiences from my own as a caregiver. While I strive to provide compassionate care, I also recognize the importance of maintaining emotional boundaries. I've learned that over-identifying with my clients' pain can lead to compassion fatigue, which ultimately impairs my ability to serve them effectively. In this sense, compassion can become a double-edged sword: it fosters deep connection and trust, yet it can also weigh heavily on our hearts if we become too entwined in others' struggles. I believe the issue is not the compassion itself, but rather the paradox at the heart of the veterinarian-client relationship: empathy can both bridge and block the wellbeing of veterinarians. By understanding this paradox, we can navigate our emotional landscape more skillfully, staying present for our clients without losing ourselves in their suffering.

Addressing Burnout among Veterinarians

Our natural tendency is to keep it all inside. It's scary to share our feelings because doing so makes us vulnerable. Shame, guilt, and embarrassment tend to stand in the way of veterinary professionals opening up about their struggles with burnout. But these fears are just that—fears.

—Kaitlyn Hensley, LMFT
(Licensed Marriage and Family Therapist)

The term "burnout" started popping up more frequently in veterinary publications in the early 2000s, decades after it was first coined by psychologist Herbert Freudenberger in 1974.[1] Freudenberger used burnout to describe the severe physical and mental exhaustion that he observed in volunteers working at a free human medical clinic. Since then, the concept has been widely used to describe a state of chronic workplace stress that can lead to physical and emotional exhaustion, along with feelings of cynicism and detachment from work. More recently, burnout was included in the 11th Revision of the International Classification of Diseases (ICD-11) as an occupational phenomenon. While not classified as an illness or medical condition, it is recognized as a reason a person might need to seek health services.

While I've undoubtedly experienced burnout several times throughout my veterinary training and career, I vividly recall symptoms that impacted my ability to work while I was a faculty member at the Ontario Veterinary College. I remember being on the clinic floor supervising fourth-year vet students, interns, and residents. We had a full caseload in the intensive care unit (ICU), including a ventilator case and two dogs in the isolation unit. It was my third week in a row on-clinics—my third consecutive week on-call—and I was feeling mentally and physically depleted. This wasn't the first time I'd felt exhausted by my work or like I was "spinning my wheels" with the caseload, but it was a time when I remember constantly feeling the urge to disconnect or detach from the cases. In other words, I no longer felt invested in what was happening with our patients, nor did I feel that I was accomplishing anything meaningful through my teaching or mentorship.

At the time, my thoughts and behaviors startled me because I didn't recognize them as symptoms of burnout. Instead, I felt like I wasn't cut out for my

DOI: 10.1201/9781003347385-30

role as an Assistant Professor and that there must be something "wrong" with me. These feelings of guilt and shame are common among veterinary team members experiencing burnout, as the culture of vet medicine has not traditionally supported seeking help. In fact, "struggling" can be seen as a sign of weakness, potentially damaging one's professional reputation. When I looked around at the other faculty members I worked alongside, I didn't hear anyone else grumbling about their clinical workload, promotion and tenure deadlines, grant proposal rejections, teaching and mentorship responsibilities, or lack of work-life balance. In fact, it looked like everyone else was happy and thriving.

The disconnect between what I was experiencing and what I perceived others to be going through led me to the conclusion that I was on the wrong path and needed to do something different. So, I did what too many burnt out veterinarians have done over the past several years—I left my job. Had I spoken more openly about my experience, taken time away from work, modified my responsibilities, or shed light on some of the systemic factors contributing to my burnout, I might still be in that role today. Yet, like so many veterinary professionals, I didn't recognize my symptoms nor did I see any other way out of my situation.

According to the Maslach Burnout Inventory, a score used commonly in scientific studies to determine whether a person has signs of burnout, there are three possible symptoms:

- Emotional exhaustion: feeling emotionally exhausted or overextended by work.

- Depersonalization (cynicism): having an impersonal response toward clients, patients, or team members.

- Low personal accomplishment: feeling incompetent at work or not accepting of personal achievements.

In hindsight, I was experiencing a form of burnout, like many veterinarians, characterized by high emotional exhaustion and depersonalization, but with an enduring sense of personal accomplishment. By that I mean, despite my struggles, I knew that I was still making a difference in the lives of my patients and their families.

The number of veterinarians experiencing burnout is difficult to quantify, given the various methods or scores used to diagnose it. However, research suggests that approximately one-third to one-half of veterinarians experience burnout. What most studies from different countries also show is that, compared to the general population, veterinarians have higher burnout scores—suggesting their experience of burnout is more frequent or severe than that of the average working person. Other interesting findings from the scientific literature include that a larger proportion of women experience burnout compared to men, and that large animal veterinarians are less likely to experience burnout compared to those working with companion animals. Of particular concern is that early-career veterinarians, or those with less experience, are more likely to exhibit burnout symptoms compared to those further along in their careers.[2–9]

Many personal and organizational factors contribute to burnout, and these have been well-documented in the veterinary literature (Box 1). For example, high levels of student debt paired with relatively low income can lead to significant financial stress, amplifying the pressure to work long hours. Perfectionism—a common trait among veterinary professionals—can result in unrealistic self-imposed expectations and a greater risk of burnout. Career stage also plays a role, as early-career veterinarians face unique challenges in establishing themselves. Poor work-life balance, often compounded by people-pleasing tendencies and the habit of prioritizing work over social connection, can likewise lead to burnout.

Box 1: Did You Know?

Many factors are associated with burnout among veterinarians.[10,11]

Personal:

- student debt
- low income
- perfectionism
- strong feelings of responsibility
- career stage
- poor work–life balance
- people-pleasing behaviors
- choosing work over social life
- personal caregiver responsibilities
- chronic physical or mental illness
- absence of social support
- absence of skills related to communication, coping, delegation, and teamwork

Organizational:

- physical hazards
- insufficient equipment or resources
- excessive workload
- frequently changing or unclear work responsibilities
- lack of autonomy
- conflict with peers or managers
- workplace bullying or cyberbullying
- high client expectations

- long work hours
- working evenings, weekends, or on-call
- lack of control over the schedule
- contradictory expectations from leadership
- competitive work environment
- perceived inequity
- bias or discrimination
- insufficient reward or recognition
- incongruent values

While research demonstrates that both personal and organizational stressors contribute to burnout, organizational factors inherently play a larger role. Exposure to physical hazards—such as fractious animals or needle sticks—can heighten stress and contribute to burnout. Inadequate equipment, such as a shortage of monitoring devices, computer workstations, or human resources, can impede workflow efficiency, increase frustration, and add to emotional strain. Excessive workloads, frequently changing or unclear responsibilities, and a lack of autonomy in decision-making can also overwhelm veterinary team members. Conflict with peers or managers, workplace bullying, and even cyberbullying can foster toxic environments strongly associated with burnout. Insufficient recognition or reword for hard work—especially when coupled with long hours, evening shifts, weekends, or on-call duties—can intensify symptoms. Addressing these challenges through organizational support, open communication, and a commitment to fostering a healthy workplace culture is essential to preventing and mitigating burnout among veterinary professionals.

Several years ago, I conducted a survey of emergency veterinary care providers—primary in the United States and Canada—to assess burnout and examine associated work-related factors. The results were published in 2023 in the *Journal of Veterinary Emergency and Critical Care*. The findings revealedthat emergency veterinary care professionals—including veterinarians, techs or nurses, and interns or residents-in-training—experience higher levels of emotional exhaustion and depersonalization, along with lower feelings of personal accomplishment, compared to their counterparts in a human emergency department. Among respondents, women, residents, those working in private- or corporate-owned referral hospitals, and those with off-shift duties reported the highest levels of burnout. Factors most closely linked to elevated burnout symptoms included feeling overwhelmed with work, lack of control over tasks, limited recognition, and perceived unfairness in resource distribution. On the other hand, those who had been in the field for more than 20 years, as well as those who were married or had children at home, reported lower burnout symptoms. Notably, workload emerged as the strongest predictor of emotional exhaustion and depersonalization, while a sense of recognition was most closely linked to feelings of personal accomplishment.[12]

The physical, mental, and emotional consequences of burnout are profound—and have undoubtedly led to some of the staffing shortages currently seen in veterinary medicine (as discussed in Chapter 38). Burnout has profound physical consequences such as fatigue, chronic inflammation, and autonomic imbalance that increase the risk of cardiovascular events, hypertension, and diabetes. Hormone imbalance caused by chronic stress has been linked to reproductive health issues in women and decreased sperm quality in men. Burnout also affects gut health via dysbiosis and immune dysregulation. Overall, it contributes to conditions like insulin resistance, type 2 diabetes, dyslipidemia, and non-alcoholic fatty liver, highlighting its far-reaching effects on physical and reproductive health.[13]

The mental and emotional health consequences are equally troubling. Burnout can impair cognition—affecting problem-solving, learning, attention, and focus—and has been shown to negatively correlate with medical knowledge, with performance drops equivalent to the loss of an entire year of residency. Neuropsychological testing reveals that individuals experiencing burnout often suffer from diminished concentration and working memory, which can compromise decision-making and increase the risk of medical errors. Emotionally, burnout can manifest as instability, detachment from work, interpersonal conflict, and desire to leave one's job. Importantly, its symptoms often overlap with those of mental health conditions such as depression, anxiety, and post-traumatic stress disorder. Left unaddressed, burnout not only impacts individual wellbeing but can ultimately compromise patient care.[13]

A 2022 paper published in *Frontiers of Veterinary Science* highlighted the economic toll of burnout in veterinary medicine (Box 2). Research conducted in collaboration with the American Veterinary Medical Association estimated that the economic cost of veterinarian burnout approaches $997 million USD annually—primarily due to turnover and reduced working hours. On average, turnover costs about $104,000 USD per veterinarian, while reduced clinical hours cost approximately $56,000 USD per vet. For veterinary technicians alone, the median cost of burnout due to turnover was estimated at $933 million USD, with each technician's turnover costing around $59,000 USD. When breaking down the impact by practice area, food animal vets have the highest median cost per veterinarian, while equine vets have the lowest. However, in terms of total industry-wide cost, companion animal vets—followed by mixed animal practitioners—contributed the most. While these estimates carry some uncertainty, they underscore the substantial financial burden that burnout places on the veterinary profession.[14]

Box 2: Did You Know?

The estimated cost of burnout in the veterinary industry is substantial, reaching about $1.93 billion USD when accounting for both veterinarians and veterinary technicians.[14]

While organizational factors associated with burnout have an undeniable impact on veterinary professionals—and arguably offer the greatest leverage for reduced burnout when addressed—individual resilience also plays a crucial role in buffering against its effects. Veterinarians with high levels of resilience demonstrate a greater ability to rebound from the challenges and stressors inherent in their demanding work. These individuals are better equipped to navigate emotionally taxing situations, maintain a positive perspective, and sustain their passion for the profession. In contrast, those with lower resilience may be more vulnerable to burnout, struggling to effectively cope with the chronic stress that often accompanies veterinary roles. Investing in strategies that enhance resilience—such as cultivating support networks, offering resources for adaptive coping, and developing strong communication skills— is essential for reducing the risk of burnout among veterinary professionals.

Research has shown that Canadian veterinarians, on average, have lower resilience scores than the general population, and those with lower resilience are more likely to experience burnout.[15] Similarly, a study of veterinarians in the US Potomac region during the COVID-19 pandemic found that late-career vets tended to have higher resilience. Contributing factors included job satisfaction, a sense of control over their work, and a work-life balance. Positive coping strategies were also associated with higher resilience. However, a common obstacle to adopting these strategies was a lack of time for self-care—highlighting one of the profession's ongoing challenges.[16]

While promoting resilience is valuable, an overemphasis on individual coping strategies can obscure the systemic roots of burnout. To create meaningful change, actionable solutions must also be implemented at the organizational level. First and foremost, veterinary workplaces must address workload management by delegating tasks appropriately, creating realistic schedules, and utilizing support staff effectively. Encouraging employees to disconnect from work during personal time—by setting clear boundaries and discouraging after-hours communication—can also help alleviate chronic stress. Improving workflow through efficient systems (e.g., user-friendly electronic medical records and dictation software) can significant reduce administrative burdens. Addressing physical discomfort through ergonomic assessments—especially for surgical staff—can also support wellbeing.

A healthy work environment is equally essential. This includes addressing bullying, fostering open communication, and ensuring psychological safety for all team members. Because financial stress is a well-documented contributor to burnout, organizations should explore compensation models that balance productivity with quality of care, and consider offering access to financial counseling. Creating a culture that supports mental health, normalizes help-seeking, and prioritizes rest breaks and recovery time can make a significantly difference to overall job satisfaction and retention.

Reflecting on my own experience with burnout, I've come to appreciate the importance of challenging the assumption that "this is just the way veterinary medicine is." Honest self-reflection—coupled with the clarity that comes with hindsight—has allowed me to better understand (and sometimes avoid) the systemic pitfalls that contribute to burnout. I now recognize how deeply these stressors are in our profession. If I'd known then what I know now, I might have found ways to remain in my academic role—better equipped to manage my wellbeing and advocate for systemic change. My hope is that by prioritizing supportive culture, manageable workloads, and open discussions around mental health, veterinary organizations can build environments in which both resilience and wellbeing are not just possible—but expected.

Finding Balance with Boundaries

I wish we would have been taught how our personal time matters, not to be a [servant] just because that's the way it's always been done. The workplace should have as much respect for my personal time away from work as much as I have respect for my work responsibilities while at work.

—Katie-Marie Buswell-Zuk, RVT
(Veterinary Surgical Technologist)

The term "boundaries" has surged in popularity over the last decade, evident from pop culture references and online trends. Google Trends data shows a more than 350% increase in searches for "what are professional boundaries," indicating growing curiosity about work-life balance.[1] Despite a brief introduction to professional boundaries during my residency training nearly 20 years ago—when I was advised during orientation not to sleep with veterinary students—the practical implications were unclear to me as a veterinarian. Of course, being raised in a household with two vet parents, I knew the importance of maintaining healthy personal boundaries. For instance, my mom's habit of sharing intimate details with clients, like my adolescent struggles or academic achievements, often left me feeling exposed and embarrassed. As a result, I've become more mindful about what personal information I share and have used this understanding to set and respect boundaries in my professional life.

While some veterinarians cherish their longstanding client relationships and see themselves almost as counselors to their patients' families, blurred boundaries within the veterinary–client relationship can cause significant distress among many vets. This is particularly evident in the context of availability, exacerbated by the increasing use of technology such as instant messaging, social media, and email between veterinarians and clients. In fact, a survey conducted over a decade ago among veterinarians in the United States found that the "expectation of being always available," was one of the most commonly cited sources of client-related stress.[2] This expectation often leads vets to feel obligated to respond to emails from clients outside of working hours, return calls on their days off, or even provide their personal cell numbers so that they can be reached by clients at any time. Moreover, many vets spend significant time on phone consults with clients without billing for their time, further blurring the boundaries between professional and personal life (Box 1).

DOI: 10.1201/9781003347385-31

Box 1: Did You Know?

A study conducted by the Veterinary Information Network (VIN) found that among nearly 1,000 veterinarians, they spent between 1 and 5 hours per week providing email and phone consultations, which are rarely billed to clients.[3]

Early in my career as a veterinary intern and resident, it was extraordinarily uncommon to exchange emails with clients. We didn't have cell phones and could only be reached by pager. This provided a buffer—or inherent boundary—to being contacted directly by clients, who had to go through the clinic or hospital on-call service to have a message passed on via the paging system. However, ten years into working as a small animal emergency and critical care specialist, I vividly recall this boundary being challenged. I'd been caring for a dog hospitalized in the intensive care unit for cluster seizures, defined as at least two seizures occurring in a 24-hour period. This situation is life-threatening and, of course, the dog's owner was concerned, given the risk that seizure activity predisposes the brain to more seizures in the future. Once the dog's condition had stabilized and he was ready to be discharged, his owner came to the hospital to take him home. She promptly demanded my cell phone number so that she could contact me directly—something, in her words, she had always done with her dog's other veterinarians.

While I had a work cell phone by this time, it was meant for internal use between those of us working in the hospital, and I had yet to cross the boundary of sharing that number with a client. I felt frustrated and resentful at the thought that this owner felt entitled to reach me anytime she wanted—a luxury I'd never dream of asking my physician or counselor. After considering the potential for her disgruntled backlash, I firmly denied her request. I told her that it was my personal rule not to share my cell phone with clients and that she'd need to go through the main hospital line to reach me, the intern, or resident on-call. I later found out when I rotated off-clinics, my colleague received the same request—to which he promptly agreed.

This underscores the diverse perceptions of healthy boundaries and the innate reluctance among many veterinarians to establish them with clients. Despite acknowledging client expectations as a common stressor, vets often hesitate to set boundaries due to fears of client backlash, guilt over potential negative outcomes for the patient, and discomfort with asserting their own needs over those of others. Through years of coaching veterinarians on boundary-setting, I've identified the top five reasons for their avoidance:

- a tendency to people-please
- fear of appearing indifferent

- anxiety about future interactions

- feeling powerless to assert boundaries

- deriving personal value from helping others, which setting boundaries seemingly compromises

These ingrained beliefs and habits often push veterinarians to give advice to neighbors on a Sunday night, accept social media friend requests from clients, or even cut into their time off for clinic visits when clients insist. Sadly, not setting healthy boundaries in these situations disrupts work-life balance, leading to burnout and job dissatisfaction. Interestingly, a study of veterinary students found that their perception of poor work-life balance among rural veterinarians increased after exposure to those vets. This suggests that the "small town vibe" of rural practice might reinforce the expectation of porous or unhealthy professional boundaries, contributing to a heightened sense of imbalance between work and personal life among students—and, potentially, future veterinarians.[4]

Financial concerns among pet owners are recognized by veterinarians in the United States and the United Kingdom as one of the most common stressors in veterinary practice, often leading to impolite interactions with clients. In situations of owner financial distress, veterinarians may face accusations such as:

- "You're just trying to make money off of pets—you don't actually care about their wellbeing."

- "I thought you were supposed to help pet owners, not bankrupt them."

- "You're just recommending these treatments to make more money."

- "It's your job to figure this out, I shouldn't have to pay for more tests."

- "If you really loved animals, you would find a way to do this for free."

These sentiments can lead vets to take on the client's financial problems as their own.

I often hear from veterinary practice owners who experience tremendous distress trying to balance the rising cost of providing veterinary care with what their clients can afford. One memorable instance involves a close friend and practice owner who had a client unable to afford treatment for her newly adopted puppy with parvoviral enteritis, a potentially life-threatening condition. In an attempt to help, my friend took the puppy home, provided necessary treatment, and nursed the dog back to health in her own bathroom - all at no cost to the owner. I can't help but wonder if some pet owners would have a different perspective on veterinarians and money if they knew about people like my friend. While this is a great example of how vets are not financially driven, actions like these also highlight the importance of setting boundaries, as they ultimately contribute to burnout.

Unhealthy boundaries among veterinarians don't just stop with clients; they also affect relationships with coworkers—and even themselves. According to a study published in the *Journal of the American Veterinary Medical Association*, abusive behaviors and confrontations among team members were noted by veterinarians as significant stressors, often persisting due to a lack of boundaries.[2] Many veterinarians have shared stories of feeling belittled or chastised by their colleagues, feeling powerless to assert their boundaries or expectations for respectful treatment. This lack of boundaries is often compounded by a lack of transparency from practice leadership regarding acceptable behavior—and a lack of psychological safety to voice concerns without fear of repercussions.

Years ago, I worked as a locum veterinarian alongside another emergency and critical care specialist at a large emergency and referral hospital. There were countless moments when the specialist would speak disparagingly to team members about me behind my back, withhold information necessary for my job, and send passive-aggressive emails regarding cases that I had managed instead of addressing concerns directly. Despite my desire to set boundaries by requesting in-person discussions about case management and face-to-face conversations to share feedback or concerns, the hospital's culture and the specialist's personality left me feeling powerless. I attempted to involve the hospital manager in conversations with the specialist, but they were new to their role and hesitant to intervene. Ultimately, the strained relationship led to a breakdown in my longstanding relief coverage at that practice—and to this day, I wouldn't feel psychologically safe to voice my concerns or assert a boundary within that environment.

Unhealthy boundaries with team members can stem from an unwavering desire to be seen as a "team player." Many veterinarians struggle to say no when asked to cover extra shifts or emergencies, fearing they'll be labeled as unhelpful or selfish—despite sometimes receiving the same favor in return. These dynamics mirror those seen in client interactions, driven by similar factors:

- A reluctance to disrupt harmony within the team
- Fear of being perceived as uncooperative
- Anxiety about future interactions with team members
- Feeling powerless, particularly when dealing with practice owners
- Deriving self-worth from helping others, making boundary-setting difficult

Setting boundaries with oneself is yet another struggle for many veterinarians, whether it involves limiting work hours, expressing needs to management, balancing work and family time, or managing technology use. Even among those who successfully establish boundaries with clients and coworkers, many falter in setting boundaries with themselves. Issues such as underutilizing paid time off, reluctance to request workplace changes, constant work-related discussions at home, and excessive screen time contribute to feelings of overwhelm and poor mental health—ultimately damaging relationships and derailing careers.

General practice veterinarians are often compared to family physicians in human medicine, facing similar challenges in ensuring consistent care. Just like doctors, veterinarians can struggle with unhealthy boundaries, leading to feelings of resentment and burnout, often due to stress and fatigue.[5] Research suggests that boundary-setting is key for healthcare workers to avoid burnout. A review on coping strategies found that establishing boundaries was linked to lower burnout levels.[6] Among human hospice and palliative care doctors, having healthy boundaries was a common way to steer clear of burnout and find satisfaction in their work.[7] Studies among human healthcare workers in places like Germany and Singapore consistently show that those who set boundaries are more resilient and less likely to burn out.[8,9]

Though there is not much research on boundaries in veterinary medicine yet, signs suggest that recognizing and respecting boundaries is gaining traction. A review of veterinary literature found mentions of boundary-setting to promote work-life balance, hinting at a possible shift toward embracing boundaries in the field.[10] As veterinarians continue navigating their roles, acknowledging the importance of boundaries could become crucial for their wellbeing and resilience.

A narrative study, *Double-Duty Caregiving*, sheds light on the experiences of women in healthcare professions who also serve as caregivers for elderly relatives, revealing the complex juggling act they perform between their professional responsibilities and personal caregiving duties.[11] Picture a female veterinarian working tirelessly at the clinic, while also tending to the needs of an aging parent or a sick pet at home. Despite their best efforts, many find themselves overwhelmed, emotionally drained, and struggling to maintain boundaries between work and personal life. For these veterinarians, it's akin to walking a tightrope—dedicating themselves to their patients while being present for their families, often blurring the lines between the two. This underscores the importance of recognizing and supporting veterinarians, especially those in the "sandwich generation," who are simultaneously caring for aging parents while also raising their own children or tending to other family obligations. Their blurred boundaries lead them to risk their own wellbeing, while striving to provide compassionate care both in and out of the clinic.

As we delve deeper into veterinary boundaries, it's evident that the landscape is nuanced and multifaceted. From navigating technological shifts to balancing professional duties with personal values, the theme of boundaries resonates deeply within the veterinary community. It's clear that respecting boundaries isn't merely a preference—it's essential for the wellbeing and sustainability of veterinary practice. By acknowledging and establishing healthy boundaries with clients, colleagues, and oneself, veterinarians can protect their mental health, foster stronger relationships, and cultivate a work environment that is both compassionate and resilient.

Unveiling the Tragedy of Veterinarian Suicide

There's an idea that veterinarians work on the belief that it's right to euthanize a hopeless case, and we are seeing ourselves, emotionally, as hopeless
cases.

—Emily Volk, DVM (Emergency Veterinarian)

The first time I became aware that suicide was a problem among veterinarians was in September 2014, not even a year after I had left my academic job.
I learned that Dr. Sophia Yin, a published author and highly regarded veterinarian specializing in animal behavior, had just died by suicide. The news
of her death was unsettling to the veterinary community; Dr. Yin was well
known for her international teachings on animal behavior and was respected
around the world for her low-stress handling practices. As an author, Dr. Yin
wrote several articles and books including my personal favorite as a veterinary
student, *The Small Animal Veterinary Nerdbook*. Every image I'd seen or could
recall of Dr. Yin in her books, published articles, or website pages was one of a
smiling and happy veterinarian, passionate about helping owners understand
dog and cat behavior so their relationships could flourish. I found it challenging to revise this image and envision her as someone who might be living with
a mental illness and struggling with thoughts of suicide.

The news of Dr. Yin's death shook the veterinary community and reig-
nited the conversation about veterinarian suicide that had begun more than
a decade prior. Several research studies published in the early 2000s highlighted concerns regarding an elevated mortality risk due to suicide among
veterinarians in comparison with the general population. This increased risk
among veterinarians in the United Kingdom was highlighted in several studies published in *The Veterinary Record*[1] and summarized in a systematic review published in *Occupational Medicine* in 2010. In that study, the authors
conducted a review of studies investigating rates and methods of suicide in
the veterinary profession and found that in the United Kingdom, the rate
of suicide among veterinarians was at least three times that of the general
population, and that self-poisoning and firearms were particularly common
methods used.[2]

DOI: 10.1201/9781003347385-32

These findings have since been mirrored among veterinarians in other countries around the world. In the United States between 1979 and 2015, male veterinarians were 2.1 times more likely to die by suicide and female veterinarians were 3.5 times more likely to die by suicide compared to the general population.[3] Among veterinarians in Australia between 2001 and 2012, rates of suicide were nearly twice as high as in the general population, with overdosing on pentobarbital being the main method of suicide.[4] Studies among veterinarians in other countries, including Canada,[5] Germany,[6] and Norway,[7] have also suggested a high suicide risk, based on an increased prevalence of thoughts or ideas of suicide among those surveyed in comparison to the general population (Box 1).

Box 1: Did You Know?

Among more than 1,400 Canadian veterinarians surveyed, 1 in 4 had thoughts of suicide over the preceding 12 months, which was substantially higher than the 1 in 10 estimated prevalence for the general population.[5]

Career differences have also been linked to varying levels of suicide risk. A study published in the *British Journal of Psychiatry* examined suicide rates across different occupations in England and Wales from 2001 to 2005 compared to the general population. Researchers utilized the Proportional Mortality Ratio (PMR), which measures the likelihood of death by suicide in a specific occupation compared to other causes, adjusting for age and gender. Their findings revealed that health professionals, including male dentists and female veterinarians, exhibited the highest suicide PMRs during this period, indicating a greater prevalence of suicide compared to other causes of death within these occupational groups. Specifically, male dentists were nearly three times more likely to die by suicide, while female veterinarians were over six times more likely, highlighting significant disparities in suicide rates within these professions.[8]

An article titled "High-Risk Occupations for Suicide" published in *Psychological Medicine* in 2013 reviewed 30 years of national occupational mortality statistics in Great Britain beginning in 1979 and ending in 2005. Between 1979–1980 and 1982–1983, veterinarians had the highest suicide rates per 100,000 population, followed by other health professionals, including pharmacists (4th), dentists (6th), and doctors (10th). But by 2001–2005, there had been significant reductions in suicide rates for each of those occupations, such that none ranked in the top 30 occupations. These professional occupations were largely replaced by manual occupations and those regarded as low-paying jobs held by individuals with low socioeconomic status.[9]

Recent data examining suicide deaths among veterinarians and other high-skilled occupations in Austria over a 35-year period (1986–2020) also revealed noteworthy findings. Among the professions studied, including physicians, dentists, veterinarians, pharmacists, notaries, lawyers, and tax advisors/public accountants, only male veterinarians exhibited a notably higher suicide risk compared to the general male population. Furthermore, among females, veterinarians, physicians, and pharmacists showed a significantly elevated suicide risk compared to the general population.[10] Interestingly, data from the Centers for Disease Control National Reporting System in the United States, published in 2016, highlighted that suicide rates are particularly high among healthcare workers (Box 2), underscoring the broader impact of mental health challenges within certain industries.[11]

Box 2: Highest Suicide Rates by Occupation among Major Industry Groups in the United States[11]

- Constructions and extractions (males and females)
- Installation, maintenance, and repair (males)
- Arts, design, entertainment, sports, and media (males)
- Transportation and material moving (males and females)
- Protective services (females)
- Healthcare (females)

The correlation between occupation and suicide risk underscores a crucial aspect: access to means of suicide. Members of many of these highlighted professions have access to substances or tools capable of causing death, such as medications for healthcare workers or firearms for those in protective services. A study evaluating access to means of suicide in Australia between 2001 and 2012 revealed that individuals in occupations with access to firearms, medications or drugs, or carbon monoxide more frequently utilized these methods compared to those without such access. Consequently, females employed in occupations with means access exhibited suicide rates three times higher than the general population, while males with means access were 1.2 times more likely to die by suicide than the general population.[12]

This information and recent research investigating access to means of suicide in veterinary medicine has ignited a conversation around the ways in which controlled substances such as narcotics or euthanasia solutions are stored in veterinary practices. A study published in the *Journal of the American Veterinary Medical Association* in 2019 investigated the mechanism of death among 73 veterinarians dying by suicide between 2003 and 2014 and found that poisoning was the cause of death in nearly half of the cases, with 77% of those deaths due to pentobarbital, the drug used to facilitate euthanasia. What was most striking about this data was that when the deaths of veterinarians due to pentobarbital were excluded from the risk analysis, vets were no more likely than the general population to die by suicide.[13]

Recently, investigators used an online survey to determine the impact of accessibility of lethal medications in veterinary workplaces on recent suicidal thoughts and the perceived likelihood of attempting suicide among veterinarians. Of the more than 300 vets who were predominantly female and working in companion animal practice, those who worked in practices where medications were unlocked during business hours were more likely to have thoughts of suicide in the preceding week and to perceive that a future suicide attempt was likely, compared to those who worked in practices where lethal medications were locked during business hours.[14] This suggests that locking potentially lethal medications has the potential to protect against suicide risk by reducing both physical and mental accessibility to the drug and, hence, the idea of suicide. Another focus group study conducted in the United States, which interviewed and surveyed more than 40 currently practicing veterinarians, found that 30% stored their pentobarbital solution unlocked at least part of the time. After engaging in the focus group discussions which centered around perceptions of factors that contribute to suicide among veterinarians, possible solutions, and barriers to improving mental health, the participants' willingness to implement storage protocol changes to pentobarbital solution increased.[15]

Given that suicide ranks as the 11th leading cause of death in the United States,[16] it's probable that most individuals will encounter its impact at some point in their lives. Recent survey research performed in Australia indicates that approximately 70% of veterinarians have known a colleague or friend who has died by suicide.[17] However, the disproportionate impact of suicide on veterinarians compared to the general population prompts the question: why? This is a common query among those affected by suicide, but the answer is multifaceted. I recall attending a Veterinary Wellbeing Summit hosted by the American Veterinary Medical Association (AVMA), where a speaker delivered a keynote on suicide. Using an analogy of a ladder, she illustrated how each factor or experience associated with suicide could pull individuals down the rungs until they reach a critical point. It's oversimplified to attribute suicide to a single cause; rather, it's the culmination of numerous factors that lead individuals to that critical point.

The American Foundation for Suicide Prevention emphasizes that suicide typically arises from a convergence of stressors and health issues, leading to feelings of hopelessness and despair. Statistics reveal that about 90% of individuals who die by suicide have a mental illness, often undiagnosed or untreated. Beyond mental health conditions, various other factors such as physical health issues, environmental changes, and family history can contribute to suicide risk (Box 2).[18] Within the veterinary profession, additional work-related factors have been identified as potential contributors to the elevated risk of suicide among veterinarians. These include work-related stressors, easy access to and familiarity with lethal substances, stigma surrounding mental illness, professional isolation, unique attitudes toward death and euthanasia, as well as the phenomenon of suicide contagion.[19]

Box 2: Risk Factors for Suicide[18]

- Mental illnesses (depression, substance use problems, bipolar disorder, schizophrenia, conduct disorder, anxiety disorders)
- Serious physical health conditions, including chronic pain
- Traumatic brain injury
- Access to lethal means such as firearms or drugs
- Prolonged stress such as harassment, bullying, relationship problems, or unemployment
- Stressful life events such as divorce, financial problems, or death of a loved one
- Exposure to another person's suicide or to graphic or sensationalized accounts of suicide
- Previous suicide attempts
- Family history of suicide
- Childhood abuse, neglect, or trauma

A recent study "Prevalence and Individual and Work-Related Factors Associated with Suicidal Thoughts and Behaviours among Veterinarians in Norway" sheds light on the alarming prevalence of suicidal feelings and thoughts among Norwegian veterinarians. The findings reveal that 27% of veterinarians felt that life was not worth living in the past year, with 5% reporting serious suicidal thoughts and 0.2% attempting suicide. Female veterinarians exhibited a significantly higher prevalence of suicidal feelings and thoughts compared to their male counterparts. Factors such as being single, negative life events, and mental distress were independently associated with serious suicidal thoughts. Interestingly, work problems emerged as the most reported contributing factor to serious suicidal thoughts, particularly among female veterinarians.[7] This underscores the need for further investigation into the gender-specific and work-related factors contributing to suicidal behavior in this profession.

A decade prior, another study examined the interview responses of over 20 veterinarians in the United Kingdom who had either attempted suicide or reported recent suicidal ideation. Participants were questioned about both work and non-work-related factors contributing to their experiences. Results showed that two-thirds of these veterinarians received a psychiatric diagnosis following their worst episode of suicidal ideation or attempts, with a similar proportion citing concurrent challenging life events alongside work-related concerns such as workplace relationships, career issues, patient challenges, work hours, and workload.[20] While the study did not specifically identify exposure to euthanasia as a contributing factor, it has been suggested by other sources. Some posit that the stress of euthanasia discussions with clients could be a factor, while others speculate whether frequent exposure to euthanasia might desensitize veterinarians to death, potentially making suicide seem more acceptable.

Researchers have delved into this relationship between veterinarians' attitudes toward animal euthanasia and human suicide. One study surveying German veterinarians found that while fearlessness about death was similar to that of the general population, lower distress about euthanasia was linked to greater fearlessness about death.[21] Another study among veterinary students in the United Kingdom found no clear links between attitudes toward convenience euthanasia and suicide, suggesting that openness to animal euthanasia does not necessarily correlate with a diminished value for human life or altered views on suicide.[22] Similarly, a study in Australia involving over 500 veterinarians revealed that the frequency of euthanasia procedures influenced the relationship between depression and suicide risk, suggesting that frequent exposure to euthanasia may serve as a protective factor against suicide.[23]

Another significant work-related factor contributing to suicide among veterinarians is the limited transferability of their skills to other professions. In a study published in 2017 titled "I've Been a Long Time Leaving: The Role of Limited Skill Transferability in Increasing Suicide-Related Cognitions and Behavior in Veterinarians", the authors investigated how difficult it is for veterinarians to switch to other jobs and how it affects their thoughts and behaviors related to suicide over a year. They did this by tracking factors like whether veterinarians wanted to leave their job, if they were feeling depressed, how they saw their skills transferring to other jobs, and if they were thinking about or exhibiting suicide-related behavior. What they found was that when veterinarians really wanted to leave their job at the start of the study, they were more likely to have thoughts and behaviors related to suicide over the year, especially if they felt like their skills would not transfer well to other jobs. Essentially, feeling stuck in their role made them feel more hopeless, which could lead to thoughts about suicide.[24]

Preventing suicide is a deeply human endeavor, one that requires us to show compassion, understanding, and a commitment to evidence-based strategies. Recent discussions within the veterinary community, particularly on social media platforms, have prompted important conversations about how we can effectively prevent suicide and support each other through the grief that follows such tragic losses. Rosie Allister, a respected researcher and manager of the Vetlife Helpline, has emphasized the critical importance of how we discuss suicide, drawing attention to the potential risks associated with certain media portrayals and narratives surrounding suicide. In an article titled "It's Good to Talk, but It Matters How We Do It" published in *The Veterinary Record* in

2021, she discussed how media coverage of suicide can influence behavior, sometimes leading to copycat suicides in vulnerable individuals (Box 3). This phenomenon, known as suicide contagion, underscores the need for responsible dialogue and reporting.[25]

Box 3: Did You Know?

Suicide contagion, often referred to as copycat suicides, occurs when exposure to media coverage or depictions of a suicide leads to an increase in suicidal behavior among susceptible individuals. Essentially, it's the phenomenon where one suicide can inspire others to attempt suicide, particularly if they are already vulnerable or impressionable.[26]

With the increasing influence of the internet and social media, there are new challenges in ensuring that discussions around suicide are handled sensitively and with care. Unfortunately, breaches of responsible media guidance are common on social platforms, heightening the risk of inadvertently causing harm to those who may be struggling with suicidal thoughts or experiences of bereavement. In the context of the veterinary profession, there are specific narratives and cultural dynamics that may further exacerbate the risk of suicide contagion, such as blaming clients for veterinarian suicide or reinforcing an oversimplified narrative that veterinarians are more likely to die by suicide. Addressing these issues requires a nuanced approach, one that respects the complexities of individual experiences while also promoting safe and supportive communication. By following guidelines that prioritize accuracy, sensitivity, and the provision of support, we can work together to reduce the risk of suicide and create a culture of understanding and empathy within our community.

Certainly, one good thing to come from increased discussion about suicide in the veterinary profession is a greater opportunity to raise awareness about prevention and postvention support. Not One More Vet (NOMV) is an organization that was founded in 2014 by Dr. Nicole McArthur in response to the suicide of Dr. Sophia Yin. Initially started as a Facebook group and social media hashtag, NOMV has since grown into a robust global community of nearly 40,000 veterinary professionals, dedicated to supporting each other in navigating the unique challenges of the veterinary profession. The organization's mission is to transform the status of mental health in veterinary medicine by providing education, resources, and peer support to ensure that no veterinary professional feels isolated. Through initiatives like the Lifeboat anonymous peer support platform, the NOMV Ambassador Program, and international outreach efforts, NOMV has become a leading advocate for mental health in veterinary medicine.

The American Veterinary Medical Association (AVMA) has also led the charge in raising awareness by creating several resources over the last several years to prevent the suicide of veterinary professionals and offer support to those who have lost a colleague or classmate to suicide. In 2022, they released a concise Suicide Prevention Resource Guide tailored for veterinary settings. This guide offers practical strategies and actionable steps for veterinary professionals to prevent suicide, covering approaches at societal, community, relationship, and individual levels. Developed with insights from suicide research and evidence-based prevention strategies, the guide provides valuable information on risk and protective factors, warning signs, and effective intervention methods. Complementing existing resources on their website (avma .org/Wellbeing), the guide underscores the preventability of suicide and is part of the organization's broader initiative to promote wellbeing and suicide prevention within the veterinary profession.[27]

Additionally, the association offers digital continuing education courses featuring wellbeing webinars, including a two-part series on preventing suicide and fostering hope and resilience within the profession. They also offer free access for all veterinary professionals to QPR training which, like CPR, is a crucial emergency response to individuals in crisis and has the potential to save lives. QPR is the most widely taught Gatekeeper training, an evidence-based program developed by the QPR Institute. QPR training typically spans less than two hours and equips participants with essential skills to recognize, intervene, and refer individuals who may be contemplating suicide. Simply, Gatekeeper training provides participants with the knowledge to question, persuade, and refer someone in crisis, as well as the resources to seek help for themselves and others. Participants also gain insights into the common causes and warning signs of suicidal behavior, empowering them to effectively support individuals in need.[28]

Vetlife, an independent charity providing complimentary and confidential assistance to members of the UK veterinary community facing emotional, health, or financial challenges, introduced comprehensive guidance tailored to veterinary workplaces dealing with the aftermath of suicide in 2022. This guidance supplements its existing suicide postvention support services, which aim to aid recovery and prevent further adverse outcomes, including subsequent suicides. The guidance is designed for individuals impacted by the suicide of a veterinary professional, their support networks, and workplace leaders committed to suicide prevention. It covers various postvention aspects, such as bereavement support and effective communication strategies, and it includes a practical checklist for immediate and ongoing support. Additionally, Vetlife's postvention service offers personalized support to practices and individuals affected by suicide through its helpline, which provides confidential guidance to UK veterinary professionals and workplaces.[29]

It is evident that the issue of suicide within the veterinary profession is multifaceted and deeply concerning. From the tragic loss of respected figures like Dr. Sophia Yin to the alarming statistics revealing elevated suicide rates among veterinarians worldwide, the need for action and support is clear. The correlation between occupation and suicide risk, compounded by factors such as access to lethal means and work-related stressors, highlights the urgency of addressing mental health within the profession. However, amidst these challenges, there is hope. Organizations like Vetlife and the AVMA, alongside other partners, have stepped up to provide vital resources, support services, and training to prevent future losses and aid those affected by suicide. By fostering a culture of care, compassion, and proactive intervention, these organizations are making positive changes and demonstrating a collective commitment to the wellbeing of the veterinary community. As we move forward, it's essential to continue these efforts, ensuring that no veterinarian feels alone in their struggles and that help is readily available to those who need it most.

If you or anyone you know are experiencing thoughts of suicide, please call 988 (Canada and United States), 0800 689 5652 (United Kingdom), or numbers available here for other countries: https://blog.opencounseling.com/suicide -hotlines/.

30

Realities and Resilience amidst the Pandemic

> As the number of patients seemed to increase, supplies decreased. We covered shifts as colleagues quarantined. We stood in the rain and snow to discuss cancer diagnoses with clients through car windows. We did our best to preserve our client relationships and our team members' health.
>
> —Scott Nolen
> (American Veterinary Medical Association Senior Reporter)

When the world shut down in mid-March of 2020, it was ten weeks before I was due to give birth to my first child. I'd spent two years trying to get pregnant on my own, so starting a family was something I'd been focused on for quite some time. But having a baby and continuing to work as a veterinarian amidst a pandemic was not on my radar at all! At the time I was traveling every few weeks, speaking at conferences or delivering workshops related to workplace wellbeing and the self-care of veterinary professionals. I was also still working in practice as a locum critical care specialist, although I knew those 12–14-hour shifts would subside once the baby arrived. What I didn't know was that everything was about to change drastically—not just for me as a parent and sole proprietor, but for veterinary medicine as a profession.

I remember it as vividly as if it was last week—the veterinary Facebook groups exploding with questions about the lockdown. Would veterinary medicine be considered an essential service or would practices have to close? Would team members be able to come to work or would they need to stay home with children who could no longer attend daycare or school? Much of that time was a blur for me, as I grappled with cancellations in all aspects of my life. My leadership and wellness workshop in Toronto at the end of March was canceled, as was my "babymoon," a weeklong wellness speaking event in Kauai for the Veterinary Emergency and Critical Care Society. At the same time my prenatal yoga classes moved online, and my postpartum doula let me know she wouldn't be able to provide support: her partner had a debilitating respiratory illness, and she was fearful of contracting COVID. To say that my world was turned upside down would be an understatement.

But my experience was miniscule compared to what most veterinary practices went through. While a few closed their doors altogether (some of them

DOI: 10.1201/9781003347385-33

permanently), most practices stayed open but adjusted their appointments to curbside. Just as what many restaurants and stores did in the early days of the pandemic, veterinary clinics and hospitals greeted clients outside wearing full personal protective equipment (PPE), took their pets inside for their exams and any necessary treatments, and spoke to the families via phone or video call. This created a tremendous amount of distress for everyone involved: team members felt bad separating animals from their families and pet owners were anxious about having to wait in their cars rather than stay with their furry family members. This was compounded in emergency situations, when pets were critically ill and needed to be hospitalized and families were not permitted to visit. Many family members went for several days or even weeks before getting to see their pets again in real life.

Perhaps the worst situations experienced by anyone during the first months of the pandemic were the low or no-contact euthanasia procedures. Depending on the hospital's policy and whether a family member was positive for or had symptoms of COVID-19, there were restrictions on the number of people (if any) who could be present for the euthanasia, the PPE they were required to wear, and the distance they had to remain from the veterinarian during the procedure. These euthanasia procedures, typically done in very close proximity in the coziest room in the hospital (often sitting side by side on a couch or sitting on a blanket together on the floor) were now done outside, or indoors wearing PPE, and with enough intravenous tubing to allow the veterinarian to remain six feet away from the pet and their family.

In some circumstances pet parents couldn't be with their animal at all; instead, they watched outside through a window or on a computer screen via Zoom—a heartbreaking situation. These low or no-contact euthanasia procedures presented unique ethical challenges to veterinary team members, who were forced to balance their safety with the emotional needs of their clients. It was clear the very protocols that were created to protect them were bound to cause fear, anxiety, and distress in the patients and families they were trying to help. What was typically an intimate setting involving the pet, family members and veterinary professionals had transformed into a physically distanced, biosecurity-focused environment that heightened the sadness of an already somber experience.

Research conducted online during the first months of the pandemic determined that limited-contact euthanasia was just one of many ethically challenging situations that veterinary team members were experiencing. Survey responses collected from more than 500 veterinary team members globally between May and July 2020 found that one-quarter of respondents regarded low or no-contact euthanasia as a common and/or stressful ethical challenge.[1] Other ethical challenges related to biosecurity, client financial limitations, animal welfare, working conditions, and client relations were identified as stressful and common, occurring at least several times per week (Box 1).[2]

Box 1: The Most Common and Stressful Ethically Challenging Situations for Veterinary Teams Early in the Pandemic[2]

Most Common Ethically Challenging Situations:

- Challenging decisions about how to proceed when clients have limited finances (64%)
- Conflict between personal wellbeing and professional role (64%)
- Conflict between the interests of clients and the interests of their animals (60%)
- Challenging decisions about what counts as an essential veterinary service (48%)
- Conflict between wellbeing of family/household members and professional role (46%)
- Challenging decisions about whether to perform non-contact veterinary visits (46%)

Most Stressful Ethically Challenging Situations:

- Conflicts between the interests of clients and the interests of their animals (50%)
- Conflicts between the interests of my employer and my own interests (43%)
- Challenging decisions about how to proceed when clients have limited finances (39%)
- Conflict between personal wellbeing and professional role (38%)
- Conflict between wellbeing of family/household members and professional role (34%)

Some of the common ethical challenges in veterinary medicine, like decision making when clients face financial constraints, were intensified during the pandemic as job loss and inability to work added further financial stress. Other situations had never been encountered before, such as determining which veterinary services were truly essential and would still be offered despite shortages of staff and PPE. For example, while most vaccines for adult companion animals can usually be delayed by weeks to months without harm, it was still deemed necessary to vaccinate puppies to prevent outbreaks of parvoviral enteritis and other communicable diseases. Likewise, masks and gowns were in short supply and there was concern that those resources available should be allocated to human hospitals. As such, veterinarians had to decide what constituted essential surgeries, including torn ligaments and dental extractions that were somewhere in the grey area between elective and urgent.

Around this time, a conversation emerged on my specialty group's email list about the practice of using human-grade respirators in veterinary intensive

care units (ICUs) to ventilate animal patients. Considering the global ventilator shortages, which compelled healthcare professionals to make challenging decisions about when and for whom to use ventilators in human ICUs, a
member of the American College of Veterinary Emergency and Critical Care
initiated the compilation of a spreadsheet listing the veterinary ICU ventilators that were accessible for local hospitals to borrow as required. Several of
the neighboring human hospitals opted to make use of these ventilators and
returned them once their COVID caseloads had subsided. While this felt like
"the right thing to do" under the dire circumstances within the human ICUs,
it created ethical challenges for those veterinary ICUs left without a ventilator
for their own animal patients. Not surprisingly, global surveys assessing ethically challenging situations found that those veterinary team members most
likely to be impacted were veterinary nurses or techs, those working with
companion animals, and those residing in the United States or Canada.[3] This
was presumably due to the high caseloads seen among these practices early on
in the pandemic and the fact that veterinary nurses and techs are often on the
front lines of communication with clients and delivery of patient care.

Another larger study published in the *Frontiers of Veterinary Science* in
2022 examined the survey responses of more than 1,100 veterinary technicians in the United States between February and March 2021. Of those responding to the survey, three-quarters reported a moderate to large effect of
the pandemic on their practice or clinic's work. More than three-quarters of
veterinary technicians agreed or strongly agreed that they were treated worse
by animal owners during COVID-19 (Box 2). Nearly half felt that PPE seemed
to frighten animals—something that was likely exacerbated by the fact that
pets were separated from their owners. Still, two-thirds of veterinary technicians felt work was easier without the family in the room during patient visit.[4]

Box 2: Did You Know?

When veterinary technicians in the United States were asked about their
greatest challenge at their practice or clinic during COVID-19, more
than half said that it was being treated worse by pet owners who did not
want to abide by curbside restrictions.[4]

A common sentiment that was beginning to unfold before the pandemic,
and that ultimately pushed the veterinary profession over the edge as
COVID-19 progressed, was understaffing. Practices that were already
struggling with a shortage of veterinarians or vet techs now faced even greater
challenges, as veterinary professionals had to balance staying home with their
children and isolating when they developed symptoms or tested positive for
COVID-19. Many clinics implemented cohorts or "pods" of team members,
consistently scheduled together, to avoid more people from having to isolate
or quarantine if they were exposed. Others mandated "full PPE" whereby all

team members wore face masks, gloves, gowns, and face shields throughout their shifts to avoid exposure to potentially infected clients and team members. What seemed like a scene out of a science fiction movie quickly became reality among many large and busy veterinary hospitals.

The staffing shortage was exacerbated by a surge in caseloads during the pandemic. Whether this was due to pet parents spending more time at home and becoming more attuned to their animals' health needs, or the result of a rise in pet purchases and adoptions, remains unclear. Research by the American Pet Products Association found that US households acquired 9 million dogs and 5 million cats during the first two years of the pandemic—meaning the number of new dogs alone was approximately equivalent to the number of people in New York City. This brought the total number of dogs and cats in the country to 108 million and 79 million, respectively.[5] While it isn't clear how many of these animals went to first-time pet owners, the pandemic puppies and COVID cats led to a surge in demand for veterinary care. A multitude of news articles throughout the pandemic highlighted difficulties in many communities in finding veterinary care for animals. Many practices stopped taking new clients altogether and others had waitlists of eight or more weeks for new pet consultations. This, of course, added yet another layer of ethical distress to veterinary team members—and frustration and anger among pet owners.

I returned to veterinary practice in July 2022 when my daughter was two years old. We were both fully vaccinated and the pandemic restrictions were beginning to ease. The caseload at that time was at a nearly all-time high, which was evident in the emergency practice where I was doing relief work. My role was predominantly mentoring interns as those working full-time on the clinic floor had caseloads too high to allow the case discussions and supervision that newly graduated veterinarians needed. I was also tasked with catching up on the backlog of phone calls to emergency clients whose pets had undergone blood testing or X-rays but had not yet received results. Some of those tests were performed several weeks prior and included results that were missed or not followed up on by the admitting emergency vet. This led many pet owners I called to express confusion, shock, and anger in response to overlooked diagnoses and delayed care.

Without a doubt, this time spent in clinical practice caused me more psychological distress secondary to ethically challenging situations than I had ever experienced before. Some of the dogs and cats waiting in the emergency room sat for more than 12 hours without a veterinarian's assessment. Seeing patients waiting so long for what would normally be addressed in just a few hours seemed morally impossible to reckon with and left me feeling desperate to help, but unable to cope. I recall fighting back tears one morning when a dog who'd been attacked by another dog waited 14 hours for a dose of pain relief. Later that day, another dog who was waiting for an exam experienced cardiopulmonary arrest and died in the triage room. The alternative for both patients was to wait at home with their families—a situation I felt was perhaps the better of two difficult options, given the intolerable circumstances created by the pandemic and veterinary staffing shortages.

Needless to say, the pandemic has left a permanent mark on the wellbeing and mental health of veterinary teams and pet owners. A research study conducted by the American Veterinary Medical Association and Merck Animal Health in 2021 found that approximately 4 of 5 of veterinarians and team members claimed their clinics were short staffed due to employee absences caused by the pandemic, and subsequently half worked longer hours than they would have otherwise. Concurrently, a larger number of veterinarians were experiencing serious psychological distress compared to pre-pandemic survey measurements.[6] Another survey conducted among faculty, staff, residents, and interns at the Ontario Veterinary College between November 2020 and January 2021 found similar links between COVID-19 and reduced wellbeing, whereby those in academia experienced increased work-related demands and work-life conflicts.[7]

Perhaps the biggest impact of the pandemic was felt among veterinary students. Interviews conducted among those at the Lincoln Memorial University–College of Veterinary Medicine demonstrated that clinical-year veterinary students had concerns about a lack of preparedness for graduation and pre-clinical students expressed concerns related to online assessments, lost opportunities for clinical experiences, and loss of social connections.[8] As someone who completed her schooling without a smartphone and with dial-up internet, I personally cannot imagine navigating the veterinary curriculum via Zoom.

Just like students, pets have also been impacted by the pandemic, in ways that we'll undoubtedly see for years to come. The aforementioned "pandemic puppies" now raise alarm bells among veterinary team members, who are rec ognizing behavior challenges among these dogs who missed their critical so-cialization period during lockdown. An Italian study published in *Veterinary Science* in 2023 compared the personalities of adult dogs who were puppies from March to May 2020 (during Italy's government-instituted lockdown) compared to adult dogs born after that time (June 2020 to February 2021). The researchers found that there was a significant increase in traits related to fear and aggression among dogs who experienced lockdown restrictions during their socialization period, suggesting that COVID-19 impacted their behavioral development.[9]

While decades of research have typically suggested the benefits of pet ownership among individuals of all ages, research investigating the benefits of having a pet during the pandemic has shown little to no benefit and, in some cases, harm. Studies among pet owners in Australia, Canada, and the United States have demonstrated lower quality of life and lower wellbeing among adults regardless of species (dogs, cats, or other), number of pets owned, quality of the human-pet relationship, or the owner's psychological characteristics.[10,11] While there were many benefits to owning and caring for a pet during the pandemic, several drawbacks were also identified (Box 3). These were impacted by the economic resources, relationship status, employment status, and whether the person had two or more children. For a person who was struggling financially or had many children living at home, the benefits of pet ownership were outweighed by the caregiving and economic burden.[12]

Box 3: Pros and Cons of Pet Ownership during the Pandemic[10,11]

Pros:

- company/companionship
- spending time together
- life purpose or meaning
- love/support
- stress relief
- routine
- distraction
- exercise

Cons:

- difficulty meeting the needs of pets
- difficulty obtaining pet supplies
- difficulty accessing veterinary care
- new and emerging behavioral issues
- fate of the pet if the owner becomes ill
- balancing responsibilities
- cost of supplies and veterinary care

The narrative of veterinary medicine during the COVID-19 pandemic unveils a tapestry of resilience, sacrifice, and ethical complexity. The profession weathered a storm of unprecedented challenges, from the poignant transformation of euthanasia procedures to the altruistic sharing of critical resources with human healthcare. The threads of understaffing, the heightened caseloads, and the surge in pet ownership intricately wove together a heavy strain, both for veterinary teams and for their clientele. As the echoes of the pandemic reverberate, it's clear that the wellbeing of veterinary professionals and the bonds between pets and their owners have been indelibly marked. Going forward, the trials faced during this challenging period will surely influence the future of veterinary practice, promoting dedication to ethical, compassionate care in a world forever changed by the global health crisis.

PART FOUR

What the Future Holds for Veterinary Medicine

31

The Rise of Veterinary Corporatization

Arguably the most notable disrupter in veterinary medicine, corporate veterinary medicine is establishing a firm foothold and appears to be gaining momentum. Every year there are more veterinary hospitals selling to corporate consolidators, and every year there are more corporations coming into the market. The corporations hold their cards close to their chests, but at the same time they are very candid about their intentions to grow and their desire to improve the veterinary community.

—Darren Osborne, MA
(Director of Economic Research for the Ontario
Veterinary Medical Association)

Having been in the veterinary space since childhood, I can attest to the fact that veterinary medicine has changed more in the last ten years than in most of the decades before. Much of this change stems from the rapid rise in corporate ownership of veterinary practices. What was once a profession dominated by solo practitioners who owned their clinics, has now been largely replaced by multi-veterinarian practices, many of which have been acquired by corporations. Whether this change is a positive one will depend on who you ask, but, without question, it's had a lasting impact on veterinary medicine.

My mom opened her companion animal practice in 1977, a year after she graduated from veterinary school. She began as a solo practitioner, and then, less than a year after opening, she hired her first associate. In the decades that followed, her practice grew to three and a half full-time associates. It was always expected that I would join my mom's practice after graduating and eventually purchase it, but that plan didn't come to fruition. After receiving offers from different corporations in the mid-2010s, my mom ultimately sold her clinic to a corporation in 2016 and retired from clinical practice a year later. In the conversations I've had with her, she's shared her happiness with this decision. She felt that the corporation did everything they could to preserve the stand-out elements of her practice and that they treated her former employees and associates with respect and care. While there's no doubt that she would have preferred to have kept it in the family, she remains confident to this day that she made the best decision for her practice.

DOI: 10.1201/9781003347385-35

Big companies started getting into vet medicine in North America back in 1987, when Veterinary Centers of America Inc. (VCA) bought its first independently owned veterinary clinic in West Los Angeles. After that, Banfield/ Medical Management International Inc. teamed up with PetSmart and started putting veterinary clinics in their stores. Then in 2007, Mars Inc., known for its iconic confectionery brands like M&Ms and pet foods like Pedigree, joined the veterinary scene by purchasing Banfield. They went on to buy BluePearl in 2015 and VCA Inc. in 2018, and they are the single largest veterinary provider in the United States today. There are now more than 60 veterinary corporations, most of which have non-veterinarian CEOs. Approximately 75% of specialty and emergency clinics and 25% of all general practices in the United States today are owned by corporations and estimates suggest that corporations control around 50% of all US veterinary hospital revenue.[1]

In the United Kingdom, a rule change in 1999 allowed non-veterinarian ownership of practices, which led to significant growth in corporate ownership. Nearly two decades later, corporatization in the United Kingdom advanced at a faster rate compared to any other European country. As of 2018, there were more than 1,700 practices owned by corporate groups, and it was estimated that more than 12,000 veterinarians and vet nurses in the United Kingdom worked for a corporate veterinary group.[2] By 2019, two companies dominated the UK veterinary care sector: Independent Vetcare (IVC), which later merged with Swedish firm Evidensia by EQT to form IVC Evidensia, and VetPartners. Since their establishment in 2011 and 2015, respectively, both companies have consistently expanded.[3] Whereas independent practices previously dominated the UK veterinary space, comprising 89% in 2013, this figure decreased significantly to approximately 45% in 2021.[4] Today six large corporate groups dominate the UK veterinary landscape (Box 1), owning 1,500 of the country's 5,000 practices.[2]

Box 1: Did You Know?

Approximately 30% of veterinary practices in the United Kingdom are owned by one of six large corporate groups: CVS, IVC, Linnaeus, Medivet, Pets at Home, and VetPartners.[2]

In 2021, IVC Evidensia announced a significant expansion into North America by acquiring the Canadian consolidator VetStrategy, boosting its global clinic count to approximately 2,000 across 17 countries. This move positioned IVC Evidensia closer to Mars Inc. as one of the largest owners of veterinary practices globally. The private equity–backed company, headquartered in Bristol, England, with Nestlé as a minority shareholder, aimed to solidify its presence in the veterinary industry with this strategic acquisition. VetStrategy, which at the time owned over 270 hospitals across nine Canadian provinces, was majority owned by Berkshire Partners, a private equity firm based in Boston, which rolled its investment into the expanded IVC Evidensia.[5] In Canada, corporations own more than 20% of all veterinary hospitals. And while there is no recorded data on the number of veterinarians employed in corporate-owned practices, the general estimate is close to 50% (Box 2).[6]

Box 2: Did You Know?

The reason that more veterinarians are estimated to work for corporate rather than privately owned practices is because corporations aim to buy larger-than-average practices with two or more veterinarian associates. This keeps acquisition costs down and minimizes their risk if a veterinarian (and income generator) leaves the practice after it is sold.

Consolidation in Australia and New Zealand has been somewhat slower compared to other developed global markets. In 2020, corporate consolidators were estimated to represent only 17%–18% of the veterinary market by revenue.[7] However, a significant transformation occurred in Australia's veterinary practice landscape in the same year when VetPartners acquired National Veterinary Care (NVC), solidifying its position as the largest practice owner in the region, surpassing Greencross.[7] By 2022, Greencross was acknowledged as the second-largest owner of veterinary practices in Australasia, operating 167 general practices and 25 specialist and emergency hospitals across Australia and New Zealand, trailing behind VetPartners, managed by US-based NVA, which boasted over 260 practices (Box 3).[8]

Box 3: Did You Know?

In the 2023 article "Is Your "Local" Vet Owned by German Billionaires?" it was revealed that many veterinary practices in New Zealand, such as Pet Doctors clinics, are owned by JAB Holding Company, a German-based private equity firm linked to the Reimann family, known for their ownership of companies like Krispy Kreme and Dr Pepper.[9] This raised concerns about transparency and continuity of personalized care for pet owners unaware of corporate ownership.

Many wonder why so many veterinary practice owners are opting to sell to corporations rather than other veterinary professionals. A lot of this comes down to the amount that corporations can pay for practices compared to private owners. In simple terms, when valuing a veterinary practice, experts look at how much money it can make. They consider factors like income, expenses, and profit, which they call Earnings Before Interest, Taxes, Depreciation, and Amortization (EBITDA). The practice's value is determined by multiplying this EBITDA by a number that represents the future income, adjusting for risks and potential growth. Before big corporations came into veterinary medicine, a veterinarian could usually sell their practice for up to five times its EBITDA. This was because banks would lend veterinarians a maximum of five times EBITDA, the same amount offered to dentists, doctors, and chiropractors. In other words, the most a veterinarian could borrow or sell for was five times EBITDA.[6]

But veterinary corporations do not rely on banks; rather, they get money from venture capitalists. So, they can offer more than five times EBITDA when buying a practice. They even offered up to 20 times EBITDA for a short time. This of course came with conditions, such as the selling veterinarian perhaps only getting part of the money upfront, having to stay on for a few years after the purchase, and meeting certain revenue targets to obtain the rest. Corporations can also afford to pay more because, once they own enough hospitals, they can negotiate better prices from veterinary suppliers by buying in bulk. This applies to any veterinarian who can get better prices if they buy more supplies. Because corporations are much larger, they get bigger discounts, which can save up to 3% of their total income. Corporations also save money by sharing resources like accountants, advertising, education, and staff among their hospitals. All these discounts and resources lead to a combined savings of approximately 6% of a hospital's total income, averaging $90,000 CAD per Canadian veterinary clinic per year.[6] There are some multiple-practice owners, as well as groups of veterinarians, who co-own one or more practices. These private owners can also take advantage of economies of scale when purchasing supplies or sharing staff between their hospitals.

While independent practice ownership isn't going away anytime soon, research suggests it is on the decline. According to studies surveying western Canadian veterinary practitioners, in 2006 80% of male veterinarians and nearly half of female veterinarians owned their practices. In a follow-up survey published in *The Canadian Veterinary Journal* in 2020, the ownership rates had dropped to just over 60% for males and one-third for female veterinarians.[10] This shift is not unique to Western Canada, it's a trend seen worldwide. In the United States, practice ownership has fallen to less than 60% for male veterinarians and less than one-third for female veterinarians.[11] While it remains unclear whether the decline in private ownership is a result of the rise in large veterinary corporations or due to other factors, what is evident is that corporations benefit significantly from this trend—as private ownership decreases and practice sale prices rise, their competitive advantage grows.

There are also some corporations that allow practice owners to swap their shares in their veterinary hospital for shares in the corporation. This has the benefit of allowing veterinarians an opportunity to continue to invest in vet medicine without the requirement of physically working in the practice. Another perk offered by corporations to vets, to keep them engaged with the practice after it's sold, is to let the veterinarian buy part of the clinic at a lower price—for example, if a corporation buys the clinic for 12 times its EBITDA, they might offer financing to a key veterinarian for the chance to own 15% of the clinic for a lower price, like nine times the EBITDA.[6]

I have several classmates, friends, and colleagues who have purchased or started their own practice during the last 20 years since my graduation. And while the number of vets who own practices is not growing, many still want to embark on practice ownership. Some have always dreamt of being a business owner, while others have opted out of employment in other private or corporate-owned practices to build their own clinic. The benefits of practice ownership are numerous and include autonomy, financial rewards, and long-term investment gains, as well as the opportunity to innovate, create a unique practice, and cultivate leadership skills. The 2021 *American Veterinary Medical Association Census of Veterinarians and Practice Owners Survey* included responses from more than 1,200 practice owners and 1,400 associate veterinarians. The results indicated that practice owners had lower burnout scores and higher compassion satisfaction scores compared to associate veterinarians.[12] This suggests that practice owners tend to experience less burnout and greater satisfaction in their role as care providers compared to their associate or employee counterparts.

Those veterinarians who do not wish to pursue practice ownership are left with the choice to work in a clinic owned by a large corporation or one that is privately owned. A historical advantage of working in a corporately owned clinic is the benefits such as health insurance, paid time off, continuing education allowances, retirement plans, and sick leave. It would make sense that if large corporations can save money, they could offer even better benefits to their employees. However, this isn't always the case—some veterinarians have reported receiving worse benefits after their clinic was acquired by a big corporation. Another perk of working for a corporation is the chance to work at different clinics under the same company. For example, at least one Canadian corporation offers "working vacations", covering travel and lodging expenses for veterinarians who work at a destination veterinary clinic in need of coverage. This allows vets to visit and explore new places without needing to take time off and is especially desirable for those with flexible lifestyles.

However, there are downsides to corporate veterinary practices, which have dominated the conversation in parts of the world. Many worry that corporate-owned practices do not listen as much to their employees compared to smaller, privately owned ones. Veterinary team members often don't have much say in how the clinic is run or in decisions about protocols or procedures. Communication with upper management and leadership can be challenging, and the clinic culture might not feel as friendly or flexible.

In some circumstances, there are also delays in getting approval for new equipment or changes in how things are done. The biggest complaint heard today is that corporations are too focused on making money, which has led to an increase in the cost of veterinary services and moral distress among those on the front lines who communicate with pet families. In fact, according to the results of the 2019 survey of veterinarians in the United Kingdom, two of the top challenges perceived within the profession were the changing structure of veterinary practice ownership and the affordability of veterinary services, each documented in 30% of respondents.[13] These concerns have prompted an investigation by the UK Competition and Markets Authority over allegations that rapid consolidation is leading to overcharging of millions of pet owners.[14]

While in retrospect it is difficult to demonstrate a cause-and-effect relationship between the rise of veterinary corporate consolidation and the cost of veterinary medicine, worries are growing among veterinary professionals and pet owners about the price of veterinary services. Some believe that this is a market correction for the decades of underpriced veterinary care and underpaid vets and veterinary team members, especially in the face of higher demand and lower supply for veterinary services. However, others believe that corporate entities have driven the cost of services higher in order to maintain their profits, especially amidst their rapid growth and accumulation of practices over the last ten years. The combination of purchasing practices at extraordinary prices and now paying veterinary professionals higher salaries than ever before has led to an increase in prices to offset these costs, putting many pet owners at risk of not being able to afford veterinary care. With privately owned practices lacking the resources and financing to offset the rising costs of veterinary supplies and salaries of their team members, they've also had to increase their prices to keep their practice doors open.

A recent study in the *Journal of the American Medical Association* published the results of a survey conducted via the Veterinary Information Network (VIN) in 2022. The responses from nearly 900 full-time associate veterinarians demonstrated clear preferences for working in private practice over corporate practice. About one-third of those surveyed were employed in private practice, while the other two-thirds worked in corporate practice. More than half expressed a preference for private practice, whereas only 1 in 10 favored corporate practice. Distinct differences emerged in terms of employment benefits. Veterinarians in corporate practice were more likely to report access to insurance coverage (e.g., health, dental, life, short-term disability), mental wellness programs (including counseling), wellness mobile phone applications, employer-sponsored VIN memberships, and funding for continuing education, compared to those in private practice. However, they also reported a heightened sense of pressure to generate revenue and see a higher volume of clients per shift. Conversely, vets in private practice indicated higher satisfaction levels regarding individual recognition by upper management, the prevailing hospital culture, the ability to terminate challenging or abusive client relationships, and the availability of mentorship opportunities.[1] Similar disparities have been noted among UK vets working in corporate versus private practice (Box 4).

Box 4: Did You Know?

Results from a 2020 Vetspanel survey revealed higher stress levels among UK veterinarians working in corporate practices compared to independently owned ones. Burnout was reported by 48% of corporate veterinarians, surpassing the figures for independent (35%) and group practice (31%) veterinarians.[15]

Large veterinary corporations are facing additional challenges as they expand. Think of it like a giant tree that grew too tall. The higher it grows, the harder it becomes to maintain and support itself. With more corporate entities, the shortage of skilled veterinary professionals and managers to hire is leading them, in some circumstances, to settle for less experienced hires. I know of several friends and colleagues working in corporate-owned practices who have seen their clinic struggle (or even close) due to ineffective management and a massive exodus of team members who have moved into privately owned practices.

For now, the acquisition of independently owned veterinary practices by large corporations is still taking place but has slowed considerably. The high purchase prices seen five to ten years ago are less common today but still exceed what most veterinarians can obtain financing for. And as long as large corporations can secure funding from investors, they are likely to keep growing. However, if economic challenges arise or the stock market faces instability, these companies might find it difficult to secure that funding. Without it, their expansion could continue to slow down, even if they don't vanish entirely.

As the veterinary profession continues to evolve under the influence of corporatization, the landscape of veterinary care is being reshaped in profound ways. While corporate ownership offers resources and benefits that can support both clinics and practitioners, it also brings challenges to maintaining the personal touch and autonomy historically valued in veterinary practice. For veterinarians, understanding the impacts of corporate consolidation will be essential in navigating their careers and making informed decisions about practice ownership or employment. And for pet owners, this shift invites greater transparency and awareness of who is providing care for their beloved animals. In the years to come, the balance between the needs of businesses, professionals, and pet owners will likely define the next chapter in the story of veterinary practice ownership.

Insights into Pet Health Insurance

As a cancer survivor myself and mom to a teenage driver, I have different feelings about insurance than I used to. When faced with catastrophic choices, it allows us to concentrate on what is best for our loved ones.
— Jessica Heard, DVM (Veterinarian)

When my daughter turned a year old, I decided that I was ready to have a dog again. Without hesitation, I knew I wanted another Standard Poodle. Since my family's first Standard Poodle, named Fergie (after Sarah Margaret Ferguson, Duchess of York), I've always had the breed, and they remain my favorite to this day due to their intelligence, athleticism, and rapt attention to the humans around them. I've often told people with full honesty that Standard Poodles can read minds. Like any breed, they're not without their downsides, including genetic or heritable disorders that can have life-threatening consequences. They have a higher risk of Addison's disease, a syndrome whereby the adrenal glands do not produce enough cortisol or hormones that regulate the body's electrolytes, as well as a predisposition to GDV (gastric dilation volvulus), in which their stomach twists on itself, requiring emergency surgery to survive.

Because I'm a veterinarian and have treated dozens of Standard Poodles for these very conditions, purchasing pet health insurance for Vivian, our new dog, was a no-brainer. As an emergency and critical care specialist, I've also seen first-hand the bills for lengthy hospitalizations for intensive care or cancer treatments that can easily reach tens of thousands of dollars. As a solo parent who is self-employed, I don't have the discretionary income to cover these potential expenses. And although I've encountered numerous clients with pet health insurance, I haven't experienced being an "owner" in this situation. So, I put out a question to a private Facebook group for Canadian veterinarians, asking which of the currently available pet health insurance companies were most favorable. The group came back strongly in favor of purchasing pet health insurance, with helpful comments regarding company differences in coverage, claims handling, and direct payment to veterinary practices versus repayment to pet owners.

Ultimately, I chose a company that covers 90% of costs related to illness or injury, which happened to be the one that I'd found most comprehensive

DOI: 10.1201/9781003347385-36

as a specialist submitting claim paperwork for my clients. Since purchasing Vivian's insurance, I've had tremendous peace of mind knowing that, should anything happen to her, I won't have to weigh the cost of her care beyond my $1,000 CAD deductible. My premiums are about $150 per month and have increased annually in the four years since I adopted her. Despite spending more than $5,000 CAD on her insurance premiums to date, I still feel that the cost justifies the relief of coverage for a potentially ten-thousand-dollar-plus bill. Indeed, after owning Vivian for just over a year, she began showing gastrointestinal symptoms, which we later determined were due to a dietary intolerance. Before coming to this conclusion, we gave her a diagnostic examination, including blood tests, Addison's disease screening, abdominal X-rays, ultrasound, and 24-hour hospitalization for intravenous fluids. My out-of-pocket cost was $1,200, much lower than the $4,000 CAD total bill.

Yet not everyone is in favor of pet health insurance, and it has taken time to garner support for it in the veterinary space. Pet health insurance first came on the market in the mid-1970s and imposed a significant administration cost to practices whose clients utilized it. At the time, most vets didn't feel that the premiums justified the current costs of veterinary care and instead recommended that pet owners save money each month upon adoption of their pet and use that "emergency fund" as needed to pay for care. As veterinary prices increased over the next two decades, and the bond between animals and their families continued to grow, more veterinarians and pet owners were considering the benefits of pet health insurance (Box 1).

Box 1: Did You Know?

In 1995, according to *DVM Newsmagazine*, a typical client in the United States would opt for euthanasia when the veterinary bill reached or exceeded $576 USD. However, for those clients with pet health insurance, the bill would typically have to exceed $2,000 before they chose to euthanize their pet.[1]

The interest in pet health insurance surged again in the late 1990s and early 2000s (Box 2). At that time, both the American and the Canadian Veterinary Medical Associations expressed their support for pet health insurance, which was slowly gaining traction in Canada and the United States and was more popular in European countries. The Canadian Veterinary Medical Association (CVMA) endorsed pet health insurance as a way to limit financial dilemmas experienced by pet owners.[2] Concurrently, the American Veterinary Medical Association (AVMA) published a guideline on pet health insurance stating: "The Association recognizes that a viable companion animal health insurance program will be important to the future of the veterinary profession's ability to continue to provide high quality and up-to-date veterinary service."[3] The

AVMA Pet Health Insurance Policy still exists today and includes recommendations for pet health insurance policies (Box 3).[4]

Box 2: Did You Know?

In 2004, just 3% of pet owners in the United States had health insurance for their animals, as reported by a survey conducted by the American Animal Hospital Association. Similarly, a survey by Ipsos Reid market research in 2001 found that pet owners in Canada insured 2% of cats and 9% of dogs. Meanwhile, a report by Datamonitor in 2005 revealed that pet owners in the United Kingdom insured approximately 12% of cats and 18% of dogs.[3]

Box 3: Did You Know?

The American Veterinary Medical Association pet health insurance policy recommendations are as follows:[4]

- Require a veterinarian-client-patient relationship.
- Allow policyholders to choose their own veterinarians, including specialists and emergency and critical care facilities.
- Never interfere with the veterinarian's fee structures.
- Be approved by the state insurance regulatory agency where the policy is sold.
- Be consistent with the Principles of Veterinary Medical Ethics and the pet health insurance industry's ethical standards.
- Use licensed veterinarians to assist in claims adjudication.
- Be clear about policy limits, pricing structures, and optional coverage (e.g., coverage for annual wellness visits) that might be available to policyholders.
- Be transparent about how the terms and conditions of plans will impact coverage and costs, including the financial obligations of policyholders such as co-pays, deductibles, and exclusions.
- Communicate clearly about the fee reimbursement process (i.e., how reimbursements are determined and how quickly reimbursements are provided to policyholders).

In 2017, I wrote a blog post titled "How Pet Health Insurance Can Improve the Mental Health of Veterinarians."[5] In the blog, I describe the high rates of mental health problems among veterinarians, explaining that some of the biggest stressors that we experience in practice stem from situations when clients cannot afford the cost of their pet's veterinary care. Many things can unfold in this scenario, and it varies from client to client. But the most difficult situation that veterinarians face is when a pet owner's financial limitations result in the euthanasia of their pet. While I am absolutely a proponent of euthanasia when it comes to reducing animal suffering and ending life in a humane way, it is morally distressing for vets when we know that we can help an animal with treatment, surgery, a procedure, or medication, yet we're unable to because the owner cannot afford it.

Around the same time, an article published in the *Journal of the American Veterinary Medical Association* presented findings from a survey conducted among small animal vets in the United States and Canada. The survey aimed to explore veterinarians' perspectives on the impact of client awareness of costs and pet health insurance on various aspects of practice. It also examined how client financial constraints could affect veterinarians' satisfaction and wellbeing, offering suggestions for addressing these challenges. Over half of the vets surveyed noted that client economic limitations influenced their ability to provide optimal care for their patients daily. Similarly, a significant proportion reported experiencing moderate to substantial burnout, with client economic limitations cited as a key contributing factor. Additionally, nearly all vets believed that increased client awareness of veterinary costs and access to pet health insurance would enhance pet care and contribute to greater satisfaction for both clients and veterinary teams.[6]

Given the escalating expenses associated with veterinary care, there is a growing emphasis on educating pet owners about the potential costs involved. For several years, I served as the resident veterinary expert on the Outdoor Journal Radio Show in Toronto, addressing common inquiries from pet owners on topics ranging from heat stroke prevention to frostbite, pet adoption, and tick-borne diseases. One recurring theme, particularly prevalent during the holiday season when listeners contemplated gifting pets to loved ones, was the considerable expense associated with veterinary care. According to Rover .com, in 2024, the initial costs for new dog owners ranged from $2,465 to $4,770 CAD (during the first year), with annual expenditures for essentials like dog food, toys, and flea medication varying from $965 to $4,020 CAD. These numbers indicate a jump in dog-owning costs of 44% compared to 2023. Optional expenses such as grooming, daycare, and kennel fees during vacations added further financial burden, averaging between $1,525 and $6,680 per year for most dog owners.[7] These figures don't include unforeseen visits to emergency clinics for illnesses or injuries, which could incur several thousand dollars in additional expenses.

The results of a survey of US pet owners were published in *The Veterinary Record* in 2021 and illustrate the importance of informing pet owners about the cost of veterinary care and how that information might impact their willingness to purchase pet health insurance. More than 300 uninsured pet parents were surveyed and given a choice experiment where they could decide whether they would purchase pet health insurance. The results showed that the uptake of pet health insurance increased by 12% after veterinary treatment cost and canine cancer risk information was provided.[8] It also seems that most American pet owners who report having health insurance for their pet are satisfied. Another survey of pet parents presenting to a small animal specialty hospital over a two-month period found that nearly 80% were satisfied with their pet health insurance plan and more than 70% would recommend it to a friend.[9]

The advantages of pet health insurance for both families and veterinary care providers revolve around the ability to prevent euthanasia due to financial constraints and opt for life-saving treatments like surgeries or chemotherapy that might otherwise be unaffordable. One study examining the impact of insurance on euthanasia rates before gastric dilation volvulus (GDV) surgery at referral hospitals in Australia revealed stunning findings: none of the insured dogs with GDV were euthanized before surgery, whereas euthanasia was the most common outcome for uninsured dogs prior to GDV surgery.[10] This underscores the critical role insurance coverage plays when owners are confronted with the urgent decision of pursuing costly surgery or resorting to euthanasia for a condition that would otherwise be fatal.

Certainly, like any other issue, pet health insurance has its upsides and downsides, affecting both pet owners and veterinary professionals. While it facilitates necessary and potentially costly medical treatments without financial constraints, mitigating the need for economic euthanasia in some cases, concerns arise regarding the escalating premiums. An article published in 2022 titled "Is Pet Health Insurance Able to Improve Veterinary Care? Why Pet Health Insurance for Dogs and Cats Has Limits" highlights the dilemma faced by pet owners with limited financial means, who struggle to afford both veterinary bills and monthly insurance premiums. This raises ethical concerns, particularly when families are unable to afford either veterinary expenses or pet health insurance coverage.[11]

Furthermore, there are concerns regarding the excessive use of diagnostic tests or overtreatment for pets covered by health insurance. In my experience as a veterinarian and specialist, I've witnessed situations when colleagues recommend performing diagnostic tests such as advanced imaging (CT scan or MRI) that could have been delayed (or avoided) with a more gradual approach to the patient's care. While we have more diagnostic modalities available to us in veterinary medicine than ever before, it's not necessary that we use those modalities in every situation. For example, while an MRI might be fully covered for an elderly dog with acute vestibular signs such as falling over or tilting the head, waiting to determine whether the signs improve with time (in cases of "old dog vestibular syndrome") may be an appropriate use of staffing resources and financial means. Alternatively, a young dog with mild gastrointestinal signs after eating a rich or fatty treat might undergo hospitalization and a battery of diagnostics for suspected pancreatitis, when close outpatient monitoring and supportive care may be sufficient. In both situations I've seen the more expensive option being elected simply because "the owner has insurance." One could argue that owners have insurance for a reason, so let's use it to pursue the very best veterinary care—but where does one draw the line between what is necessary or excessive?

An online questionnaire that was distributed to more than 600 veterinarians in the United Kingdom, Austria, and Denmark surveyed attitudes about pet health insurance and shared case examples used to determine whether coverage by insurance might influence treatment decisions. The results published in *The Veterinary Record* in 2022 showed that many veterinarians in Austria and the United Kingdom thought that insurance could lead to overtreatment. In fact, in response to the case examples provided, vets surveyed were more likely to suggest a CT scan to a client with an insured animal in comparison to a client who said they had financial limitations. Likewise, vets in the United Kingdom were more likely to suggest a CT scan to a client with an insured animal, when compared to a client without insurance.[12] These findings raise the ethical concern that pet health insurance could create differential access to clinical care for animals and undoubtedly increase the demand for more cost-intensive veterinary care.

While I do find myself exhaling a sigh of relief upon discovering that a patient in the emergency room or ICU has insurance, I don't consciously perceive it as affecting the care I provide. From my perspective, it eases the discomfort of presenting families with expensive estimates following unexpected or uncertain diagnoses. It also allows for more flexibility in the number and speed of tests we can conduct to reach a diagnosis, reducing the need for a cautious, financially constrained approach. While I strive to maintain a step-by-step approach with all my patients, I acknowledge the possibility that the presence of insurance subconsciously influences my decisions, leading to choices I might not otherwise make if the pet were uninsured.

Pet insurance is gaining popularity worldwide, with the highest adoption rates observed in the United Kingdom and Europe, particularly among dog owners (Box 4).[13] In the United States[14] and Canada,[15] only about 1% of cats and 4% of dogs are insured, while in Australia, the figure stands at approximately 7% of pets.[16] In stark contrast, a substantial proportion of pets in the United Kingdom—41% of cats and 54% of dogs—are insured.[17] Regarding the cancellation or non-renewal of pet health insurance policies, the primary reasons cited by pet owners are high costs, perceived low necessity, and the need to reduce expenses.[18]

Box 4: Did You Know?

In a study published in *Frontiers of Veterinary Science* in 2023 titled "Do People Really Care Less about Their Cats Than about Their Dogs?" researchers found that among pet owners in Denmark, Austria, and the United Kingdom, more dogs than cats were insured in all three countries.[13]

In the intricate world of veterinary care, a debate swirls around whether individuals should own pets if they can't shoulder the financial weight of potential veterinary expenses, particularly emergencies or surgeries that could soar into the thousands. Navigating the delicate discussion around the financial aspects of pet care as a veterinarian, I've found solace in the evolving landscape of pet health insurance. Encouraging friends and family to embrace this safeguard, I've witnessed a shift from viewing it as a mere expense to recognizing it as a vital tool for responsible pet ownership. The relief that washes over veterinary team members when owners have insurance not only acts as a financial safety net but also eases the moral distress often felt in veterinary care, potentially alleviating burnout and compassion fatigue among practitioners. Much like universal healthcare in human medicine, pet health insurance holds the promise of making veterinary care more accessible, thereby lightening the psychological load for those dedicated to the wellbeing of our beloved pets.

33

Transformative Technologies, Including Telemedicine

In a world in which the largest hospitality brand (Airbnb) owns no hotels and the largest taxi company (Uber) operates through the use of private vehicles, veterinarians must proactively embrace technology and innovation. To stay competitive, they must evolve their traditional business model and become "brick-and-click" veterinarians.

—Shlomo Freiman, DVM
(Veterinary Business Owner and Thought Leader)

Technology has come a long way since I began helping out in my mom's practice in the 1980s. Back then, medical records were kept in paper files, clients were alphabetized on a Rolodex, appointments were booked in a paper scheduler, and X-rays were taken on plain films. Our most advanced piece of technology at that time was probably the fax machine that was hooked up to our phone line. I still remember when we switched from the manual credit card imprinter to the point-of-sale credit card terminal; we'd have to turn off the fax machine to complete a transaction because they shared the same phone line! The rise in computer use meant a switch to an electronic appointment scheduler and electronic invoices. But the change from paper to electronic medical records didn't come until years later.

Throughout the hospital—not just at the reception desk— technology has also advanced. Digital X-rays for full body and dental images have replaced the plain films that were once developed in a dark room. Automated laboratory machines have replaced manual techniques for blood and urine analysis. Advanced monitoring devices such as oscillometric blood pressure monitors, capnography, and pulse oximetry have replaced "old school" methods of feeling pulses and checking gum color. Electrocardiograms (ECGs / EKGs), which were once cumbersome to use and could only be transmitted to a specialist by telephone, can now be measured with a smartphone or other handheld device and streamed wirelessly to a computer for interpretation. In the ICU, point-of-care ultrasound has largely replaced auscultation with a stethoscope and ECG leads that once tangled with IV lines been replaced by wireless telemetry systems.

DOI: 10.1201/9781003347385-37

The healthcare industry is thought to be on the forefront of technology. Whether using electronic health records, digital medical imaging, or data analytics to streamline processes, healthcare in general is relatively quick to use technology to advance patient care. Yet, while the many ways in which technology has bettered medicine are endless, veterinary medicine would not fall into the category of "early adopter" when it comes to new tech. With many practices still using paper medical records and others only recently implementing digital radiography, practices are often slow to adopt technologies that could enhance patient and client care.

This resistance to change was put to the test when the pandemic began in 2020. Because many veterinary practices closed their doors to clients or had families whose health inhibited them from being face to face in exam rooms, vets had to adjust, which meant leveraging telehealth more than they ever had before. While still a relatively new concept in the veterinary space, telehealth is the use of digital information and communication technologies to deliver health information, education, or care remotely. It's an overarching term, divided into categories depending on who is involved in the exchange of information or communication (Box 1). Telehealth uses technology such as mobile devices, apps, video conferencing, email, audio or video recordings, text messages, and wearable monitoring devices to share information that enhances the care of the patient in some way.

Box 1: Did You Know?

Telehealth exists in many categories, including:

- teladvice and teletriage (non-client to veterinarian or veterinary technician / nurse)
- teleconsulting (specialist or consultant to veterinarian)
- telesupervision (veterinary team to veterinarian)
- telemonitoring (animal to veterinarian or veterinary technician / nurse)
- telemedicine (client to veterinarian)
- e-prescription (pharmacy or distributor to veterinarian)

Since the start of the pandemic, companies around the world have emerged to offer telemedicine services for routine care or non-urgent concerns when pet owners are unable to schedule a timely appointment with their regular veterinarian. Additionally, new companies that offer teletriage services can respond to client calls in or outside of regular practice business hours to screen animals for life-threatening emergencies and direct them to the nearest veterinary hospital, or back to their regular practice if the circumstance is not urgent. There are also companies that are leveraging technology to lessen the workload or improve efficiency in practices amidst the ever-present staffing shortage. These include software programs that automate call-backs to clients, as well as voice-to-text transcription services that expedite electronic medical record-keeping. There are also companies of veterinary specialists who liaise with veterinarians to interpret digital imaging, such as X-rays or CT scans, and offer advice and support for challenging patients that require advanced level care (Box 2).

Box 2: Did You Know?

An online survey of veterinarians in the United States conducted between March and June 2020 revealed that the percentage of practices offering telehealth services, including teleadvice, telemedicine, e-prescription, teletriage, or telemonitoring increased from 12% before the pandemic to 38% during the pandemic.[1]

Due to the explosion in e-commerce around the world, one would assume animal owners would be keen to make use of telehealth and its related technologies. But a 2022 survey of more than 2,000 dog and cat owners in Austria, Denmark, and the United Kingdom found that very few dog (12%) or cat (6%) owners have used telemedicine. Moreover, three-quarters of those surveyed who have not previously utilized telemedicine expressed uncertainty about using it in the future or indicated that they would not consider using it.[2] And among more than 700 mostly Canadian pet owners surveyed in 2021, the majority had experience with veterinary care via telephone, while only 5% had used live videoconferencing. When asked about preferred interactions with their veterinarian, face-to-face (in-person) interactions were the preference, followed by telephone, and then live video conferencing. Pet owners expressed less confidence in communication during virtual consultations and, for those who had experienced virtual consultations in the past six months, participants were divided on recommending them.[3] Despite some hesitation toward telemedicine, one study's findings suggest that pet owners may place a higher value on virtual consultations with familiar or local veterinarians (Box 3).[4]

Box 3: Did You Know?

A recent study showed that dog and cat owners are willing to pay $38 USD more for a telemedicine consultation with their regular veterinarian and $13 USD more for a telemedicine consultation with a veterinarian in their community (who was not their veterinarian) when compared to a veterinarian from outside their community.[4]

Another 2020 survey study of veterinarians, vet nurses, and cat owners, predominantly in the United Kingdom, indicated that telephone consultations were their preferred method of telemedicine, favoring it over email or video consultations. Interestingly, vets and vet nurses expressed a higher preference for sharing photos compared to the cat owners surveyed, with some cat owners citing technical issues as a potential drawback to telemedicine. The cat owners also identified telemedicine as particularly well suited for monitoring, advice, and repeat prescription consultations, rather than for new concerns or problems. Both the cat owners and veterinary professionals identified that telemedicine appointments reduced stress for both the cat and the owner, by avoiding travel time, handling, and waiting room experiences. But despite those benefits, there was a shared consensus on the drawbacks of telemedicine, with the inability to conduct a physical examination being the most frequently mentioned concern. Both owners and veterinary professionals expressed worries about the potential for delayed or incorrect diagnoses.[5]

Dr. Lori Teller, former president of the American Veterinary Medical Association and clinical professor at Texas A&M University College of Veterinary Medicine & Biomedical Sciences, advocates for telemedicine as a valuable tool in veterinary care but stresses the importance of establishing an in-person Veterinary–Client–Patient Relationship (VCPR) first. Teleadvice and teletriage, which provide basic answers and determine urgency without requiring a VCPR, are distinct from telemedicine, which involves patient-specific recommendations and follow-up. Dr. Teller warns against relaxing VCPR laws, emphasizing the risks of misdiagnosis and inappropriate treatment without an initial in-person visit, as mandated by federal requirements from the United States Food and Drug Administration and Department of Agriculture (Box 4). While telemedicine can enhance access to care once a VCPR is established, Dr. Teller highlights the necessity of addressing acute issues through in-person visits, particularly for animals lacking regular care such as those in remote communities.[6]

Box 4: Did You Know?

The United States (US) Food and Drug Administration (FDA) has said veterinarians need to do an in-person examination before prescribing medications not labeled for veterinary use. Currently, 43 US states use language from the FDA and 22 US states have language prohibiting VCPR from being established virtually.[6]

Telemedicine has the benefit of increasing access to veterinary care across many client demographics and patient populations. A recent study at the University of Pennsylvania School of Veterinary Medicine explored the use of telemedicine through the Pets for Life program, which offered free virtual telehealth visits to pet families in underserved areas. Surveys from the pet families revealed that one-quarter would have faced transportation challenges, and more than half would have been unable to afford in-person veterinary appointments. Thus, telehealth appears to be a viable alternative with both clients and students reporting overwhelmingly positive experiences.[7] Additionally, telehealth can allow owners of rare animals such as exotics (small mammals, reptiles, birds, and fish) or found wildlife to receive rapid medical care when in-person veterinary care for that species is unavailable.[8]

Telehealth also has the capacity to enhance veterinary student education. A study in the United States recruited veterinary practitioners to conduct telehealth case rounds for veterinary students at Kansas State and Texas A&M Universities. The virtual sessions, held monthly over two academic years, aimed to expose students to a broader range of clinical cases and assess the feasibility and acceptance of telehealth as a teaching tool. Veterinarians presented routine cases from their practice, covering clinical decision points, diagnosis, treatment, management, and ethical or communication issues. The project successfully increased the quantity and diversity of cases for students, with over 95% reporting increased clinical confidence and competence. Presenting practitioners expressed unanimous interest in participating in similar telehealth instruction in the future.[9]

While many veterinary practices are slow to adopt technological advances, including those involved with digital presence such as websites and social media platforms, recent research makes a business case for doing so. A survey was conducted among nearly 250 veterinary practices in Bosnia and Herzegovina, focusing on their digital presence, use of information technologies, and business performance. The results revealed that only 10% of the surveyed practices had a business-related website, and just over half were present on at least one social media platform. When comparing digital marketing strategies and online presence to annual profits, the study found that effective digital marketing strategies, especially Google advertisements, website search engine optimization, and social media advertisements, increased annual profits the most, while web presence, Google Business account utilization, and consistent social media management also positively impacted annual profit.[10] While restrictions in certain jurisdictions prevent mainstream advertising of veterinary services, maintaining an online and social media presence is essential to sustaining or growing veterinary practices.

With the addition of artificial intelligence (AI), there are a growing number of new tools and solutions to improve the quality and efficiency of veterinary care. Some ways AI is being used in veterinary medicine, albeit controversial in certain circumstances, include:

- Diagnostic Imaging: AI is utilized to enhance the analysis of diagnostic images such as X-rays, MRIs, and CT scans. Machine learning algorithms can assist in the early detection of conditions such as tumors, fractures, or arthritis.

- Pathology and Histology: AI is applied in veterinary pathology to analyze tissue samples and identify abnormalities. Automated systems can assist pathologists in diagnosing diseases and conditions, leading to faster and potentially more accurate results.

- Predictive Analytics: Machine learning algorithms can analyze large sets of data to identify patterns and trends. In veterinary medicine, predictive analytics can help in forecasting disease outbreaks, identifying at-risk populations, and optimizing preventive care strategies.

- Telemedicine and Remote Monitoring: AI-powered telemedicine platforms and remote monitoring solutions are becoming more prevalent in veterinary care. These technologies enable pet owners to connect with veterinarians for remote consultations, and wearable devices can provide real-time health data for monitoring.

- Natural Language Processing (NLP): NLP technology is used in veterinary practice management software to extract information from clinical notes, reports, and other unstructured data. This can help streamline administrative tasks and improve data accessibility.

- Behavior Analysis: AI is applied to analyze animal behavior through video monitoring or wearable devices. This can aid in the early detection of behavioral issues or health problems, providing insights into preventive care.

- Drug Discovery: AI is playing a role in drug discovery for veterinary medicine. By analyzing vast datasets, machine learning algorithms can identify potential drug candidates and predict their efficacy in treating specific animal diseases.

- Robotics in Surgery: While not yet widespread, robotic-assisted surgery is being explored in veterinary medicine. AI-controlled robotic systems can assist veterinarians in performing precise and minimally invasive surgical procedures.

- Computer Vision: A field of AI that has shown promise in detecting signs of human skin disease has recently been investigated in veterinary dermatology. Computer vision tools have the potential to differentiate healthy dog paws from paws that are infected or have cancer.[11]

The pandemic not only transformed veterinary practices and patient care, but also reshaped the way I conducted my business. Previously, I delivered lectures and workshops in person, but, as restrictions grew, I transitioned nearly all my offerings to Zoom, including online programs and one-on-one coaching. My clinical practice underwent a remarkable shift as well. As a veterinary specialist, I'd always worked on the clinic floor, with minimal phone interaction with pet owners. However, the pandemic propelled my clinical practice into the virtual realm, where I began providing specialist advice through teleconsultations—a prospect that would have seemed implausible to the veterinarian I was 20 years ago. Yet, amidst staffing shortages and the rapid spread of COVID-19, this became the new reality in the early 2020s.

As someone who regularly manages emergency shifts with up to 20 cases in a 12-hour window, I've also come to rely on AI scribe software to handle the extraordinary caseload. This technology streamlines my workflow by transcribing medical records as I go, allowing me to focus more directly on patient care without compromising thorough record-keeping. Not only does this enhance efficiency, but it also reduces the mental load, helping me stay sharp and focused during intense shifts. The technological advances in veterinary medicine brought on by the pandemic, from teleconsultations to AI-drive documentation, have reshaped the profession in ways that will only grow in the years to come.

Striving for Diversity, Equity, and Inclusion

Diversity, equity, and inclusion are more than concepts or words—they are the foundation of compassionate, effective care. To truly care for animals, we must first understand and honor the diversity of the people who love and care for them. This guiding principle bridges our mission with the ability to deliver exceptional outcomes for every client, patient, and community we serve.

—Avery Alston (Director, People Experience & DEI)

Veterinary practice is a multigenerational workplace, where baby boomers through Gen-Z's work together to care for animals and their owners. But despite the wide range of ages represented by employees in veterinary practice, the discipline is the least diverse of all medical professions. Since its inception in the late 1700s through the early 1980s, veterinary medicine has been composed of predominantly Caucasian/White male professionals. And while there has been great progress in recent decades to attract women to the profession, people of color, persons with disabilities, and other groups remain heavily underrepresented. In developed countries where the population is changing quickly, the demographics of pet owners are changing along with what people expect from veterinarians. To keep up, a more diverse group of veterinary professionals is required so that we can meet the needs of everyone.

The demand for vets is increasing, especially in underserved areas. To address this, there's a need for a professional body that brings diverse perspectives to veterinary education, regulatory medicine, and clinical practice. Ensuring broad representation in vet medicine, a crucial field for global health and food safety, begins well before students enter veterinary schools. Using the United States as an example, over the next 40 years, the population is expected to undergo significant changes. Asian and Hispanic/Latino communities are growing faster than other groups, with the Asian population projected to increase by 79% and the Hispanic/Latino population expected to double by 2050. In contrast, the non-Hispanic/Latino Caucasian/White group is anticipated to decrease by 6%.[1] Despite these shifts, the educational landscape, especially in higher education, has not kept pace. According to Zippia, the

DOI: 10.1201/9781003347385-38

most common ethnicity of current doctoral students in the United States is White (54%), followed by Hispanic or LatinX (18%), Asian (12%), and Black or African American (11%).[2]

Certainly, many students choose not to apply to vet medicine for reasons that include not being fully prepared academically, financial restrictions, life situations, or having other interests. However, it's unlikely that vet colleges can continue to rely on the same pipeline of applicants as before, given the increase in demand for veterinary professionals alongside the concurrent changing needs of clientele. Schools need to focus on increasing diversity in science, technology, engineering, and math (STEM) fields to ensure future enrollment in their programs. While vet medicine may not be growing as rapidly as some other STEM occupations, there's still a large projected increase in the demand for vets due to factors like retiring baby boomers and emerging needs in areas such as food safety, public health, and biomedical research.

Unfortunately, there's a significant lack of diversity in STEM fields, particularly in vet medicine, with underrepresentation of both women and men from racial and ethnic backgrounds (Box 1). The number and share of science and engineering degrees earned by underrepresented minorities (URMs) increased at all degree levels between 2011 and 2020 with associate's degrees earned by URMs growing at the highest rate (from 31% in 2011 to 43% in 2020). However, the increase is much less pronounced at higher degree levels, especially for science and engineering doctorates, where the share of degrees earned by URMs increased from 13% to 16%.[3] This presents a significant issue, because obtaining a Bachelor of Science degree serves as a crucial pathway to acquiring the Doctor of Veterinary Medicine degree and pursuing further professional and graduate degrees. Ensuring underrepresented students have access to STEM education at the undergraduate level is essential. Equally important is guaranteeing their success in college, to prevent the perpetuation of an unrepresentative vet student body compared to the diversity of the animal-owning population.

Box 1: Did You Know?

In 2013, *The Atlantic* listed veterinary medicine as #1 among the "33 Whitest Jobs in America."[4]

Recent data from the 2021 United States Bureau of Labor Statistics reveals that 93.3% of US veterinarians are White, with 5.6% Asian, 4.7% Hispanic/Latinx, and 1.2% Black.[5] This lack of diversity is also evident among vet students, wherein 75.9% of 2020 veterinary school graduates were White, 7.5% Latinx/Hispanic, 5.5% Asian, 3% Black, and 4% multiracial. Populations including Black, Latinx, Asian, Native American, Alaska Native, and Native Hawaiian and Pacific Islander are considered underrepresented in vet medicine, constituting 22% of the 2019–2020 US veterinary student enrollment. Additionally, male (18.1%) and first-generation college students (26.3%) are also considered URMs in vet medicine by the American Association of Veterinary Medical Colleges.[6] To establish a sustainable pipeline of applicants for vet schools in the United States and other developed countries, it's crucial to implement recruitment strategies focusing on diversity across the entire K-20 education system. Creating a more diverse applicant pool, especially in STEM and agriculture disciplines, is vital for the future of the veterinary profession.[7]

The lack of diversity in vet medicine can lead to unwelcoming or even hostile learning environments, as highlighted in the video "A Profession in Crisis: Discrimination in Veterinary Medicine", released near the beginning of the Black Lives Matter movement. This video shares experiences of people of color facing derogatory comments, microaggressions, and reprimands, shedding light on the challenges present in the profession.[8] I remember the first time I watched the video and how surprised I was by the experiences that were shared. Then I spoke with some of my friends and colleagues who are URMs and learned that the microaggressions and backhanded comments are not only very real but also deleteriously common. Examples include a Black vet student being told, "You're so articulate!" after giving a presentation or a Latinx veterinarian misperceived as a vet assistant. Microaggressions also impact pet owners whereby clients from marginalized groups might only receive information about low-cost veterinary care, based on assumptions about their socioeconomic status. This can perpetuate harmful stereotypes. While often unintentional, these microaggressions can cause serious harm to those experiencing them.

The lack of diversity, equity, inclusion, and belonging (DEIB) in veterinary medicine not only affects the profession but also impacts animal health. In food animal medicine, having fewer underrepresented veterinarians, along with a higher number of Black and Latinx workers, can make it hard to communicate effectively about animal care. And when it comes to taking care of pets, individuals with disabilities, families of mixed races, and individuals whose gender identity is non-binary struggle to find veterinary care that understands and respects their backgrounds, no matter where they live. The demographics of people who own pets are changing, which makes it crucial for veterinary care to be inclusive and accessible to diverse groups of pet owners.

Efforts to promote diversity and inclusion in veterinary medicine have been ongoing since the 1970s. In 2005, the Association of American Veterinary Medical Colleges launched the DiVersity Matters program, a nationwide initiative focused on diversity issues. Then in 2017, the American Veterinary Medical Association (AVMA) Council on Education (COE) updated curriculum standards to include cultural competency. This involves assessing students' ability to "demonstrate ethical and professional conduct, including those that show an understanding and sensitivity to client diversity and individual circumstances as a core competency." And most recently, in 2021, the AVMA COE, which also happens to be the only accrediting body for vet schools in the United States and Canada, updated their accreditation standards for veterinary medical colleges to incorporate: "Opportunities throughout the curriculum for students to gain and integrate an understanding of the important influences of diversity and inclusion in veterinary medicine, including the impact of implicit bias related to an individual's personal circumstance on the delivery of veterinary medical services."[9] The revised standards underscore the significance of integrating social justice education into veterinary curricula.

Several vet schools are taking the lead on creating DEIB initiatives within their curriculum for students, faculty, and staff. Recognizing the need for a more inclusive culture, the Ohio State University College of Veterinary Medicine (OSU-CVM) has integrated DEIB as a foundational principle in its strategic plan. The college has appointed a Chief Diversity Officer, established DEIB committees involving faculty, staff, and students, and created an external DEIB Council to provide guidance. To enhance diversity in student admissions, OSU-CVM has implemented a holistic review process, emphasizing non-cognitive factors and providing diversity and bias training for everyone involved in the admissions process. Efforts to increase diversity extend to faculty and staff recruitment, with an emphasis on mentoring, training, and increasing staff diversity to better reflect the broader community. The college has also implemented programs such as the Community of Inclusion Certificate Program and Safe Zone training to foster a supportive environment. Affinity groups, discussions on timely topics, and addressing ableism are part of OSU-CVM's commitment to creating an inclusive and welcoming campus. The college is also actively working to counter microaggressions and is engaged in curricular redesign to embed DEIB principles within the education framework. OSU-CVM commitment to DEIB is recognized through its receipt of the Health Professions Higher Education Excellence in Diversity Award for five consecutive years.

Over the last several years, OSU-CVM has been actively engaged in recruitment efforts, reaching over 10,000 individuals from kindergarten through grade 12 and undergraduate students. This initiative aims to build a diverse pipeline of future veterinarians, providing exposure to the profession and creating role models for underrepresented students. The results are evident in the growing diversity of OSU-CVM applicants. From 2009 to 2010, only 6% of applicants identified as URMs, but by 2020 to 2021, this percentage increased significantly to 26.3%. The racial/ethnic diversity of incoming classes followed suit, rising from 7.1% in 2009–2010 to an impressive 35.2% in 2020–2021. These positive trends occurred alongside a threefold increase in total applicants, a 13-fold increase in URM applicants, and a fivefold increase in URMs accepting seats in the class. OSU-CVM has also made significant strides in diversifying its student body. In 2019, the national pool of US veterinary school applicants comprised 13.1% males and 24.4% URMs. In comparison, students entering OSU-CVM in the same year represented a more diverse cohort, with 26% males and 35% URMs. In the 2020–2021 academic year, national enrollment statistics showed 18.2% males and 22.8% URMs, while OSU-CVM enrolled 23.4% males and 27% URMs. Alongside this increasing diversity, OSU-CVM students have maintained high academic standards, boasting similar average GPAs and matriculation/graduation rates as previous classes.[10]

The College of Veterinary Medicine at North Carolina State University, where I completed my residency, is also actively fostering a culture of diversity and inclusion through various initiatives. Notably, the college hosts the Veterinarians as One Inclusive Community for Empowerment group (VOICE), a student-led organization, as well as the Faculty Committee on Diversity and Inclusion, which has student and staff representation. Other college-wide efforts focus on integrating cultural competency programming for veterinary students, with mandatory training by the National Coalition Building Institute during the first-year orientation. Veterinary students are also required to undertake three diversity-focused experiences annually as part of their curriculum, including a one-week diversity elective developed and instructed by two academic staff members. Similar professional development opportunities are extended to faculty, staff, and graduate students throughout the academic year.[11]

National and international veterinary organizations are also taking steps to grow their DEIB initiatives and programming. In 2014, the Multicultural Veterinary Medical Association was created with the goal of making veterinary medicine more diverse, equitable, and inclusive. Along with other groups such as the AVMA, they have taken steps to address racism in the veterinary profession. These include assessing the situation, making resources more accessible, being accountable and transparent, increasing membership, committing to diversity, investing in the cause, and engaging with the community. The hope is that these same steps can be used as a guide to include anti-racism efforts in vet school, making the profession more diverse and responsive to the needs of different communities.[12]

In 2021, the Royal College of Veterinary Surgeons in the United Kingdom released their Diversity and Inclusion Group Strategy with the following Statement of Intent: "We need diverse and inclusive veterinary professions, where everyone can flourish and be themselves, both professionally and personally. Bias, discrimination and harassment exists within our professions: we need to identify it, reject it and change our culture for the better."[13] Following that in 2022, the AVMA named their inaugural chief DEIB officer to "advance [their] commitment to creating diverse, equitable, and inclusive work and educational environments across veterinary medicine."[14]

Other smaller organizations and groups are following suit, including my own specialty college, which formed the American College of Veterinary Emergency and Critical Care DEI Committee in 2020. Now functioning alongside the Veterinary Emergency and Critical Care Society DEI Committee,[15] their goals are to (1) inspire and encourage underrepresented populations/identities as members of ACVECC and in veterinary medicine as a whole; (2) create a safe environment in which to engage in conversations around race, diversity, and equity; (3) promote diversity and inclusion education and resources regarding anti-racist, LGBTQIA, women's rights, and religious and disability justice education; and (4) create an environment where people feel safe, heard, valued, and respected.[16] In addition to offering mentorship to URMs interested in vet medicine, they also sponsor one URM vet student to attend the International Veterinary Emergency and Critical Care Society meeting each autumn and promote DEIB initiatives through their active social media account @CriticallyDiverse. And through the Credentials Committee that oversees the board certification of residents-in-training, they require all residents to engage in at least one of five options for diversity and inclusion training, ranging from completing certificate programs to attending lectures or discussions at the annual conference.[17]

The American Association of Veterinary Clinicians (AAVC) has taken significant strides toward enhancing DEIB within clinical post-DVM graduate training programs and academic faculty. Through the establishment of a Diversity, Equity, and Inclusivity working group and the development of a strategic plan, the AAVC has prioritized the recruitment and selection of talented and diverse candidates for intern and resident positions. By incorporating holistic approaches that go beyond traditional metrics like grades and class rank, the AAVC aims to build a more resilient and inclusive workforce in veterinary medicine.[18] This initiative aligns with broader efforts to address the lack of diversity within the profession, recognizing the importance of representation in improving innovation, patient outcomes, and overall workforce satisfaction. Recommendations include standardized assessment criteria, consideration of non-academic experiences, and ongoing evaluation and revision of selection processes to ensure equitable opportunities for all candidates. Additionally, a commitment to DEIB must be embedded within the organizational culture of veterinary institutions, supported by leadership, shared governance, and equitable compensation practices.

The gender disparity in veterinary leadership roles is just one facet of the broader issue of DEIB within the profession. Despite the increasing feminization of vet medicine, which has seen a significant rise in the number of women entering the field, gender equality remains elusive (Box 2). From the gender pay gap and the "motherhood penalty" to the underrepresentation of women in leadership roles within vet schools, systemic biases continue to hinder female advancement and prosperity. This gender gap is evident not only in academic leadership, where female deans remain a minority (Box 3), but also in corporate settings, with animal health and wellness companies exhibiting predominantly male executive teams.

While strides have been made in some organizations toward gender parity, the overall landscape underscores persistent challenges in promoting diversity at all levels of veterinary practice. Factors contributing to this disparity extend beyond gender alone and intersect with issues of race, ethnicity, socioeconomic status, sexual orientation, age, religion, ability, neurodivergence, and other dimensions of identity. Initiatives aimed at addressing DEIB issues in veterinary medicine must recognize the intersectionality of these challenges and work toward creating inclusive environments that foster the advancement of all individuals, regardless of their identities and experiences. By promoting diversity in leadership and embracing inclusive practices, the veterinary profession can better serve the needs of its diverse clientele and contribute to the overall health and wellbeing of both animals and humans.

Box 2: Did You Know?

Female veterinarian specialists in private practice make 25%–29% less than their male counterparts and female veterinarians in academia earn 8%–10% less than their male colleagues.[19]

Box 3: Did You Know?

More than 80% of the class of 2025 in veterinary schools is female,[20] yet 75% of veterinary school deans are male.[21]

35

Redefining Veterinary Education for a Dynamic Profession

> Students learn how to take care of patients, but they need to learn how to take care of themselves. I want to see it become standard in the curriculum that students are taught how to take care of their health and welfare.
>
> —Nienke Endenburg, PhD
> (Clinical Psychologist and Associate Professor)

Early in my career, I faced a pivotal moment that opened my eyes to the emotional challenges of veterinary medicine. It was during an overnight emergency shift when a man came in with his 19-year-old cat—a long-time patient with chronic kidney disease, diabetes, and other ongoing issues. He was clearly devoted to his furry companions and had done everything he could to care for them. But as he tearfully handed me his beloved cat, I could tell this visit was different. Something about the way he looked at my side this wasn't just another check-up—it was serious. Even though I had the medical training to make a diagnosis and explain the treatment options, I realized I wasn't prepared to handle the emotional weight of the situation. I didn't know how to support him in that moment, and I felt the heaviness of his grief and the tough decisions he was facing. That night made me step back and really think about what it means to be a veterinarian—and how much more there is to the role than just treating animals.

That experience really opened my eyes to a gap in my veterinary training. I had all the clinical knowledge and hands-on skills to diagnose and treat medical issues, but I hadn't been taught how to handle the emotional and ethical side of things—especially when it came to end-of-life decisions. I found myself struggling to balance what I knew medically with what the owner was feeling and valuing. It was a turning point for me. I began to understand just how essential communication, empathy, and ethical decision-making are in this profession. That moment sparked a commitment in me to keep growing in those areas—to not only be a skilled veterinarian, but also someone who can truly support pet owners through the hardest parts of the journey.

In 1999, an article titled "The Current and Future Market for Veterinarians and Veterinary Medical Services in the United States" published in the *Journal of the American Veterinary Medical Association* highlighted a concern that veterinarians lacked business management and communication skills considered

DOI: 10.1201/9781003347385-39

key for success in practice.[1] Since that time, veterinary schools around the world have striven to incorporate business and communication training into their curricula to varying degrees and in different formats. When I completed vet school, we had two half-days dedicated to practice management and communication, delivered to our entire class in a lecture-style format. A small part of this training involved a client simulation that a couple of my classmates participated in, while the rest of us observed from our seats—not terribly helpful when you consider the need for experiential learning among adults.

Since then, the curriculum of my former vet school has drastically changed to include a core veterinary business class offered throughout one semester for each of the three pre-clinical years of training. Within the class, concepts covered include interest rates, lending, investing, retirement planning, financial statements, business structures, contracts, liability, practice valuation, and practice management. These concepts have the potential to help the financial literacy and wellbeing of all aspiring veterinarians, regardless of whether they intend to own a practice or other business someday. Likewise, communication training is now robustly embedded in the curriculum, including a yearlong course during third year focusing on history-taking, euthanasia conversations, and disclosure of medical errors and including lectures and laboratories with opportunities to practice communication skills in a simulated environment.

My communication training while on faculty at the Ontario Veterinary College was rooted in the Calgary-Cambridge model. It was transformative, immersing me in role-playing scenarios that enhanced my rapport-building skills like agenda setting and empathy statements. Teaching in the Art of Veterinary Medicine course further solidified these skills, demonstrating their real-world application in client communication. Despite the evidence demonstrating the benefits of such training in boosting communication skills and confidence,[2] some veterinarians still find it inadequate (Box 1), suggesting improvements like using practicing vets as client actors for more realistic simulations. Concerns also arise about the peer feedback process during simulations, with some feeling uncomfortable being judged by their classmates. Additionally, time constraints within the curriculum often limit simulations to specific scenarios like history-taking and euthanasia conversations, leaving little room for addressing other challenging situations like financial constraints or angry clients.

Box 1: Did You Know?

A report published in the *Journal of Veterinary Medical Education* in 2015 revealed that 98% of veterinarians surveyed in the United Kingdom and the United States agreed that communication skills were as important or more important than clinical knowledge. Yet only 35% said their communication skills training during veterinary school prepared them well or very well for communicating with clients about the health of their pets.[3]

Not only do many veterinarians feel unprepared for practice when it comes to their communication skills, many also feel ill-equipped for most day-to-day clinical requirements. Advances in companion animal medicine and surgery require general practitioners to be competent in a wide range of surgical techniques, from spay-neuter surgeries for puppies and kittens to cystotomies for bladder stone removal, laceration repairs, skin growth removals, intestinal obstructions, cruciate (knee ligament) ruptures, fracture repairs, and dental extractions. Students are lucky to watch, never mind practice, most of these procedures during veterinary school, leaving them reliant upon mentorship and trial-and-error once they arrive in general practice. A general practice veterinarian once shared with me that, despite receiving four hours of lectures on dentistry in school (which was more than the one hour I had!), she still felt completely unprepared for the many dental procedures she was expected to perform starting in her very first week on the job.

Debate as to what to include in the vet school curriculum has existed for decades and has led to regular recommendations published by organizations, such as the Pew National Veterinary Education Program and the European Association of Establishments for Veterinary Education. These often lead to curriculum reviews and redesigns to better align with their recommendations. A 20-year review of the veterinary medical curriculum published in the *Journal of Veterinary Medical Education* in 2008 suggested that modern vet programs must prioritize not just knowledge acquisition, but also the development of skills, values, and attitudes. It also highlighted repeated shortcomings in areas like business management, effective interpersonal communication, and problem-solving. It concluded that future curricula should facilitate greater diversification and specialization among vet students, offering ample opportunities to focus on areas like public health, population medicine, and issues such as food safety and bio- and agro-terrorism. The paper also emphasized instilling a culture of active learning, fostering strong lifelong learning skills and attitudes among students.[4]

That same year, the American Association of Veterinary Medical Colleges convened the North American Veterinary Medical Education Consortium (NAVMEC), bringing together the broadest spectrum of stakeholders of veterinary medical education assembled to date. Their three goals were to (1) recognize shifting societal demographics and anticipate the demands placed on the veterinary medical profession by these changes; (2) establish a collective understanding of the essential skills and qualities that every veterinarian should embody upon graduation, irrespective of their chosen specialization; and (3) determine the necessary adaptations in veterinary medical education to align with emerging societal requirements, ensuring that graduating veterinarians are equipped with the identified core competencies. In their document "Roadmap for Veterinary Medical Education in the 21st Century: Responsive, Collaborative, Flexible" they listed core competencies that they believed pertinent for all vet medicine graduates, considering animal-owning clients and society (Box 2). One of the concepts mentioned to help develop these competencies was to "teach commonly seen clinical conditions uncommonly well" focusing on primary care, wellness, and prevention.[4]

Box 2: Core Competencies Recommended for All Veterinary Medical Graduates

- Multispecies knowledge plus clinical competency in one or more species or disciplines
- One health knowledge: animal, human, and environmental health
- Professional competencies
- Communication
- Collaboration
- Management (self, team, system)
- Lifelong learning, scholarship, value of research
- Leadership
- Diversity and multicultural awareness
- Adapt to changing environments

During my time in veterinary school in the early 2000s, the curriculum was focused almost entirely on seven species—dogs, cats, horses, cows, sheep, pigs, and chickens—with a brief introduction to small exotic animals such as ferrets, rabbits, and pet birds in third year. There were no opportunities within the curriculum to focus on species of interest, except when choosing third-year externship experiences or fourth-year clinical rotations. Even then, I was required to take at least two large animal rotations during my fourth year, even though I knew with 100% certainty that I wouldn't be stepping foot anywhere near a horse or cow as a practicing veterinarian. While the inclusion of the seven species helped me to pass my North American Veterinary Licensing Examination (NAVLE), it in no way prepared me to be a better companion animal vet.

Most vet schools now offer tracked curricula allowing students to specialize in more common species of interest, with some offering additional tracks like exotic species or public health. While initial responses to tracking varied, with concerns about limiting post-graduation opportunities, many (myself included) see its benefits in avoiding unnecessary species-specific learning. Feedback from graduates suggests that the majority specialize in narrow areas of vet medicine after graduation, challenging the notion of a generalized pre-clinical education (Box 3).[5] However, concerns persist among general practice veterinarians that the vet school experience does not fully prepare them for the realities of practice, particularly in settings with different caseloads and financial constraints. Despite efforts to expose students to community practice settings, much of their clinical experience still revolves around cases managed by specialists, limiting exposure to challenging client conversations about financial limitations and alternative treatment options.

Box 3: Did You Know?

A study comparing graduates from the Ohio State University (broad-based learning) and University of California–Davis (tracked learning) found that over 90% of veterinarians specialize in a narrow area of veterinary medicine after graduation. It also showed strong support for hiring associates with specific training in the species seen at the practice.[5]

Spectrum of care (SpOC) in veterinary medicine refers to a range of evidence-based treatment options available to pet owners across different socioeconomic backgrounds. It encompasses the diverse needs and financial constraints of pet owners, emphasizing the importance of providing comprehensive veterinary care regardless of financial limitations. Training vets to deliver SpOC from the onset of their careers is advocated as a crucial addition to veterinary education, ensuring graduates possess the necessary competencies to address the varying needs of pet owners. The Ohio State University College of Veterinary Medicine has introduced an innovative curriculum aimed at preparing new graduate vets for clinical practice, which emphasizes a SpOC approach to address affordability and accessibility of veterinary services. Through a blend of clinical and didactic training, students receive comprehensive instruction, with a focus on communication, collaboration, professional identity development, and integrated problem-solving. The curriculum incorporates hands-on clinical experiences across all four years, ensuring students are equipped to provide a broad range of treatment options for diverse clientele.

Medical knowledge has undergone a significant transformation over the years, with the doubling time decreasing from 50 years in 1950 to a mere 0.2 years (or 73 days) by 2020.[6] This rapid expansion poses considerable challenges for education, patient care, and research in both human and veterinary medicine. Similarly, vet medicine has seen substantial advancements in recent years, such as once rare surgeries like subcutaneous ureteral bypass becoming commonplace, alongside routine procedures like mechanical ventilation and dialysis for animals in the intensive care unit becoming daily occurrences. These changes highlight the need for updates to vet school curricula, prompting critical reflections on what content should be prioritized amidst the emergence of new procedures and protocols.

The ongoing debate regarding the inclusion of basic biomedical science training in veterinary school curricula has gained fervor. Conversations with classmates and colleagues often involve reminiscing about hours spent in histology labs or embryology classes, questioning their relevance to everyday clinical practice. However, experts emphasize the indispensability of biomedical sciences in understanding the physiological and pathological mechanisms crucial to animal health and disease. They advocate for integrating biomedical knowledge into veterinary education to enhance critical thinking, communication skills, and the ability to apply theoretical concepts to practical clinical scenarios, thereby elevating the quality of animal care and veterinary practice.[7] While a complete removal of the "ology" subjects seems unlikely, striving to integrate their concepts throughout veterinary training appears to be a sensible approach.

When I ask other veterinarians what they feel was missing from their vet school training, the answer I receive the most pertains to their mental health and wellbeing. Veterinarians report feeling underprepared when it comes to managing their stress, utilizing effective coping strategies, engaging in self-care, mitigating perfectionism, and maintaining an identity outside of their veterinary role. Across the board they also express that they wish they had learned concepts such as boundary setting and work-life separation during vet school, rather than decades later (if at all, for some of them). They describe the many traumas in veterinary practice such as witnessing animal abuse or neglect, dealing with distraught owners, or navigating cyberbullying from clients as situations they were wholly unprepared for. While veterinary medical training (or any medical training for that matter) cannot prepare individuals for every situation they might encounter in clinical practice, a commitment to incorporating mental health and wellbeing training into the curriculum is a must moving forward.

During the last few years, some schools have introduced components of wellbeing into the core and elective curriculum. Nearly ten years ago, my pharmacology professor at the Western College of Veterinary Medicine began offering a Mindful Veterinary Practice elective for third-year students.[8] This class focused on mindfulness in the context of veterinary practice, whereby mindfulness-based strategies were used to enhance interpersonal communication, reduce stress, and improve attention and working memory, all with the intended goal of enhancing patient care and career satisfaction. Unfortunately, elective rotations do not carry the same weight as those incorporated into the core curriculum whereby students may not prioritize the content or skip classes altogether. This has led researchers to recommend embedding mindfulness and other wellbeing classes into the core curriculum such that they are given the weight and recognition that they deserve, which is what the University of Murdoch did with its mindfulness program.[9]

The Be Well initiative at the Ohio State University College of Veterinary Medicine offers a comprehensive and integrated approach to health and wellbeing for students, staff, and faculty. Programs under the Be Well umbrella include Health Athlete Training, which provides workshops and seminars on stress management, time management, and work-life balance, as well as the MINDSTRONG program that offers evidence-based cognitive-behavioral skills-building to enhance resilience and promote self-protective factors for overall wellbeing. Additionally, Be Well $: Financial Day is a biannual financial summit exposing vet students to essential financial topics like debt management, taxes, and investing. These initiatives aim to foster a culture of wellbeing and inclusivity, empowering individuals to thrive academically, professionally, and personally within the veterinary community and beyond.[10]

Reflecting on the experiences shared and the evolving landscape of veterinary education, it's evident that there are significant areas where traditional curricula have fallen short in preparing veterinarians for the multifaceted demands of modern practice. From communication skills and business acumen to mental health and specialized clinical training, there's a growing recognition of the need for comprehensive education to produce competent, confident, and resilient graduates. Fortunately, proactive initiatives and reforms are underway across vet schools worldwide to bridge these gaps. By integrating robust communication training, immersive clinical experiences, and holistic wellness programs into core curricula, educators are striving to equip aspiring vets with the skills and support they need to thrive in diverse practice settings. As we continue to refine and innovate veterinary education, let us remain committed to nurturing a new generation of veterinarians who not only excel in clinical proficiency, but also embody empathy, resilience, and lifelong learning.

Exploring Veterinary Frontiers
Outside Clinical Practice

Too many times I describe my work outside of practice and people will ask me whether I miss being "a real vet." Knowing my identity as a vet is not tied to the traditional clinical role has been powerful in not getting bogged down by these misperceptions.

—Vanessa Tonn, DVM, BSc (Industry Veterinarian)

When I tell people I'm a veterinarian, they almost always ask, "where do you practice?" What many people don't realize is that veterinarians can have jobs outside of clinical practice while still utilizing their Doctor of Veterinary Medicine (DVM) degree. I witnessed this firsthand, my veterinarian mom owning and working in a small animal practice while my veterinarian dad worked in government, focused on the welfare of farm animals and food safety. But for the longest time, and certainly throughout vet school, I believed there were only a handful of career trajectories destined for those graduating as a DVM.

This perspective is not unique to me; many others in the profession share it. For those who ultimately land in clinical practice, the only question about their career thereafter is whether they wish to own a practice someday. I recall very few conversations about alternative career paths, such as becoming a public service veterinarian or an industry representative for a pet food or pharmaceutical company. The reality is that there are many jobs that a person with a DVM degree can have—jobs that are in dire need of filling thanks to the current shortage of veterinarians.

Veterinarian and best-selling author of *All Dogs Go to Kevin,* Jessica Vogelsang, wrote an article for *DVM360* in 2016 titled "37 Ways to Use a DVM Degree."[1] In it, Dr. Vogelsang highlights the fact that most vet students perceive their post-graduate choices to be either (1) starting work right away or (2) applying for an internship. She then highlights the various career paths that a veterinarian can pursue, including what she refers to as "The obvious" (practice owner, private practice association, corporate practice associate, locum, practice manager), "The specialties" (rehabilitation, acupuncture or chiropractic, cat-only, zoo medicine, laboratory medicine, forensics), "The niches" (behavior, hospice, mobile, vaccine-only, wildlife, military, government, telemedicine, law), "The nonprofits" (animal rescues, shelters, animal

DOI: 10.1201/9781003347385-40

welfare, disaster response), "The teaching" (professor, speaker, media source, social media influencer, consultant, coach, writer, editor), and "The industry" (technical services veterinary, diagnostic laboratories, entrepreneur). Even this exhaustive list of options doesn't fully encompass everything that a DVM degree qualifies a person to do.

An article published in 2020 in *Veterinary Sciences* identified at least 16 different roles that veterinarians in the United States can fill, as collated from publicly available resources on the American Veterinary Medical Association website (Box 1).[2] Examples include caring for zoo, wildlife, non-domestic, pet, farm, or aquatic animals; working in animal shelters or rescues organizations; studying the effects of pesticides and pollutants on both animals and humans; evaluating the safety and efficacy of medical products and pet foods; ensuring the safety of the human food supply; and participating in disease surveillance and antiterrorism protocols. These roles can be applied to most countries (with different titles or government agencies of course), and they are a testament to the vast number of opportunities for veterinarians that often get overlooked by the public and those working within the profession.

Box 1: Did You Know?

There are nearly 20 roles that a veterinarian in the United States can have, including the following[2]:

- Care for zoo/wildlife/non-domestic animals and aquatic animals and fish residing in aquariums, wildlife sanctuaries, and other parks
- Care for pet animals
- Work in Centers for Disease Control and Prevention (CDC) to protect human populations from disease
- Work in animal shelters and rescue operations
- Work in USDA Animal and Plant Health Inspection Service (APHIS) to monitor the development of vaccines for safety and effectiveness
- Care for farm animals, including those entering the food system (e.g., cows, pigs, chickens, turkeys, sheep, etc.)
- Work in the National Institutes of Health (NIH) and its National Library of Medicine
- Work in the US Air Force Biomedical Science Corps as public health officers
- Work in private industries providing animal care and conducting research in animal and human health
- Work in US Army Veterinary Corps providing protection from bioterrorism and care of government-owned animals and their interests

- Work in USDA Agricultural Research Service (ARS) and the National Institute of Food and Agriculture (NIFA) for research, research administration, and animal care
- Work in the Environmental Protection Agency (EPA) studying the effects of pesticides, industrial pollutants, and other contaminants on animals and humans
- Work in the US Food and Drug Administration (FDA), evaluating the safety and efficacy of medicines, medical products, pet foods, and food additives
- Work in the USDA Food Safety and Inspection Service (FSIS) to ensure safety of the human food supply
- Work in the US Department of Homeland Security developing disease surveillance and antiterrorism procedures and protocols
- Work in USDA Animal and Plant Health Inspection Service (APHIS) for disease surveillance to prevent foreign animal diseases from entering the country

When I graduated in 2004, nearly all my 70-ish classmates went into food animal, companion animal, or equine practice. More than a few of us, myself included, pursued advanced training through internships or research programs, but the vast majority went straight into what most people picture when they think of a veterinarian. For those of us who did not enter clinical practice after veterinary school, a couple are no longer working in the veterinary profession and the rest who completed internship programs went on to residencies and became board-certified specialists. Incidentally, some of us who became specialists are no longer in clinical practice full-time: one is working as a relief specialist and another as director of teleconsulting for a large veterinary corporation. The point being, aside from a few exceptions, the public perception of what a veterinarian does for work is reflected in the career trajectories of my graduating class.

The authors of the article "Public Perceptions of Veterinarians from Social and Online Media Listening" captured more than 1.7 million mentions of terms such as veterinarian, #veterinarian, veterinary medicine, and others between September 2017 and November 2019.[3] The results revealed a striking absence of terms pertaining to veterinary roles beyond caring for household pets and companion animals. This highlights the disparity between how the general population perceives veterinarians' roles in society in comparison to the diverse career opportunities that are available, many of which influence the health and wellbeing of humans.

The reason it's important to highlight the discrepancy between the public's perception of what a veterinarian does and the reality of what they can do is so that a diverse pool of applicants can be attracted to vet medicine to fulfill the many vacancies open for vets in so-called alternative career paths. Likewise, it's important for current vets to recognize the different options available to them as they move through their careers. Burnout, job dissatisfaction, injuries, parenting responsibilities, and a myriad of other factors can lead a person to choose to leave their clinical practice role. However, many who make that shift are left with the unsettling feeling that there's "nowhere else to go" or "nothing else to do" beyond their traditional clinical role.

This is precisely why social media groups such as *DVMoms: GAIN*, a veterinary group for veterinarian mothers with government, academic, industry, and non-clinical careers, have emerged in recent years.[4] The private group, created in 2020, now has more than 4,600 members—and continues to grow. In the group, you'll find posts from veterinarians—all of whom also identify as moms— who have left full-time clinical practice to pursue careers in government (e.g., emergency preparedness, public health, US Food and Drug Administration), academia (e.g., teaching in community colleges, veterinary schools, universities, or even high schools), industry (e.g., technical services roles with major pet food or pharmaceutical companies), and a wide range of other roles, including consulting, telemedicine, writing, and more. At least one or two jobs are posted to the page weekly with questions shared pertaining to transitioning from practice to non-clinical careers.

Similarly, *Vets: Stay, Go, Diversify* was founded in 2018 by Ebony Escalona, a UK-based veterinarian working for an international equine charity. It began as a private Facebook group aimed at supporting veterinarians in staying within the profession, exploring diverse career paths, or transitioning out of vet medicine entirely, and has grown into a thriving online community. With more than 25,000 members, it continues to provide an inclusive platform where veterinarians can connect, share job opportunities (mostly outside of clinical practice), and seek guidance on topics such as contract negotiation, interviews, resume writing, and starting a business.[5] This continued engagement in this community is a testament to the growing awareness that veterinary professionals are not limited to a single career path—and that many fulfilling alternatives exist both within and beyond the walls of a clinic.

The limited career path envisioned by many vet students hasn't gone unnoticed—government agencies and corporations have recognized the need to educate and attract veterinarians into fields like biomedical research and public health. In response to this need, the Cornell Leadership Program for Veterinary Students was developed to provide a unique summer research experience for prospective veterinarians who want to influence the profession through a science-based career, outside of traditional practice roles. In addition to the research experience gained during the 10-week program, students also receive career counseling and exposure to graduate training opportunities that promote career paths as scientists or public health professionals. In addition to having a strong interest in research, applicants from across the

United States must have completed their first year of vet school and be at least six months from graduation at the time the program begins.[6]

A study published in 2020 in the *Journal of Veterinary Medical Education* evaluated surveys collected between 1990 and 2016 from more than 600 alumni of the Cornell Leadership Program for Veterinary Students. The authors aimed to determine whether the inspiration and experience of the program translated to a commitment to a career in science. What they found was that the career ambitions expressed by students while participating in the program differed greatly from their actual outcomes. For example, one-third of a surveyed cohort aspired to a career in academia, but less than half ultimately achieved that goal. In contrast, more than 60% of those who had no clear career objective ended up working in clinical practice.[7,8] As is the case for many vet students, those without a definitive career plan often find themselves in a practice setting by default.

The journey from the conventional narrative of veterinary medicine to the uncharted territory of alternative career paths challenges long-held assumptions. Reflecting on my own path and the evolving landscape of the profession, I'm continually amazed by the expanding range of roles veterinarian can fill—far beyond traditional clinical practice. Discovering that veterinarians can serve as public health leaders, industry innovators, government stewards, or educators underscores the incredible versatility of a DVM degree. The gap between public perception and the breadth of available opportunities is more than a passing observation—it's a call to action. It invites aspiring veterinarians to consider the many pathways open to them, and it encourages those already in the field to rethink their career trajectories. The rise of supportive online communities like DVMoms: GAIN and Vets: Stay, Go, Diversify reflects a growing recognition that there is no single "right" path in veterinary medicine. By challenging the narrow career mold often perpetuated in veterinary training, we open the door to a more diverse, innovative profession—one better positioned to make a meaningful impact on both animal and human wellbeing.

The Unsung Heroes of Veterinary Medicine

The Taco Bell near my apartment was paying $1 less per hour than I was making as an RVT after I graduated. I was nursing patients and on my feet 12 or more hours per day, calculating complex infusions, dealing with aggressive patients, putting in central lines, taking arterial blood samples, and more. All for $1 more per hour than if I was rolling burritos.

—Leilani Mustillo, RVT (CEO, Animal HealthLink)

I couldn't do the clinical work I do as an emergency and critical care specialist without the support of my veterinary technicians/technologists (VTs). Referred to as veterinary nurses in some countries, VTs are, in my opinion, the backbone of clinical practice. In general companion animal clinics, these dedicated professionals perform essential tasks such as taking X-rays, collecting blood samples, administering medications, and assisting with anesthesia, dentistry, and surgery. They also play a vital role in educating pet owners on topics like nutrition, deworming, dental care, and environmental enrichment.

In the intensive care unit (ICU), where I spend most of my clinical practice time, the work of my VTs is absolutely crucial to the care our patients receive. They monitor vital signs, perform blood draws and run cage side tests, place nasal oxygen cannulas and feeding tubes, insert indwelling catheters into arteries and veins, assess patients for pain, and assist during patient assessments or advanced procedures such as abdominocentesis (belly tap) or chest tube placement. At this point in my career, I've truly lost count of the number of times a VT has saved a patient by alerting me to a sudden change— worsening vitals, labored breathing, or signs of deterioration. I rely on my VTs to be my eyes and ears in the ICU while I juggle client phone calls, update medical records, and review lab work or imaging.

VTs work in various settings, including general practices, referral hospitals, academic institutions, research facilities, zoos, and animal shelters. The schooling that VTs receive varies from a two-year to a four-year degree, but, in most jurisdictions, VTs must take a credentialing exam to become registered, licensed, or certified, depending on the requirements of the state or province in which they work (Box 1). The titles "RVT" (Registered Veterinary Technician or Technologist), "LVT" (Licensed Veterinary Technician), "CVT"

DOI: 10.1201/9781003347385-41

(Certified Veterinary Technician), and "VN" (Veterinary Nurse) all refer to professionals in the field of veterinary technology who have completed the necessary education and training to provide medical care to animals under the supervision of a licensed veterinarian. The specific title and requirements can vary geographically, but, in general, the term "VN" is used in the United Kingdom, Australia, and New Zealand, and "VT" is used in the United States and Canada.

Box 1: Did You Know?

According to the US Bureau of Labor Statistics, VTs are among the 30 fastest growing occupations, with one of the highest projected percent changes in employment anticipated between 2022 and 2032.[1] In 2022, there were nearly 123,000 jobs for VTs, and the outlook for 2032 shows an increase of 21%, which is seven times higher than the national average of 3% across all occupations.[2]

In the United States, the National Association of Veterinary Technicians in America (NAVTA) launched the Veterinary Nurse Initiative in 2015 to begin the conversation about changing the title of "veterinary technician" to "veterinary nurse." This motion was met with strong resistance from the American Nurses Association (ANA), which would not endorse the proposed change. The ANA stated that the title "nurse" is protected and should be used only for the care of humans. Instead, they suggested that NAVTA unite under one of their preexisting titles for VTs.[3] Because I strongly believe that the work my VTs do under my supervision in the ICU is equivalent to the care provided for sick and hospitalized human patients, I often refer to my VTs as VNs when speaking to pet owners. This terminology helps convey to families the full scope of care that VTs provide for their pets, whereas terms like "technologist" or "tech" might lead many to think of software development or data analysis. In short, I feel that the designation of "nurse" gives VTs the respect and recognition they truly deserve.

Like the prospect of veterinarians becoming specialists in particular fields, VTs can also become a veterinary technician specialist (VTS), which involves obtaining specialized certification in a specific area of veterinary medicine, such as emergency and critical care, dentistry, internal medicine, or anesthesia (Box 2). To achieve this designation, candidates must have graduated from a VT program and passed the Veterinary Technician National Examination (VTNE). They then need to complete rigorous advanced training and education that involves gaining hands-on experience in their chosen specialty for a minimum number of years, applying to a recognized academy, passing a specialized exam, and maintaining certification through continuing education. VTS certification signifies a high level of expertise and dedication within a particular field of veterinary technology, allowing VTs to excel in their chosen specialization. I have had the honor and great pleasure of working with many VTS(ECC) VTs who spent years obtaining their certification as a specialist in emergency and critical care. Their advanced skills and knowledge in my area of specialization make them invaluable assets to the ICU patient care team.

Box 2: Veterinary Technician Specialties Recognized by the National Association of Veterinary Technicians in America[4]

- Academy of Veterinary Emergency and Critical Care Technicians and Nurses
- Academy of Veterinary Dental Technicians
- Academy of Internal Medicine Veterinary Technicians (specialties in Cardiology, Neurology, Small Animal, Large Animal, and Oncology)
- Academy of Veterinary Technicians in Anesthesia and Analgesia
- Academy of Veterinary Zoological Medicine Technicians
- Academy of Veterinary Technicians in Clinical Practice (specialties in Small Animal [Canine/Feline], Small Animal [Feline], Exotic Companion Animal, and Production Medicine)
- Academy of Laboratory Animal Veterinary Technicians and Nurses (specialties in Research Clinical Nursing [Traditional], Research Clinical Nursing [Non-Traditional], Research Surgeon, and Research Anesthetist)
- Academy of Veterinary Behavior Technicians
- Academy of Veterinary Clinical Pathology Technicians
- Academy of Dermatology Veterinary Technicians
- Academy of Equine Veterinary Nursing Technicians
- Academy of Physical Rehabilitation Veterinary Technicians
- Academy of Veterinary Nutrition Technicians
- Academy of Veterinary Ophthalmic Technicians
- Academy of Veterinary Surgical Technicians
- Academy of Veterinary Technicians in Diagnostic Imaging

It might seem unlikely that those who work directly with animals most of their days would experience struggles similar to, or even exceeding, those of veterinarians (Box 3). Yet, the American Animal Hospital Association reports that the attrition rate for VTs is approximately 25%, meaning that one out of every four VTs either leaves or transitions to a new veterinary job at any given time.[5] Why? This statistic shows that year after year, hundreds—if not thousands—of individuals choose careers as VTs, only to opt out within just a few years. Is it the demands and risks of the job? The fact that they are paid much less than their human nursing counterparts? Or both?

Box 3: Did You Know?

In the United States[6] and Australia,[7] studies show that VTs have a higher risk of suicide, with standardized mortality ratios ranging from 1.25 to 5 times higher than the expected number of suicide deaths in the general population. *If you or someone you know are experiencing thoughts of suicide, help is available.* Please call 988 (USA or Canada) or 0800 689 5652 (United Kingdom). Other suicide support lines can be found here: https://blog.opencounseling.com/suicide-hotlines/.

There's no disputing that the job of a VT can be physically demanding, requiring lifting and restraining pets, long hours standing, and exposure to animal-related injuries. Two decades ago, researchers in Australia investigated the occupational hazards faced by VTs and published their survey results in the *Australian Veterinary Journal.* Of the nearly 150 responses collected, there was a high prevalence of exposure to X-rays (97%), anesthetics (96%), disinfectants (96%), formaldehyde (76%), and pesticides or insecticides (71%). Acute injuries were incredibly common, including dog or cat bites or scratches (98%), needle stick injuries (71%), and lacerations (43%). More than half of the VTs reported chronic neck or back pain, and 39% reported allergies of some kind.[8] A different study surveying veterinarians and VTs in Ohio found a 12-month prevalence of musculoskeletal discomfort of 60% respondents, affecting the neck, low back, and legs or feet, with 43% of the work performed by VTs rated as high or very high risk, compared to just 9% of activities performed by veterinarians.[9] In other words, VTs are truly doing the "heavy lifting" in veterinary practice.

In addition to the physical toll of veterinary work, VTs also experience tremendous emotional stress in dealing with ethically challenging situations and difficult interactions with pet owners or team members. I see my VTs as the true "frontline" workers of veterinary practice, as they're usually the first to speak with the client and examine the pet during emergency or wellness visits. As such, they often bear the brunt of the emotional backlash from pet owners, especially in response to distressing medical situations or large financial estimates. It's also not uncommon for pet owners to be dismissive or demeaning to VTs, only to be sweet as pie once the veterinarian enters the room—a situation that makes my skin crawl. I have zero tolerance for clients who fail to treat every veterinary team member with the same respect. On rare occasions, I've had to reprimand clients who do not treat my VTs with the dignity and compassion they deserve.

When it comes to client complaints in particular, recent research demonstrates that VTs are heavily affected. A study published in 2022 in *Veterinary Medicine and Science* reviewed more than 550 questionnaires from veterinary support staff, including VTs. Approximately one-third reported being subject to a client complaint in the previous six months, with the cost of care being the primary reason (79%). About half reported feeling depressed because of the client complaint and more than one-quarter considered changing their career because of it.[10] Perhaps surprisingly, clients are not the only individuals to impact the mental wellbeing of VTs. Research from Japan, published in the *Open Veterinary Journal* the same year, demonstrated that of the more than 100 survey responses collected from VTs, 41% reported experiences of verbal or physical violence or sexual harassment, with staff members implicated as the most common perpetrators.[11] Unfortunately, I've witnessed verbal harassment from veterinarians toward VTs in the workplace, ranging from muttered insults to yelling and swearing. While in most veterinary settings these behaviors are few and far between, the toll they take cannot be overstated.

Given that workplace stressors, including conflict and poor interpersonal dynamics, are strongly linked to job dissatisfaction, it may come as no surprise that burnout is a growing problem among VTs. Research conducted by Merck Animal Health and the American Veterinary Medical Association in 2021 demonstrated that, compared to one-third of veterinarians, half of staff respondents (including VTs) reported high levels of burnout.[12] Similarly, a report published in *Veterinary Anaesthesia and Analgesia* in 2023 showed that, among nearly 400 anesthesia team members completing the survey worldwide, less than half of anesthesia specialists met criteria for burnout, compared to 80% of anesthesia VTs. Astoundingly, nearly 90% of the anesthesia VTs working in North America who responded to the survey met criteria for burnout.[13]

The relationship between work-related demands, resources, and wellbeing among VTs was first explored in a 2016 study published in the *New Zealand Veterinary Journal*. Researchers found that VTs with high job demands—such as heavy workloads, emotional strain, or complex tasks—or limited job resources were more likely to experience emotional exhaustion, a core symptom of burnout. The study also identified key job resources that helped reduce attrition, including opportunities for skill development, task predictability, and recognition. Positive team relationships were also highlighted as essential workplace resources.[14]

Similar themes emerged in a 2020 study published in *Frontiers in Veterinary Science*, which analyzed more than 1,600 survey responses from practicing VTs around the world to assess burnout. More than half of the respondents had scores indicating burnout. Job resources that were predictive of lower burnout scores included schedule control, a sense of adding value to the practice, and opportunities for professional development.[15] These findings mirror the countless conversations I've had with VTs over the years. They simply want to enjoy the people they work with, feel supported by those they work for, have some control over their schedules and tasks, and know that they have the chance to progress in their careers.

And while you might assume that VTs fare better than human nurses when it comes to burnout, research suggests otherwise. A study of more than 250 VTs employed at veterinary teaching hospitals in the United States and Canada revealed that their burnout scores were actually higher than those reported among human trauma nurses. The primary factors associated with burnout in these VTs included fear or anxiety related to supervisor communications, perceptions that patient loads were too high to allow for excellent care, and a lack of available assistance during sudden increases in workload.[16] This research has prompted many veterinary hospital managers worldwide to strive for patient-to-VT ratios that align with the severity of illness and level of care required. Still, ongoing VT shortages and high veterinary caseloads continue to place many VTs remain at a greater risk of burnout than ever before.

Another testament of the dedication of VTs to the animals they care for—and to the veterinary profession—is the fact that most are paid little more than a living wage. According to the US Bureau of Labor Statistics, the median pay for a VT in May 2022 was $38,240 USD per year, or $18.38 USD per hour.[2] Low pay has been consistently cited as a major concern among VTs in the United States surveyed by the NAVTA.[17] Similarly, in in the United Kingdom, the median pay for a VN in March 2022 was £24,227. A 2019 Survey of the Veterinary Nurse Profession revealed that 25% of VTs said they were planning to leave the profession within five years, with 77% citing low pay as the main reason.[18] In Canada, while the national median and hourly wage have gradually increased, the gains have been minimal when adjusted for inflation. In 2015, the average hourly wage for a VT was $19 CAD, and by 2019, it had only increased to $20.45 CAD when inflation-adjusted.[19]

I personally know of more than a dozen extremely talented, intelligent, and dedicated VTs who have made the heartbreaking decision to leave the profession in pursuit of better-paying careers. Most often, these are young professionals who dream of starting a family and buying a house, but quickly recognize that a VT salary makes these goals difficult—if not imossible—especially if they are single or relying solely on their income. Many transition to similar hands-on professions such as human nursing, ultrasound or X-ray technology, or physical therapy. Others choose to go back to school to become veterinarians.

Thankfully, I've started to see positive shifts in the profession. More practices and hospitals are utilizing VTs to their full scope of practice and paying them more accordingly. Some have committed to paying a salary that allows for a decent standard of living, while others offer bonuses, equity opportunities, or unlimited continuing education to help VTs pursue certifications, specializations, or advanced practitioner or leadership roles.[18,20] The VTs I've had the privilege of working alongside absolutely deserve to be paid more—

and systemic steps must be taken throughout across the profession to support their retention and satisfaction.

VTs are the unsung heroes of veterinary medicine. Though they often work in the shadows, they play a pivotal role in patient care. Their responsibilities, expertise, and compassion make them indispensable members of the veterinary team. Yet the challenges they face—from physical strain to emotional stress and financial hardships—are immense and must be addressed. For the profession to thrive, a concerted effort must be made to provide VTs with the recognition, compensation, and support they deserve. This includes advocating for standardized titles, promoting specialized training, and creating healthier, more respectful workplaces. By truly valuing and empowering VTs, we not only improve their wellbeing—we elevate the quality of care for our patients, strengthen client relationships, and support the sustainability of the veterinary profession as a whole.

38

Responding to the Veterinary Workforce Crisis

The pandemic staffing shortages had a huge effect on the ER / specialty clinic where I work. We lost a number of staff during the pandemic, and we struggled for years post-pandemic to get back to minimum staffing numbers. We could not be open 24/7, and our ER was closed for 2 days each week. During that time, even when the ER was open, we were often closed to outpatients since we had reached capacity with the current numbers of inpatients. The staffing shortage prevented our team from working efficiently and from seeing the number of pets that we normally could. This situation had a significant impact on the veterinary care that we were able to provide for our community.

—Katharine Woods, DVM, DVSc, DACVIM
(Small Animal Internal Medicine Specialist)

In recent decades, there has been a significant rise in pet ownership worldwide, leading to a greater demand for veterinary services. Countries like Canada, the United States, the United Kingdom, China, and Australia have all experienced an increase in dog and cat ownership. This trend predates the pandemic but saw a substantial boost in 2020 when millions of people globally adopted pets (Box 1). Several factors, including demographic shifts, increasing income levels, and the impact of the pandemic, have contributed to this trend. In the United States, millennials, who tend to delay having children, work remotely or in hybrid setups, and possess higher incomes and education levels, make up a significant proportion of pet owners. Additionally, a growing middle class, fueled by rising wages, is also likely driving pet purchases and adoptions.[1] This surge in pet ownership has had a significant impact on the veterinary profession, where more than three-quarters of practitioners provide companion animal care. With more households seeking veterinary care, the demand for such services in the United States has grown by over 6% annually, even after adjusting for inflation.[2]

DOI: 10.1201/9781003347385-42

Box 1: Did You Know?

During the pandemic lockdowns, more than 2 million people adopted a pet in the United Kingdom and more than a million pets were adopted in Australia.[1]

Unfortunately, the supply of veterinary professionals has not kept up with the growing demand, leading to a staffing strain throughout the industry. In Canada, for example, the population of about 13,000 veterinarians must rise by at least 4% per year to meet the growing demand. But Canada's five veterinary colleges graduate only about 450 practitioners per year—enough to cover essentially only those retiring from the profession.[3] Likewise, for decades, there has been a shortage of veterinarians in certain sectors of the profession – particularly food animal, equine practice, and public health—and in recent years, this shortage has increasingly extended to academia, shelters, emergency, and specialty practice.[4] The low supply of companion animal practitioners, coupled with high demand, has led to a dramatic increase in salaries for traditionally termed small animal veterinarians. As a result, other sectors of veterinary medicine are experiencing increased strain, now seen as less attractive alternative career paths.[5]

The scarcity of specialist veterinarians, compounded by shortages in other essential roles such as emergency veterinarians, technicians/nurses, and support staff, presents a significant challenge within the veterinary profession. As a board-certified specialist in emergency and critical care, I'm acutely aware of this increasingly pervasive issue. Practices struggle to maintain stable client care teams, with turnover occurring every two to three months in some cases. These shortages have dire consequences for pet owners, resulting in prolonged wait times for appointments and more severe illnesses upon presentation. Overwhelmed general practice teams are often forced to refer cases to specialists or emergency clinics due to limited capacity, exacerbating the strain on the entire veterinary care system. Pet owners face the frustrating reality of extended wait times—or even being turned away—highlighting the urgent need for solutions to address staffing shortages and improve access to veterinary care.

The impact of veterinary shortages has been widely reported since 2021, with numerous news articles and reports highlighting the challenges faced by pet owners worldwide. Stories have emerged detailing long wait times for existing clients, difficulties in finding veterinarians for new pet owners, and limited or no access to care in rural or remote areas. Even veterinary teaching hospitals—typically considered the pinnacle of emergency and referral medicine—have been affected. Reports in 2022[6] and 2023[7] revealed that two veterinary schools in Canada had to close their emergency services overnight due to staffing shortages, forcing pet owners to travel long distances for care.

Urban emergency hospitals have also been forced to close temporarily or permanently due to a lack of veterinarians and support staff.[8]

Recent analyses by Mars Veterinary Health reveal a significant surplus of open positions for specialist veterinarians compared to the available candidates in the current job market, with up to four times more openings than expected candidates. This surplus raises concerns, particularly for academic veterinary medicine, where up to 50% of the faculty are trained in recognized clinical specialties.[9] The indispensable roles that specialists play in teaching and research within this sector could result in a prolonged shortage of graduating veterinarians, disproportionately affecting access to veterinary care and impeding scientific advancements in veterinary medicine for years to come.

According to projections by Mars Veterinary Health, up to 55,000 additional veterinarians will be required to meet the demands of companion animal healthcare in the United States by 2030. Despite the existence of 33 veterinary schools in the United States and over a dozen more in various stages of development, with some graduating their first classes in 2023 and beyond, Mars Veterinary Health predicts a shortage of up to 24,000 companion animal veterinarians by 2030. Moreover, they anticipate that more than 30 years' worth of credentialed veterinary technicians will need to graduate to fulfill the projected ten-year industry need.[10]

These figures are in stark contrast to the American Veterinary Medical Association's (AVMA's) stance, which argues that the number of veterinarians providing services for companion animals will grow by more than 20% between 2022 and 2030, primarily due to historical increases in veterinary school class sizes and the development of additional schools. The AVMA also highlights the challenge of predicting graduating veterinarian preferences for areas or species of work, as well as changes in work hours and other aspects of veterinary medicine.[4] These conflicting studies highlight the complexity of projecting the demand for veterinarians in the United States and globally.

Considering these conflicting projections, a recent report "Demand for and Supply of Veterinarians in the US to 2032" takes a different approach, starting with broad economic projections and utilizing ten-year forecasts of occupational growth and turnover from the US Bureau of Labor Statistics. Their analysis projects a total growth and turnover need of more than 70,000 new veterinarians through 2032, while only 76% of this demand is expected to be met by the projected 53,000 veterinary graduates. This shortfall, which may not be evenly distributed geographically, could be addressed by reducing veterinarian turnover, improving efficiency, and increasing the supply of graduates. Recommendations include prioritizing veterinarian mental health, leveraging technology for efficiency gains, and expanding the role of veterinary technicians and nurses. Additionally, there may be a need for further expansion of veterinary programs to meet the evolving demand for veterinarians.[11]

Because the veterinary workforce shortage has reached unprecedented levels, particularly in companion animal practice, national veterinary organizations have begun to prioritize the issue and seek long-term solutions. In 2022, the British Veterinary Association's (BVA's) senior vice president, Dr. Justine Shotton, identified the workforce problem as the profession's most significant challenge and committed to taking action to mitigate its worsening impact.[12] Similarly, organizations such as the Canadian Veterinary Medical Association (CVMA)[3] and the Australian Veterinary Association (AVA)[13] have recognized the workforce shortage as a critical issue, leading to the establishment of committees, task forces, and recommendations aimed at addressing the shortage of veterinary professionals. The CVMA's Veterinary Workforce Project, for instance, has developed Priority Pathways focusing on a multipronged approach to meeting the supply of veterinary professionals (Box 2).[3]

Box 2: Priority Pathways Established by the CVMA Veterinary Workforce Project[3]

- protocols for recruiting internationally trained veterinary team members
- strategies for enhancing retention among veterinary team members
- tools for navigating the immigration process when hiring internationally trained veterinarians
- addressing the shortage of veterinarians in rural and remote areas
- developing and implementing pathways for restricted or limited licensure for Canadian and internationally trained veterinarians
- increasing the national examination capacity for internationally trained veterinarians
- increasing capacity at Canadian veterinary colleges
- increasing university programs tailored to internationally trained veterinarians
- developing wellbeing and mental health resources for veterinary professionals
- implementing a workforce shortage public awareness campaign speaking to the value and roles of veterinarians

---

The AVMA similarly advocates for a multifaceted approach to solving the veterinary workforce shortage. They emphasize the importance of both recruiting and educating new veterinarians, but they highlight that the retention of current professionals is equally crucial. Retention has long been a serious issue for many veterinary practices, with turnover rates often surpassing those of other industries. For instance, a 2020 report by the American Animal Hospital Association found an annual turnover rate of 23% in veterinary practice—significantly higher than the average turnover rate of 12%–15% in the hospitality industry nationwide.[14] In some practices I've worked in, the annual turnover rate for certain positions has approached 50%, indicating that half of the team members leave their roles within a year. These high turnover rates place tremendous strain on practices, and, in cases of particularly negative experiences, some veterinary professionals may even leave the profession altogether.

It's striking how a lack of mentorship can profoundly impact veterinarians' career trajectories. For example, a friend from my veterinary school class, more than a year after graduating, revealed that she had left her first job out of veterinary school to work in a bakery. This was someone who had long aspired to be a veterinarian, so her decision to abandon veterinary medicine shocked me, especially considering her amiable nature, pragmatic approach to medicine, and natural ability to connect with others. As we discussed her experience, it became clear that her dissatisfaction stemmed from unrealistic expectations and the absence of mentorship and support from her practice management and team. Sadly, her story is not unique. Many of our classmates faced similar situations, arriving at their first jobs with expectations of mentorship and guidance, only to find themselves left to navigate the complexities of practice on their own. Some persevered, determined to provide the support they wished they had received, while others sought opportunities elsewhere that offered the mentorship and training they desired.

Numerous veterinary organizations and companies recognize the importance of mentorship and coaching to enhance job satisfaction and retention of newly graduated veterinarians. In the United Kingdom, for instance, the Veterinary Graduate Development Programme (VetGDP) was established to support the skills development of new veterinarians in alignment with their specific roles. Under VetGDP, each new vet is paired with a workplace coach, referred to as an Advisor, who undergoes comprehensive training in educational and social theories, as well as the latest coaching and feedback research in medical education. Utilizing an online learning platform, Advisors provide tailored support to new vets during the program. VetGDP is widely implemented across the United Kingdom and is accessible to all recent graduate veterinarians. To ensure program quality and engagement, the Royal College of Veterinary Surgeons (RCVS) oversees its implementation through the RCVS Code of Professional Conduct and performs regular checks. Ultimately, the program aims to facilitate optimal professional growth for new vets and foster positive learning environments within their workplaces.[15]

In the United States, MentorVet, a veterinary mentorship and professional development program dedicated to enhancing early career wellbeing, collaborated with the AVMA to launch MentorVet Connect in 2023. This initiative offers a free mentoring program to any AVMA member who graduated from veterinary school within the past five years. MentorVet Connect partners early career veterinarians with trained mentors from outside their workplace, to provide them with emotional and career support, and act as advisors and sounding boards for various inquiries over a six-month period.[16] MentorVet has also piloted MentorVetTech, aimed at supporting veterinary technicians.

Both MentorVet and MentorVetTech demonstrate improvements in wellbeing and reductions in burnout among their program participants, marking significant strides toward reducing attrition within the veterinary community.[17]

While numerous recommendations and programs are aimed at mitigating the shortage of veterinarians, a critical gap remains in addressing shortages among other vital members of the veterinary team. In my conversations with veterinary practice owners and managers, a recurring concern emerges: while there may be an adequate number of veterinarians, there's often a shortfall in the number of technicians or assistants essential for facilitating veterinarians' work efficiently. This shortage translates into delays in crucial procedures like lab work, X-rays, emergency surgeries, and other essential tasks due to insufficiently trained veterinary technicians or technologists available. Although many veterinary technician and technology schools are increasing their graduate numbers to meet the growing demand, the persistently high attrition rates among these professionals underscore the need for comprehensive measures to attract and retain them in the profession long term.

Considering the current state of the veterinary profession, it's clear that while some progress has been made, significant challenges remain. Initiatives like the Veterinary Workforce Project and MentorVet Connect have provided valuable support, but there's still much to be done. Looking ahead, a collaborative effort among veterinary organizations, educational institutions, and industry stakeholders is essential to develop effective solutions. This involves prioritizing mentorship programs, improving retention strategies, and addressing shortages in vital support roles. By taking proactive steps, we can ensure a sustainable and thriving veterinary profession, meeting the needs of both animals and their owners.

Paving a Path to Self-Care and Self-Compassion

> With time and life experience, I have learned to offer myself the same empathy and understanding I strive to give others. In the end, we are all humans trying to do our best. We just need to remember to give ourselves the same care we bestow upon our patients.
>
> —Bobbie Deschamps, RVT, VTS (ECC)
> (Veterinary Nurse)

You would think that veterinarians, regarded as some of the most compassionate caregiving professionals, would find it easy to extend compassion and care toward themselves. Yet, for many veterinarians I know and speak to, the opposite holds true. While they express kindheartedness for the animals they care for and the families who deeply love their pets, veterinarians often inflict on themselves a criticism so fierce, they wouldn't extend it to their worst enemy. I remember lecturing at a regional veterinary teaching conference to more than 50 faculty members—people who dedicate their time to educating and inspiring veterinarians of the future. When I brought up the notion of self-compassion, those in attendance immediately expressed resistance, stating vehemently that their self-criticism was necessary to achieve their goals and avoid making mistakes.

The same resistance is apparent when I encourage veterinarians to practice self-care. Amidst eye-rolling and shoulder shrugs, they make comments like:

"Taking care of myself seems like an indulgence."
"Putting myself first? That just feels wrong."
"I'm too busy taking care of others to worry about myself."
"Self-care feels like a luxury for people with more time."
"Taking time for me? I'd rather be productive."
"Self-care seems selfish when there's so many animals who need my help."
"I feel guilty when I prioritize my own needs."
"Self-care feels like a way to avoid responsibilities."

The sentiment is that self-care seems like a frivolous waste of time, and they'd rather focus on providing care for their patients and clients.

DOI: 10.1201/9781003347385-43

Unfortunately, whether veterinarians see the benefit or not, experts suggest that veterinarians and other caregiving professionals have an ethical duty to take care of themselves. In fact, the Green Cross Academy of Traumatology, a non-profit organization comprised of licensed mental health professionals and other care providers, created Standards of Care Guidelines. The purpose of creating the guidelines was twofold: first, to remind practitioners in any caregiving field to avoid harming themselves while fulfilling their duty to help others; and second, to attend to their own physical, social, emotional, and spiritual needs as a way of ensuring quality care for those they support. The guideline's ethical principles of self-care state that it is "unethical not to attend to your self-care as a practitioner because sufficient self-care prevents harming those we serve."[1]

I can attest to this when I reflect on times in my career when I made a mistake with a patient simply because I wasn't taking care of myself. I remember working a locum shift at a busy specialty referral and emergency hospital, where a dog in severe pain from an undiagnosed condition needed relief in the form of a narcotic drip. A shortage of opioids in our hospital meant that I had to use a drug I was less familiar with, and that I wasn't in the habit of prescribing on a regular basis. Leading up to this shift, I'd over-extended myself and wasn't practicing self-care. By this I mean that my daily routine of getting eight hours of sleep, exercising for 45 minutes, walking my dog outside for half an hour, and prioritizing activities like meditation and healthy eating, had all taken a backseat to a marathon stint of shifts, late nights on the couch watching Netflix, and a caffeine and snack food combo to keep me fueled during the day. Consequently, I made a mistake with my patient's drug calculation resulting in a tenfold overdose of a morphine-like drug. This meant that I returned to work the next day to find a dog that was minimally responsive and nearly comatose.

It's in this sort of situation that I'm personally reminded of the importance of self-care in my quest to help animals and their owners. When I try to impart the magnitude of this priority to other veterinarians, I use the flight attendant analogy. When you wait comfortably (or uncomfortably, depending on your seat selection) on the plane for takeoff, you're subjected to the pre-flight spiel from the flight crew. This includes instructions to put on your own oxygen mask *first* before assisting others. The rationale is to prevent you from passing out before you have the chance to help someone else. When I think of my adorable five-year-old, and how difficult this would be for me as a parent in an emergency on an airplane, I can see both the logic in this recommendation and the challenge of putting it into action in real life. I, too, have felt this hesitation and resistance in my career as a veterinarian and acknowledge the difficulty in having to potentially turn away from a patient who needs my help, so that I can first take care of myself.

I often heard this from veterinarians at the beginning of the pandemic, when it seemed like everyone's self-care went out the veterinary clinic window. With team member shortages due to illness, isolation requirements, and childcare responsibilities, those still working were left to manage their usual caseloads—which only grew as pet ownership surged during the pandemic. During these excruciating years, veterinarians often told me they felt they had no choice but to keep going. Taking time off for rest or self-care felt impossible, knowing how few others were available to help and how great the demand had become. This, of course, led to a rise in burnout among many veterinarians, some of whom ultimately took time off, left clinical practice, or exited the profession entirely.

When I share the need for self-care with other veterinarians, I lead with my own experiences of burnout and how my absence of self-care contributed to it. Granted, burnout is a consequence that results from many factors, some of which are systemic or organizational and completely unrelated to self-care. However, I will say that I had experiences of burnout brought on by my own inability to look after myself, which now stand out as reminders that caring for myself must come first so I can properly and compassionately care for others. Examples include:

- Taking breaks: during shifts and between shifts to rest, refuel, and rehydrate

- Practicing mindfulness: tuning into my thoughts, feelings, and bodily sensations to manage my stress and enhance my emotional regulation

- Seeking support: connecting with colleagues, friends, family members, and mental health professionals to discuss work and non-work stressors

- Prioritizing hobbies: getting to the mountains for a hike or rollerblading on the riverwalk to remind myself of who I am and what I do outside of vet medicine

- Setting boundaries: recognizing my limits in the number of shifts I can comfortably work in a row and not letting work bleed into my home life in the form of emails, texts, and other work-related tasks

- Connecting with others: prioritizing my non-work relationships with friends and family to sustain a sense of community and belonging

Importantly, nowhere on my personal list of self-care strategies is lounging on the couch streaming shows and drinking wine. While these are activities I've enjoyed from time to time, I've learned that they're distinctly different from self-care and more aptly termed unhealthy coping strategies. For so many people, myself included, unhealthy coping strategies in the form of substance use, social media scrolling, online shopping, and TV watching function as reflexive distractions or "numbing agents" that, while comforting in the short term, erode wellbeing in the long term. It has helped me to shift my mindset to accepting that not all self-care activities are enjoyable (case in point: go to bed early versus watch another episode), but they are *necessary* for me to show up rested, regulated, and ready to practice vet medicine.

Debbie Stoewen, a veterinarian and licensed mental health professional in Canada, wrote in a 2021 review article in *The Canadian Veterinary Journal*: "Are you practicing medicine? Then you have to practice self-care." She reminds veterinarian readers to balance the activities of life that cause fatigue with other activities that refuel or refresh.[2] These and other sentiments have led me and other researchers to investigate the benefits of self-care practices among veterinary professionals. A few years ago, along with colleagues at the University of Calgary, we investigated associations between self-care practices among pre-clinical veterinary students and their mental health. The results of that survey research, published in 2023 in *The Canadian Veterinary Journal*, revealed that several daily activities were associated with lower depression, anxiety, or stress scores among pre-clinical veterinary students. These included spending at least 15 minutes outside or exercising, spending less than 30 minutes on social media, and sleeping six to eight hours. Additionally, students who felt that self-care techniques "often" managed their stress had lower depression and anxiety scores than those who felt self-care "rarely" managed their stress.[3] Henceforth, understanding the importance of self-care in managing stressors appears to have beneficial effects on mental health when incorporated into a self-care practice.

Another recent study highlighted the importance of self-care conversations among veterinary students later in their training. While education related to self-care across veterinary schools is minimal, if it exists at all, those institutions that do include self-care in the curriculum tend to do so during the pre-clinical years. Researchers at Kansas State University College of Veterinary Medicine strayed from the norm and introduced "authentic conversations about self-care" for fourth-year veterinary medical students as a mandatory part of one of their clinical rotations. Final year students were mandatory to complete a one-on-one session with a behavioral scientist about their stressors and how they coped. The goal of the session was to enhance students' awareness of their existing strengths and "identify simple, actionable steps for improving self-care." This was achieved by asking the students to share how they responded to stress and describe coping strategies generally associated with healthy outcomes. When students described an unhealthy response to stress, the behavioral scientist emphasized the need for change and collaborated with the student to brainstorm small steps to achieve their goal. By the time the study was published in the *Journal of Veterinary Medical Education* in 2022, nearly 700 veterinary students had completed this requirement, which remains a required part of clinical training at that school.[4]

In addition to being aware of the importance of self-care and receiving support in identifying and implementing activities that promote health and wellbeing, an important component of self-care is self-compassion. Dr. Kristin Neff, co-founder of the Center for Mindful Self-Compassion, defines self-compassion as "healthy ways of relating to oneself in times of suffering, whether suffering is caused by failure, perceived inadequacy, or general life difficulties." Self-compassion allows people to accept themselves as humans, with inherent limitations and imperfections. It helps people better tolerate difficult emotions such as anxiety or shame, which are often experienced by veterinarians who recognize the need for self-care but worry that neglecting their own needs could harm the patients they're trying to help. I frequently speak to veterinarians who feel anxious at the thought of taking a day off from work to tend to themselves, fearing that their clients will have nowhere else to turn. Similarly, some vets feel shame, believing they are a "bad veterinarian" or "not good enough at their job" because they must occasionally step away from work to take care of themselves.

Self-compassion is a helpful tool for those who default to self-criticism or consider themselves unworthy of engaging in self-care. It's been a game-changer in my own life, since I first read Dr. Neff's book *Self-Compassion: The Proven Power of Being Kind to Yourself.*[5] In her book, Dr. Neff details the three components of self-compassion, which include:

- Self-kindness (versus self-judgment): embracing warmth and under-standing for ourselves while suffering, failing, or feeling inadequate, instead of disregarding our pain or subjecting ourselves to self-criticism

- Common humanity (versus isolation): acknowledging that suffering and feeling inadequate are part of the human experience and something we all go through

- Mindfulness (versus over-identification): adopting a balanced approach to our negative emotions to ensure that our feelings are neither repressed nor magnified

Along with her detailed explanations of self-compassion and the research studies that demonstrate its benefits for wellbeing, Dr. Neff offers many ex-ercises and activities to strengthen the skill. These include self-compassion journaling, creating a self-compassion mantra, and engaging in self-talk that mirrors how we might speak to a close friend or child, rather than the usu-al self-criticism we direct at ourselves. Over the years, I've engaged in more frequent and deliberate self-compassion practices including listening to self-compassion meditations, journaling about my most shameful experiences as a veterinarian, and even creating my own self-compassion mantra. As a result, I've discovered an improved ability to bounce back from challenging situa-tions and a lessened stress response during difficult times.

Research among veterinary students further supports the idea that practic-ing self-compassion can enhance resilience. A 2017 study published in the *Journal of Veterinary Medical Education* surveyed nearly 200 vet students from six schools in Australia. The researchers measured resilience using the Brief Resilience Scale (Box 1) and self-compassion using the Neff Self-Compassion Scale.[6] The study found, not surprisingly, that vet students with higher self-compassion scores also had higher resilience scores.[7] In other words, those who demonstrated higher levels of self-compassion were better able to recover from setbacks.

Box 1: Did You Know?

The Brief Resilience Scale is used to score a person's ability to recover following setbacks.[8] To calculate the score, each of the following statements are given a Likert-scale of 1 (strongly disagree) to 5 (strongly agree). Scores are added up to give a range of 6 to 30 and then divided by 6 to give an average score out of 6.

- I tend to bounce back quickly after hard times.
- I have a hard time making it through stressful events.
- It does not take me long to recover from a stressful event.
- It is hard for me to snap back when something bad happens.
- I usually come through difficult times with little trouble.
- I tend to take a long time to get over setbacks in my life.

And while, to date, there's no published research specifically measuring self-compassion among veterinarians, a study of more than 360 palliative care nurses and doctors in Australia, published in the *International Journal of Palliative Nursing* in 2018, found a positive correlation between self-compassion and self-care ability. This means that palliative care providers who scored higher for self-compassion were also more likely to practice self-care.[9] It's a compelling reminder that self-compassion and self-care are inextricably linked. For veterinarians, embracing self-compassion could potentially make it easier to engage in self-care practices we know are essential for long-term wellbeing.

My self-care practice is unlikely to let up anytime soon, given the benefits I've seen in my personal and professional life. Whether it's lessening my distress after making a mistake while caring for a patient or giving myself permission to take a break from clinical work when I'm feeling overwhelmed, self-compassion is the throughline that allows me to show up as the best version of myself—for the animals and the people I strive to help. Moreover, fostering a culture of self-care and compassion within the veterinary community can lead to a more resilient profession, better equipped to handle the challenges and pressures of veterinary medicine. By prioritizing our wellbeing, we not only strengthen our ability to provide excellent care, but also help create a supportive and sustainable environment for future generations in the field.

40

Reshaping Veterinary Culture to Value Team Wellbeing

> There's no doubt a veterinary life can be tough at times. We all exist on a sliding scale of wellbeing, from good to poor. While the fluctuations on this scale vary in frequency and intensity for each of us, we all experience low times and need mechanisms to recover. But who is responsible for helping us cope with the challenges and providing and delivering the means of recovery?
>
> —Liz Barton, MA VetMB, MRCVS (Cofounder, WellVet)

When I first worked in my mom's companion animal practice, veterinary medicine was still very much rooted in the adage "the client is always right." Team members often had to deal with clients who were belligerent, rude, or otherwise challenging—and these behaviors were frequently tolerated at the expense of staff wellbeing. Health and other extended benefits were also uncommon for veterinary professionals employed in privately owned practices. While employers might cover costs like licensing and continuing education, they rarely offered health insurance or contributed to retirement plans.

Times have changed. Veterinary team members are now recognized as a precious resource. The old mentality of "the customer comes first" has largely been replaced by zero tolerance policies and no-nonsense responses to behaviors that jeopardize the mental health or wellbeing of the team. In fact, many veterinary corporations now market themselves with slogans like "taking care of the people who take care of the pets," emphasizing their commitment to supporting professional wellness and career longevity. More than ever, veterinary businesses and organizations are realizing that without their employees, they can't provide services—prompting a deeper look at what they're doing to support their people.

An area that has seen a significant improvement is in the benefits offered to new graduate veterinarians. According to the Students of the Canadian Veterinary Medical Association New Graduate Survey results published in June 2023 and including data from the graduating class of 2022, 98% of new veterinarians had their licensing fees paid. Additionally, 94% received coverage for continuing education, 91% had their health insurance premiums paid, 85% had malpractice insurance coverage, 81% had dental insurance premiums

DOI: 10.1201/9781003347385-44

paid, and 59% received sick or compassionate leave coverage.[1] In contrast, among the graduating class of 2020, only 87% had their licensing fees paid, 88% received coverage for continuing education, 69% had health insurance premiums paid, 59% had malpractice insurance coverage, 60% had dental insurance premiums paid, and 37% received sick or compassionate leave coverage.[2]

Similar changes have been seen among veterinary technicians. According to a 2022 survey by the National Association of Veterinary Technicians in America, benefits for vet techs have increased significantly since 2016. At least 60% of employers were providing coverage for vacation, federal holidays, health insurance, sick days, continuing education, travel expenses, retirement plans, and pet care. Additional benefits—such as vision and dental insurance, as well as overtime pay—were also reported and hadn't been mentioned in previous suveys.[3]

The good news for both veterinary employers and employees is that mental health benefits are now more available and affordable than in the past. Two of the most common supports are health insurance that covers mental health treatment and participation in an Employee Assistance Program (EAP). An EAP (or EFAP, which includes coverage for immediate family members) offers support for employees dealing with personal or work-related challenges that could affect their job performance, physical and mental wellbeing, or emotional health. While these programs were once rare in veterinary settings, they're now widely offered through third-party benefit providers.

According to the 2021 Merck Animal Health Veterinarian Wellbeing Study, more than half of surveyed veterinarians reported having medical insurance that covered mental health treatment. However, over one-third were unsure whether their insurance included this coverage. Likewise, nearly half said their employer did not provide an EAP and one-quarter weren't sure.[4] This lack of access—or lack of awareness—underscores the importance of clear communication around available support, so that veterinary team members can easily access the help they need.

The most recent Merck Animal Health Veterinary Team Wellbeing Study conducted in 2023 revealed a similar trend among veterinary support staff: nearly one-third of veterinary technicians, assistants, and receptionists said they did not know whether their health insurance covered mental health counseling or treatment. The study also highlighted significant disparities in EAP and mental health coverage between corporate and privately owned veterinary practices (Box 1).[5]

Box 1: Did You Know?

According to survey responses collected from US veterinary team members in 2023, 61% said that their corporate practice offered EAP compared to 16% of those in non-corporate practice.

In some provinces and states, veterinary medical organizations now offer EAPs or EFAPs to their members as part of membership or licensing dues. This has improved access to mental health support across the profession, making it more consistent for those dealing with personal or work-related challenges. EAPs typically provide free and confidential evaluations, short-term counseling, referrals, and ongoing support services. Many also offer 24/7 assistance, access to a nationwide network of therapists, online wellness platforms, guidance for supervisors, and other services. These programs are designed to help employees cope with stress, substance use, grief, or relationship problems. EFAPs may also cover an employee's dependents and extend support to non-work issues such as legal or financial concerns, as well as assistance in finding elder or childcare.[6]

In the United Kingdom, VetLife is a fee and confidential helpline available by phone or email, offering 24/7 support to veterinarians, veterinary nurses, and vet students (Box 2). The service supports individuals experiencing stress, anxiety, depression, substance use problems, or disordered eating. Its team includes crisis workers, psychiatrists, mental health nurses, and therapists. VetLife Financial Support also provides financial assistance, including emergency aid, debt management help, and sometimes grants or one-time payments for those in need. These efforts—along with others from the Royal College of Veterinary Surgeons' MindMatters initiative—highlight the growing commitment among veterinary organizations to support the health and wellbeing of professionals in the field.[7]

Box 2: Did You Know?

The Vetlife Helpline was first established in 1992 to aid struggling veterinarians in the United Kingdom. In 2021 alone, helpline volunteers responded to 3,390 contacts by email and telephone—an average of 10 contacts per day—offering support related to mental health concerns, stress, work-related troubles, work-life balance, and more.[8]

In 2017, the American Veterinary Medical Association (AVMA) hired a veterinary social worker to serve as Director of Veterinary Wellbeing and Diversity Initiatives, aiming to strengthen mental health and wellness support for veterinarians in the United States. Since then, the AVMA has launched several initiatives, including a dedicated website with resources for suicide prevention, substance use, and crisis support, as well as a robust library of webinars on topics like conflict management, setting boundaries, dealing with rude behavior at work, and coping with burnout. The AVMA has also introduced certificate programs focused on promoting workplace wellbeing, which features modules on workplace culture, self-awareness, social awareness, and communication skills. A strong emphasis has also been placed on suicide prevention, with offerings such as free QPR (Question, Persuade, Refer) Gatekeeper Suicide Prevention Training and resource guides tailored for individuals, organizations, and academic settings for preventing and coping with suicide.[9]

Australia has also recently launched a wellness initiative called THRIVE, aimed at fostering satisfying, prosperous, and healthy careers for veterinarians and veterinary team members. All THRIVE initiatives align with the Australian Veterinary Association (AVA) policy on protecting and improving the mental health of veterinary professionals. This policy highlights of the need to address work-related stressors and implement interventions that promote wellbeing at the individual, team, leadership, and organizational levels. The overarching goal is to develop comprehensive industry frameworks and guidelines that prioritize mental health and wellness throughout the profession. THRIVE is built on three co-pillars: (1) prevention of mental health problems, (2) promotion of mental health and a thriving profession, and (3) protection for individuals experiencing mental health challenges. In addition to offering suicide prevention resources, THRIVE provides a graduate mentoring program, a webinar series, and training in psychological health and safety and mental health first aid. Veterinary professionals and their families also have access to free 24/7 counseling through the AVA Counseling Service, and a wellness app to help optimize health and wellbeing.[10]

Thoughtful, comprehensive, and, frankly, necessary initiatives like these are becoming more common worldwide. In 2024, the Canadian Veterinary Medical Association (CVMA) appointed a Director of Wellbeing and Diversity, Equity, and Inclusion to lead the development of similarly structured programs that complement their existing wellness offerings. These include mental health videos, webinars, and resources, as along with discounted access to The Working Mind, an evidence-based program for employees and managers that promotes mental health and reduces stigma around mental illness in the workplace. Thanks to the CVMA, veterinarians across Canada also have free access to Togetherall, an online peer support platform that offers a safe, 24/7 space to connect, share, and discuss thoughts and experiences. The platform is monitored by licensed mental health professionals who step in when there are concerns about self-harm or suicide.[11]

In addition to the steps taken by veterinary medical associations to better support the mental health and wellness of their members, large veterinary practices and corporations are also offering benefits such as extended coverage for mental health appointments, paid time off specifically for mental health, access to meditation applications like Headspace, discounted gym memberships, robust health spending accounts, and policies to encourage disconnecting from work on days off. While these benefits do not entirely eliminate some of the toxic cultures or challenging work conditions that still present in certain practices, they do help employees feel valued and supported in terms of their mental health and overall wellbeing.

Support for veterinary professionals is also expanding before they even enter the workforce. It's becoming more common for veterinary schools to include components in their curriculum that focus on professional skills. These classes emphasize strategies for maintaining mental and physical health, fostering professional wellbeing, and promoting financial security for long, fulfilling careers. Additionally, it's increasingly common for students to have access to a dedicated social worker or psychologist at their school, helping to overcome some of the historical barriers to mental health support, such as scheduling difficulties due to demanding course loads or the challenge of accessing main campus counseling services. Hopefully these supports will foster a culture of help-seeking and mental health awareness that will benefit veterinarians throughout their careers.

Many of the larger veterinary corporations are also employing social workers to support their teams (Box 3).[12] The role of social workers in these settings can vary, ranging from providing mental health support to veterinary team members to assisting clients who are grappling with end-of-life decisions for their pet or experiencing complicated grief after the death of their animal. There are countless situations in which a veterinary social worker can be helpful. I've had the privilege of working in practices where social workers were available, and I took full advantage of their services whenever possible. One practice had a social worker visit once a week to follow up with families whose pet had been euthanized the week before. In those cases, I'd make sure to notify the social worker of any particularly upsetting euthanasia situations where I was concerned that the owner might experience complicated grief and need additional support. I've also worked in practices with a full-time veterinary social worker who was available in-hospital to communicate with clients when the veterinary team felt a mental health professional was needed. I remember one instance when an owner told me they had nothing to live for if their pet died in the hospital. I immediately contacted the social worker, who intervened and helped the owner access the mental health support they needed.

Box 3: Did You Know?

The University of Tennessee College of Veterinary Medicine and College of Social Work established the first veterinary social work program in the United States in 2002. Since then, hundreds of social workers have completed the Veterinary Social Work Certificate Program (VSW-CP), which offers training in four key areas: the link between human and animal violence, grief and loss, animal-assisted interactions, and compassion fatigue management. With a focus on integrating animals into social work practice ethically, the program aims to equip professional social workers with the skills needed to navigate human-animal relationships across various settings and practice methods.[13]

Not only are social workers and other mental health professionals helpful during crisis situations involving veterinary team members or clients, but they also play a vital role in proactively supporting team wellbeing and workplace dynamics. I know several social workers who lead workshops on self-care, offer coaching around boundaries, and facilitate mediation during times of conflict to help teams function more healthfully. In my experience, simply knowing I have a mental health professional I can call upon alleviates some of the moral stress or anxiety I might otherwise feel when navigating a difficult situation on my own.

A significant shift in the profession's priorities begin in July 2018, when the AVMA and the RCVS collaborated through the Mind Matters International initiative to issue a joint statement on mental health and wellbeing. Since then, this statement has since been endorsed by numerous veterinary organizations around the world[14]:

- Canadian Veterinary Medical Association (August 2019)
- Federation of Veterinarians of Europe (August 2019)
- World Small Animal Veterinary Association (August 2019)
- American Association of Veterinary State Boards (December 2020)
- Veterinary Council of New Zealand (May 2021)
- Federation of European Companion Animal Veterinary Associations (May 2021)
- American Association of Veterinary Medical Colleges (July 2021)
- Australian Veterinary Association (December 2021)
- Veterinary Medical Association Executives (April 2022)

These collective efforts mark a meaningful step forward for the veterinary profession. The adoption of mental health as a shared priority, and the implementation of concrete support initiatives reflect a growing awareness of the need to nurture the wellbeing of veterinary professionals. Still, while the progress is encouraging, the journey is far from over. Continued advocacy, education, and the expansion of supportive programs are essential to maintaining this positive momentum. By fostering a culture of care and compassion, we can build a profession in which veterinary professionals feel truly supported, valued, and empowered. This, in turn, will enhance not only their wellbeing, but also the quality of care they provide to the animals and the people who depend on them.

Author's Note

Thank you for taking the time to read this book and explore the multifaceted world of veterinary medicine with me. I hope it has provided insight into both the joys and the challenges of our profession.

If you feel inspired to take action and support positive change within veterinary medicine, consider learning more about organizations dedicated to advancing and supporting our field. These organizations play crucial roles in advocating for veterinary professionals, promoting wellbeing, and shaping the future of veterinary care.

Here are just a few of the many websites where you can find more information:

- American Animal Hospital Association: https://www.aaha.org/for-veterinary-professionals/wellness-for-veterinary-professionals

- American Veterinary Medical Association (AVMA) Advocacy: https://www.avma.org/advocacy

- Association of Asian Veterinary Medical Professionals (AAVMP): https://www.aavmp.org

- AVMA Wellbeing Resources: https://www.avma.org/resources-tools/wellbeing

- Australia Veterinary Association Thrive: https://www.ava.com.au/Thrive

- BlackDVM Network: https://www.blackdvmnetwork.com

- BlendVET: https://www.blend.vet

- Canadian Veterinary Medical Association (CVMA) Mental Health and Wellness Resources: https://www.canadianveterinarians.net/veterinary-resources/veterinary-health-and-wellness-resources

- Diversify Veterinary Medicine Coalition (DVMC): https://www.diversifyvetmed.org

- Happy Vet Project: https://www.happyvetproject.org

- iMatter: https://www.i-matter.ca
- LatinX Veterinary Medical Association (LVMA): https://latinxvma.org
- MentorVet: https://www.mentorvet.net
- Multicultural Veterinary Medical Association (MCVMA): https://www.mcvma.org
- Not One More Vet (NOMV): https://www.nomv.org
- Pride Veterinary Medical Community (PrideVMC): https://www.pridevmc.org
- Reviving Veterinary Medicine: https://www.revivingvetmed.com
- Veterinary Hope Foundation: https://www.veterinaryhope.org
- VetLife: https://www.vetlife.org.uk
- Vet Mind Matters: https://www.vetmindmatters.org
- WellVet: https://www.wellvet.co.uk

These organizations offer valuable insights and opportunities to get involved, whether through advocacy, education, or support initiatives. Together, we can work toward a sustainable and fulfilling future for veterinary professionals and the animals we care for.

Thank you once again for your interest and support!

Warmly,
Marie

Acknowledgments

Writing this book has been an incredible journey, and I couldn't have done it without the support and encouragement of many wonderful people.

First and foremost, I want to thank my family and friends. To my parents, Elly and Bob Holowaychuk, your dedication to veterinary medicine inspired me from a young age—without you I might never have written this book. To my dog Vivian, your unwavering presence kept me going through countless days and nights of researching and writing. And to my family and friends who championed my efforts to write a book about veterinary medicine, your support propelled me forward.

I am deeply grateful to my mentors, Bernie Hansen, Dorothee Bienzle, Linda Martin, Rita Hanel, Steve Marks, and Terri DeFrancesco, whose guidance and wisdom have been invaluable throughout my career.

Special thanks to my editor, Alice Oven of Taylor & Francis/CRC Press, for your keen insights and suggestions for my manuscript. You provided me with the animal-loving perspective that I was hoping for. And thank you to my assistant, Alexis Kelly, for your invaluable help with research, quotations, and fact-finding, and to my photographer, Amber Clearsky, for capturing the beautiful cover photo.

To my colleagues in the veterinary wellbeing space, notably my dear friends Jen Brandt, Josh Vaisman, and Sonja Olson, thank you for your steadfast camaraderie and support.

I also wish to extend my appreciation to the institutions that have shaped my journey, including the University of Alberta, University of Saskatchewan Western College of Veterinary Medicine, Washington State University College of Veterinary Medicine, North Carolina State University College of Veterinary Medicine, and University of Guelph Ontario Veterinary College.

A heartfelt thank you to the veterinarians, veterinary professionals, and beta readers who shared their stories and provided feedback. Your insights brought depth and authenticity to this book. Special thanks to the members of my closed Facebook community, whose support and thoughtful contributions throughout the writing and editing process have been invaluable.

Lastly, to my readers and the wider veterinary community, thank you for your dedication and compassion. I hope this book resonates with you and sparks meaningful conversations about the future of our profession.

References

CHAPTER 1

1. TradeSchools.Net. (2020). What do you want to be when you grow up? Trade Schools, Colleges and Universities. https://www.trade-schools.net/learn/childhood-aspirations (accessed March 29, 2023).
2. Neufeld, J. (2019). First veterinary class celebrates 50 years. WCVM Today, Western College of Veterinary Medicine. https://wcvmtoday.usask.ca/articles/2019/06/first-veterinary-class-celebrates-50-years.php (accessed March 29, 2023).

CHAPTER 2

1. Burns, K. (2019). Census of veterinarians finds trends with shortages, practice ownership. American Veterinary Medical Association. https://www.avma.org/javma-news/2019-07-15/census-veterinarians-finds-trends-shortages-practice-ownership (accessed March 29, 2023).
2. Siqueira Drake, A.A., Hafen Jr., M, Rush, B.R., & Reisbig, A.M.J. (2012). Predictors of anxiety and depression in veterinary medicine students: a four-year cohort examination. *Journal of Veterinary Medical Education*, 39, 322–330.

CHAPTER 3

1. National Institute for Occupational Safety and Health. (2020). Risks from Not Getting Enough Sleep: Impaired Performance. CDC Archive. http://cdc.gov/niosh/emres/longhourstraining/impaired.html (accessed May 30, 2024).
2. Greenhill, L.M. & Young, K. (2020). 2020 Intern salaries offered through the VIRMP. Association of American Veterinary Medical Colleges. https://www.aavmc.org/assets/Site_18/files/Data/2020%20Intern%20Salaries-Final.pdf (accessed July 12, 2021).
3. Morello, S. L., Shiu, K. B., & Thurston, J. (2021). Comparison of resident and intern salaries with the current living wage as a quantitative estimate of financial strain among postgraduate veterinary trainees. *Journal of the American Veterinary Medical Association*, 260(1), 124–132.

CHAPTER 4

1. Scharf, V. F., McPhetridge, J. B., & Dickson, R. (2022). Sleep patterns, fatigue, and working hours among veterinary house officers: a cross-sectional survey study. *Journal of the American Veterinary Medical Association*, 260(11), 1377–1385.

2. Chigerwe, M., Barter, L., Dechant, J. E., Dear, J. D., & Boudreaux, K. A. (2021). A preliminary study on assessment of wellbeing among veterinary medical house officers. *PloS One*, 16(6), e0253111.

3. American Association of Veterinary Medical Colleges. (2021). Veterinary Intern & Resident Wellbeing Study I. AAVMC Clinical Wellbeing Initiative. https://www.aavmc.org/wp-content/uploads/2022/10/AAVMC-Wellbeing-InternResident-Study-02.pdf (accessed April 3, 2023).

4. Jaworski, J.L., Thompson, L.A., & Weng, H. (2022). Quality of life of veterinary residents in AVMA-Recognized Veterinary Specialty Organizations using the WHOQOL-BREF instrument. *PLoS One* 17(5), e0268343.

5. American Association of Veterinary Medical Colleges. (2022). AAVMC Guidelines for Veterinary Intern & Resident Wellbeing. https://www.aavmc.org/wp-content/uploads/2022/10/AAVMC-Wellbeing-InternResident-Guidelines.pdf (accessed April 3, 2023).

CHAPTER 5

1. QS Top Universities. (2024). QS World University Rankings by Subject: Veterinary Science 2024. https://www.qschina.cn/en/university-rankings/university-subject-rankings/2024/veterinary-science (accessed May 30, 2024).

2. Morello, S. L., Colopy, S. A., Bruckner, K., & Buhr, K. A. (2019). Demographics, measures of professional achievement, and gender differences for diplomates of the American College of Veterinary Surgeons in 2015. *Journal of the American Veterinary Medical Association*, 255(11), 1270–1282.

CHAPTER 6

1. Statistics Canada. (2023). Census Profile, 2021 Census of Population. https://www12.statcan.gc.ca/census-recensement/2021/dp-pd/prof/index.cfm?Lang=E (accessed March 29, 2023).

2. Know Alberta. (2022). How Many Lakes in Alberta? https://www.knowalberta.com/how-many-lakes-in-alberta/ (accessed March 29, 2023).

3. Government of Ontario. (2022). About Ontario. https://www.ontario.ca/page/about-ontario (accessed March 29, 2023).

4. Leonard, J. (2023). How do you know if you're having a panic or anxiety attack? Medical News Today. https://www.medicalnewstoday.com/articles/321798#signs-and-symptoms (accessed May 30, 2024).

5. Veterinary Committee on Trauma. (2022). Request Registry Use. https://vetcot.org/request-registry-use/ (accessed May 30, 2024).

CHAPTER 7

1. Morley, P. (2014). Too many veterinarians, or a bubble market? Veterinary Practice News. https://www.veterinarypracticenews.ca/too-many-veterinarians-or-a-bubble -market/ (accessed March 29, 2023).
2. Segal, D. (2013). High debt and falling demand trap new vets. The New York Times. https://www.nytimes.com/2013/02/24/business/high-debt-and-falling-demand-trap -new-veterinarians.html (accessed March 29, 2023).
3. American Veterinary Medical Association. (2021). Veterinary specialists in the U.S. https://www.avma.org/resources-tools/reports-statistics/veterinary-specialists-2021 (accessed April 3, 2023).
4. Janson, K., & Cote, F. (2019). Entrepreneurs and mental health study. Canadian Mental Health Association. https://cmha.ca/news/entrepreneurs-and-mental-health -study/ (accessed March 29, 2023).

CHAPTER 8

1. Zimlich, R. (2014). A farewell to Dr. Sophia Yin. DVM360. https://www.dvm360.com /view/farewell-dr-sophia-yin (accessed March 20, 2023).
2. Anthony, K. (2023). EFT Tapping. Healthline. https://www.healthline.com/health/eft -tapping (accessed March 14, 2024).
3. Chiesa, A., & Serretti, A. (2009). Mindfulness-based stress reduction for stress management in healthy people: a review and meta-analysis. *Journal of Alternative and Complementary Medicine (New York, N.Y.)*, 15(5), 593–600.

CHAPTER 9

1. Fraser, C. (2024) What Is the Cost of Veterinary School in Canada? 2024 Facts & Statistics. PetKeen. https://petkeen.com/cost-of-veterinary-school-canada-facts -statistics/#8_61_of_veterinary_graduates_are_female_while_only_38_are_male (accessed May 30, 2024).
2. Douglas, J. & Johnson, J. (2020). Number of Applicants to Veterinary Medical Colleges Soars 19 Percent Year-Over-Year. American Association of Veterinary Medical Colleges. https://www.aavmc.org/news/number-of-applicants-to-veterinary-medical -colleges-soars-19-percent-year-over-year/ (accessed May 30, 2024).
3. Veterinary Schools Council. (2021). Admissions processes and entry requirements for UK veterinary schools. https://www.ed.ac.uk/files/atoms/files/vsc_admissions _guide_2022.pdf (accessed May 30, 2024).
4. University of Saskatchewan. (2024). Veterinary Medicine - Doctor of Veterinary Medicine (DVM) Western College of Veterinary Medicine. Admissions. https:// admissions.usask.ca/veterinary-medicine.php (accessed May 30, 2024).
5. Royal Veterinary College University of London. (2024). Bachelor of Veterinary Medicine Entry Requirements. https://www.rvc.ac.uk/study/undergraduate/bachelor -of-veterinary-medicine#panel-graduate-applicants (accessed May 30, 2024).

6. UC Davis Veterinary Medicine. (2024). Criteria for Admission. https://www.vetmed .ucdavis.edu/admissions/criteria-admission (accessed May 30, 2024).
7. NC State University. (2024). Frequently Asked Questions DVM Admissions. College of Veterinary Medicine. https://cvm.ncsu.edu/academics/admissions/faq/#:~:text =We%20admit%20an%20incoming%20class,residents%20and%2023%20non %2Dresidents (accessed May 30, 2024).
8. American Veterinary Medical Association. (2024). Accredited Veterinary Colleges. https://www.avma.org/education/center-for-veterinary-accreditation/accredited -veterinary-colleges (accessed May 30, 2024).

CHAPTER 10

1. Chieffo, C., Kelly, A. M., & Ferguson, J. (2008). Trends in gender, employment, salary, and debt of graduates of US veterinary medical schools and colleges. *Journal of the American Veterinary Medical Association*, 233(6), 910–917.
2. Bain, B., Ouedraogo, F., Hansen, C., Radich, R., & Salois, M. (2020) 2020 Economic State of the Veterinary Profession. American Veterinary Medical Association. https:// ebusiness.avma.org/ProductCatalog/product.aspx?ID=1905 (accessed May 30, 2024).
3. Bain, B., Salois, M., Ouedraogo, F., Hansen, C., & Dutton, B. (2018). 2018 AVMA & AAVMC Report on the Market for Veterinary Education. American Veterinary Medical Association. https://www.avma.org/sites/default/files/resources/2018-econ -rpt1-veterinary-education.pdf (accessed May 30, 2024).
4. Bain, B., Lefebvre, S. L., & Salois, M. (2021). Characteristics of and comparisons between US fourth-year veterinary students graduating with and without educational debt from 2001 through 2020. *Journal of the American Veterinary Medical Association*, 260(5), 559–564.
5. Burns, K. (2022). Starting salaries up, debt down for new veterinarians. AVMA News. https://www.avma.org/news/starting-salaries-debt-down-new-veterinarians (accessed May 30, 2024).
6. Canadian Veterinary Medical Association. (2023). SCVMA New Graduate Report Class of 2022. https://www.canadianveterinarians.net/media/qnkmyla3/2022-scvma -grad-report_final_en.pdf (accessed May 30, 2024)
7. Bain, B., Lefebvre, S. L., & Salois, M. (2021). Characteristics of and comparisons between US fourth-year veterinary students graduating with and without educational debt from 2001 through 2020. *Journal of the American Veterinary Medical Association*, 260(5), 559–564.
8. BeMo Academic Consulting. (2024). Vet School Rankings: The Ultimate Guide. https://bemoacademicconsulting.com/blog/vet-school-rankings (accessed May 30, 2024).
9. RocApply. (2020). Cost of living in Saint Kitts and Nevis. https://www.rocapply.com /study-in-saint-kitts-and-nevis/about-saint-kitts-and-nevis/cost-of-living-in-saint -kitts-and-nevis.html (accessed May 30, 2024).
10. AGCAS Editors. (2023). Veterinary surgeon job profile. Prospects. https://www .prospects.ac.uk/job-profiles/veterinary-surgeon (accessed May 30, 2024).

11. Veterinary Jobs Marketplace. (2024). Veterinary Salary Survey Australia. https://www.veterinaryjobsmarketplace.com.au/resources/veterinarian-salary-survey-australia/ (accessed May 30, 2024).

12. Chisholm-Burns, M. A., Spivey, C. A., Stallworth, S., & Zivin, J. G. (2019). Analysis of educational debt and income among pharmacists and other health professionals. *American Journal of Pharmaceutical Education*, 83(9), 7460.

13. Volk, J. O., Schimmack, U., Strand, E. B., Vasconcelos, J., & Siren, C. W. (2020). Executive summary of the Merck Animal Health Veterinarian Wellbeing Study II. *Journal of the American Veterinary Medical Association*, 256(11), 1237–1244.

14. Volk, J. O., Schimmack, U., Strand, E. B., Reinhard, A., Vasconcelos, J., Hahn, J., Stiefelmeyer, K., & Probyn-Smith, K. (2022). Executive summary of the Merck Animal Health Veterinarian Wellbeing Study III and Veterinary Support Staff Study. *Journal of the American Veterinary Medical Association*, 260(12), 1547–1553.

15. Bain, B., & Lefebvre, S. L. (2022). Associations between career choice and educational debt for fourth-year students of US veterinary schools and colleges, 2001–2021. *Journal of the American Veterinary Medical Association*, 260(9), 1063–1068.

CHAPTER 11

1. Wikipedia. (2024). Academic honor code. https://en.wikipedia.org/wiki/Academic_honor_code (accessed May 30, 2024).

2. Roder, C. A., & May, S. A. (2017). The hidden curriculum of veterinary education: mediators and moderators of its effects. *Journal of Veterinary Medical Education*, 44(3), 542–551.

3. Stanek, A., Clarkin, C., Bould, M. D., Writer, H., & Doja, A. (2015). Life imitating art: depictions of the hidden curriculum in medical television programs. *BMC Medical Education*, 15, 156.

CHAPTER 12

1. American Veterinary Medical Association. (2022). Veterinary specialties. https://www.avma.org/education/veterinary-specialties (accessed April 3, 2023).

2. Veterinary Internship & Residency Matching Program. (2023). Match Data. https://www.virmp.org/Statistics (accessed April 3, 2023).

3. Jandrey, K. E., Goggs, R., Kerl, M., Guillaumin, J., & Kent, M. S. (2018). Analysis of the first-time pass rate of the American College of Veterinary Emergency and Critical Care certifying examination (2010-2015). *Journal of Veterinary Emergency and Critical Care*, 28(3), 187–191.

4. American Veterinary Medical Association. (2022). Reports and statistics. https://www.avma.org/resources-tools/reports-statistics (accessed April 3, 2023).

5. Lloyd, J.W. (2022). Pet healthcare in the US: Are there enough veterinary specialists? Is there adequate training capacity? https://news.vin.com/apputil/image/handler.ashx?docid=10897708 (accessed April 3, 2023).

6. Morello, S. L. (2023). Resident and intern salaries: can tracking our progress help us understand our future? *Journal of the American Veterinary Medical Association*, 261(5), 758–765.

CHAPTER 13

1. ASPCA. (2022). Which Lilies Are Toxic to Pets? https://www.aspca.org/news/which -lilies-are-toxic-pets (accessed May 30, 2024).
2. American Society of Veterinary Nephrology and Urology. (2022). Hospitals Offering Advanced Renal and Urinary Treatments. https://www.asvnu.org/facilities (accessed May 30, 2024).
3. Sabino, C. V., Holowaychuk, M., & Bateman, S. (2013). Management of acute respiratory distress syndrome in a French Bulldog using airway pressure release ventilation. *Journal of Veterinary Emergency and Critical Care*, 23(4), 447–454.

CHAPTER 14

1. Koudounaris, P. (2023). The Rainbow Bridge: The True Story Behind History's Most Influential Piece of Animal Mourning Literature - If you meet your pet in the afterlife, thank Edna Clyne-Rekhy. The Order of the Good Death. https://www .orderofthegooddeath.com/article/the-rainbow-bridge-the-true-story-behind -historys-most-influential-piece-of-animal-mourning-literature/ (accessed June 10, 2024).
2. Quain, A. (2021). The gift: Ethically indicated euthanasia in companion animal practice. *Veterinary Sciences*, 8(8), 141.
3. Matte, A. R., Khosa, D. K., Coe, J. B., & Meehan, M. P. (2019). Impacts of the process and decision-making around companion animal euthanasia on veterinary wellbeing. *The Veterinary Record*, 185(15), 480.
4. Ashall, V. (2018). Ethical dilemmas encountered by small animal veterinarians: challenging the status quo? *The Veterinary Record*, 182(19), 546–547.
5. Moses, L., Malowney, M. J., & Wesley Boyd, J. (2018). Ethical conflict and moral distress in veterinary practice: A survey of North American veterinarians. *Journal of Veterinary Internal Medicine*, 32(6), 2115–2122.
6. Hartnack, S., Springer, S., Pittavino, M., & Grimm, H. (2016). Attitudes of Austrian veterinarians towards euthanasia in small animal practice: impacts of age and gender on views on euthanasia. *BMC Veterinary Research*, 12, 26.
7. Gates, M. C., Kells, N. J., Kongara, K., & Littlewood, K. E. (2023). Euthanasia of dogs and cats by veterinarians in New Zealand: protocols, procedures and experiences. *New Zealand Veterinary Journal*, 71(4), 172–185.
8. Scotney, R. L., McLaughlin, D., & Keates, H. L. (2015). A systematic review of the effects of euthanasia and occupational stress in personnel working with animals in animal shelters, veterinary clinics, and biomedical research facilities. *Journal of the American Veterinary Medical Association*, 247(10), 1121–1130.

9. Tran, L., Crane, M. F., & Phillips, J. K. (2014). The distinct role of performing euthanasia on depression and suicide in veterinarians. *Journal of Occupational Health Psychology*, 19(2), 123–132.

10. Dow, M. Q., Chur-Hansen, A., Hamood, W., & Edwards, S. (2019). Impact of dealing with bereaved clients on the psychological wellbeing of veterinarians. *Australian Veterinary Journal*, 97(10), 382–389.

11. Tran, L., Crane, M.F., Phillips, J.K. (2014). The distinct role of performing euthanasia on depression and suicide in veterinarians. *Journal of Occupational Health Psychology*, 19(2), 123–132.

12. Rohlf, V., & Bennett, P. (2005). Perpetration-induced traumatic stress in persons who euthanize nonhuman animals in surgeries, animal shelters, and laboratories. *Society & Animals*, 13(3), 201–219.

13. Whiting, T. L., & Marion, C. R. (2011). Perpetration-induced traumatic stress - A risk for veterinarians involved in the destruction of healthy animals. *The Canadian Veterinary Journal*, 52(7), 794–796.

CHAPTER 15

1. Judd, A. (2021). B.C. floods: Thousands of pigs, cows, chickens and likely bees died in Fraser Valley. Global News. https://globalnews.ca/news/8421653/bc-floods-animals-killed-fraser-valley/ (accessed June 10, 2024).

2. Pohl, R., Botscharow, J., Böckelmann, I., & Thielmann, B. (2022). Stress and strain among veterinarians: a scoping review. *Irish Veterinary Journal*, 75(1), 15.

3. Campbell, M. L. (2013). The role of veterinarians in equestrian sport: a comparative review of ethical issues surrounding human and equine sports medicine. *Veterinary Journal*, 197(3), 535–540.

4. Batchelor, C. E., & McKeegan, D. E. (2012). Survey of the frequency and perceived stressfulness of ethical dilemmas encountered in UK veterinary practice. *The Veterinary Record*, 170(1), 19.

5. Moses, L., Malowney, M. J., & Wesley Boyd, J. (2018). Ethical conflict and moral distress in veterinary practice: A survey of North American veterinarians. *Journal of Veterinary Internal Medicine*, 32(6), 2115–2122.

6. Williams, J. M., Wauthier, L., Scottish SPCA, & Knoll, M. (2022). Veterinarians' experiences of treating cases of animal abuse: An online questionnaire study. *The Veterinary Record*, 191(11), e1975.

7. Canadian Veterinary Medical Association. (2018). Responsibility of Veterinary Professionals in Addressing Animal Abuse and Neglect. Position Statements. https://www.canadianveterinarians.net/policy-and-outreach/position-statements/statements/responsibility-of-veterinary-professionals-in-addressing-animal-abuse-and-neglect/ (accessed June 10, 2024).

8. Gallagher, B., Allen, M., & Jones, B. (2008). Animal abuse and intimate partner violence: researching the link and its significance in Ireland - a veterinary perspective. *Irish Veterinary Journal*, 61(10), 658–667.

9. Williamson, V., Murphy, D., & Greenberg, N. (2022). Experiences and impact of moral injury in U.K. veterinary professional wellbeing. *European Journal of Psychotraumatology*, 13(1), 2051351.
10. Williamson, V., Murphy, D., & Greenberg, N. (2023). Veterinary professionals' experiences of moral injury: A qualitative study. *The Veterinary Record*, 192(2), e2181.
11. Kipperman, B., Rollin, B., & Martin, J. (2021). Veterinary student opinions regarding ethical dilemmas encountered by veterinarians and the benefits of ethics instruction. *Journal of Veterinary Medical Education*, 48(3), 330–342.
12. Brscic, M., Contiero, B., Schianchi, A., & Marogna, C. (2021). Challenging suicide, burnout, and depression among veterinary practitioners and students: text mining and topics modelling analysis of the scientific literature. *BMC Veterinary Research*, 17(1), 294.
13. Quain, A., Mullan, S., & Ward, M. P. (2022). "There was a sense that our load had been lightened": evaluating outcomes of virtual ethics rounds for veterinary team members. *Frontiers in Veterinary Science*, 9, 922049.
14. Ashall, V. (2023). Reducing moral stress in veterinary teams? Evaluating the use of ethical discussion groups in charity veterinary hospitals. *Animals*, 13(10), 1662.
15. Rosoff, P. M., Moga, J., Keene, B., Adin, C., Fogle, C., Ruderman, R., Hopkinso, H., & Weyhrauch, C. (2018). Resolving ethical dilemmas in a Tertiary Care Veterinary Specialty Hospital: adaptation of the Human Clinical Consultation Committee Model. *The American Journal of Bioethics*, 18(2), 41–53.

CHAPTER 16

1. Robinson, D. & Hooker, H. (2006). The UK veterinary profession in 2006: the findings of a survey of the profession conducted by the Royal College of Veterinary Surgeons. https://www.rcvs.org.uk/news-and-views/publications/rcvs-survey-of-the-professions-2006/ (accessed May 30, 2024).
2. Bartram, D. J., Yadegarfar, G., & Baldwin, D. S. (2009). Psychosocial working conditions and work-related stressors among UK veterinary surgeons. *Occupational Medicine (Oxford, England)*, 59(5), 334–341.
3. Gardner, D. H., & Hini, D. (2006). Work-related stress in the veterinary profession in New Zealand. *New Zealand Veterinary Journal*, 54(3), 119–124.
4. Shibly, S., Rodl, C.A., & Tichy, A. (2014). Vet – a 'dream job'? Survey of work-related satisfaction and possible emotional stressors of veterinarians in a university setting. Wiener Tierärztliche Monatsschrift – Veterinary Medicine Austria. https://www.wtm.at/smart_users/uni/user94/explorer/43/WTM/Archiv/2014/WTM_03-04-2014_Artikel_1_Art.1318.pdf (accessed May 30, 2024).
5. Kersebohm, J. C., Lorenz, T., Becher, A., & Doherr, M. G. (2017). Factors related to work and life satisfaction of veterinary practitioners in Germany. *Veterinary Record Open*, 4(1), e000229.
6. Clise, M. H., Matthew, S. M., & McArthur, M. L. (2021). Sources of pleasure in veterinary work: A qualitative study. *The Veterinary Record*, 188(11), e54.

7. Nett, R. J., Witte, T. K., Holzbauer, S. M., Elchos, B. L., Campagnolo, E. R., Musgrave, K. J., Carter, K. K., Kurkjian, K. M., Vanicek, C. F., O'Leary, D. R., Pride, K. R., & Funk, R. H. (2015). Risk factors for suicide, attitudes toward mental illness, and practice-related stressors among US veterinarians. *Journal of the American Veterinary Medical Association*, 247(8), 945–955.

8. Stetina, B. U., & Krouzecky, C. (2022). Reviewing a decade of change for veterinarians: past, present and gaps in researching stress, coping and mental health risks. *Animals: An Open Access Journal from MDPI*, 12(22), 3199.

9. Polachek, A. J., & Wallace, J. E. (2018). The paradox of compassionate work: a mixed-methods study of satisfying and fatiguing experiences of animal health care providers. *Anxiety, Stress, and Coping*, 31(2), 228–243.

CHAPTER 17

1. Irwin, A., Hall, D., & Ellis, H. (2022). Ruminating on rudeness: Exploring veterinarians' experiences of client incivility. *The Veterinary Record*, 190(4), e1078.

2. Vande Griek, O. H., Clark, M. A., Witte, T. K., Nett, R. J., Moeller, A. N., & Stabler, M. E. (2018). Development of a taxonomy of practice-related stressors experienced by veterinarians in the United States. *Journal of the American Veterinary Medical Association*, 252(2), 227–233.

3. Irwin, A., Silver-MacMahon, H., & Wilcke, S. (2022). Consequences and coping: Investigating client, co-worker and senior colleague incivility within veterinary practice. *The Veterinary Record*, 191(7), e2030.

4. Nett, R. J., Witte, T. K., Holzbauer, S. M., Elchos, B. L., Campagnolo, E. R., Musgrave, K. J., Carter, K. K., Kurkjian, K. M., Vanicek, C. F., O'Leary, D. R., Pride, K. R., & Funk, R. H. (2015). Risk factors for suicide, attitudes toward mental illness, and practice-related stressors among US veterinarians. *Journal of the American Veterinary Medical Association*, 247(8), 945–955.

5. Gordon, S., Gardner, D. H., Weston, J. F., Bolwell, C. F., Benschop, J., & Parkinson, T. J. (2019). Quantitative and thematic analysis of complaints by clients against clinical veterinary practitioners in New Zealand. *New Zealand Veterinary Journal*, 67(3), 117–125.

6. Bryce, A. R., Rossi, T. A., Tansey, C., Murphy, R. A., Murphy, L. A., & Nakamura, R. K. (2019). Effect of client complaints on small animal veterinary internists. *The Journal of Small Animal Practice*, 60(3), 167–172.

7. Gibson, J., White, K., Mossop, L., Oxtoby, C., & Brennan, M. (2022). 'We're gonna end up scared to do anything': A qualitative exploration of how client complaints are experienced by UK veterinary practitioners. *The Veterinary Record*, 191(4), e1737.

8. Rogers, C. W., Murphy, L. A., Murphy, R. A., Malouf, K. A., Natsume, R. E., Ward, B. D., Tansey, C., & Nakamura, R. K. (2022). An analysis of client complaints and their effects on veterinary support staff. *Veterinary Medicine and Science*, 8(2), 925–934.

9. McCafferty, C. & Yankowicz, S. (2022) Veterinary hospital reports threats over puppy's emergency case. DVM360. https://www.dvm360.com/view/veterinary-hospital-reports-threats-over-puppy-s-emergency-case (accessed May 30, 2024).

CHAPTER 18

1. Moore, I. C., Coe, J. B., Adams, C. L., Conlon, P. D., & Sargeant, J. M. (2014). The role of veterinary team effectiveness in job satisfaction and burnout in companion animal veterinary clinics. *Journal of the American Veterinary Medical Association*, 245(5), 513–524.

2. Pizzolon, C. N., Coe, J. B., & Shaw, J. R. (2019). Evaluation of team effectiveness and personal empathy for associations with professional quality of life and job satisfaction in companion animal practice personnel. *Journal of the American Veterinary Medical Association*, 254(10), 1204–1217.

3. Moore, I. C., Coe, J. B., Adams, C. L., Conlon, P. D., & Sargeant, J. M. (2015). Exploring the impact of toxic attitudes and a toxic environment on the veterinary healthcare team. *Frontiers in Veterinary Science*, 2, 78.

4. Vande Griek, O. H., Clark, M. A., Witte, T. K., Nett, R. J., Moeller, A. N., & Stabler, M. E. (2018). Development of a taxonomy of practice-related stressors experienced by veterinarians in the United States. *Journal of the American Veterinary Medical Association*, 252(2), 227–233.

5. Connolly, C. E., Norris, K., Martin, A., Dawkins, S., & Meehan, C. (2022). A taxonomy of occupational and organisational stressors and protectors of mental health reported by veterinary professionals in Australasia. *Australian Veterinary Journal*, 100(8), 367–376.

6. Wojtacka, J., Grudzień, W., Wysok, B., & Szarek, J. (2020). Causes of stress and conflict in the veterinary professional workplace - a perspective from Poland. *Irish Veterinary Journal*, 73(1), 23.

7. Chigerwe, M., Barter, L., Dechant, J. E., Dear, J. D., & Boudreaux, K. A. (2021). A preliminary study on assessment of wellbeing among veterinary medical house officers. *PLoS One*, 16(6), e0253111.

8. Irwin, A., Silver-MacMahon, H., & Wilcke, S. (2022). Consequences and coping: Investigating client, co-worker and senior colleague incivility within veterinary practice. *The Veterinary Record*, 191(7), e2030.

9. American Psychological Association. (2024). The American workforce faces compounding pressure - APA's 2021 Work and Well-being Survey results. https://www.apa.org/pubs/reports/work-well-being/compounding-pressure-2021 (accessed June 10, 2024).

10. Kustritz, M. V., & Nault, A. J. (2010). Professional development training through the veterinary curriculum at the University of Minnesota. *Journal of Veterinary Medical Education*, 37(3), 233–237.

11. Gardner, D. H., & Rasmussen, W. (2018). Workplace bullying and relationships with health and performance among a sample of New Zealand veterinarians. *New Zealand Veterinary Journal*, 66(2), 57–63.

12. Merck Animal Health. (2024). Creating a Positive, More Energized Veterinary Team. https://www.merck-animal-health-usa.com/offload-downloads/2023-vet-team-wellbeing-presentation (accessed June 10, 2024).

CHAPTER 19

1. Kogan, L., Schoenfeld-Tacher, R., Carney, P., Hellyer, P., & Rishniw, M. (2021). On-call duties: the perceived impact on veterinarians' job satisfaction, well-being and personal relationships. *Frontiers in Veterinary Science*, 8, 740852.
2. Adam, K., Baillie, S., & Rushton, J. (2015). Retaining vets in farm animal practice: a cross-sectional study. *The Veterinary Record*, 176(25), 655.
3. Arbe Montoya, A. I., Hazel, S. J., Hebart, M. L., & McArthur, M. L. (2021). Risk factors associated with veterinary attrition from clinical practice: a descriptive study. *Australian Veterinary Journal*, 99(11), 495–501.
4. Routly, J. E., Taylor, I. R., Turner, R., McKernan, E. J., & Dobson, H. (2002). Support needs of veterinary surgeons during the first few years of practice: perceptions of recent graduates and senior partners. *The Veterinary Record*, 150(6), 167–171.
5. Jelinski, M. D., Campbell, J. R., Naylor, J. M., Lawson, K. L., & Derkzen, D. (2009). Factors associated with the career path choices of veterinarians in western Canada. *The Canadian Veterinary Journal*, 50(6), 630–636.
6. Chambers, R., & Belcher, J. (1994). Predicting mental health problems in general practitioners. *Occupational Medicine (Oxford, England)*, 44(4), 212–216.
7. Dowell, A. C., Hamilton, S., & McLeod, D. K. (2000). Job satisfaction, psychological morbidity and job stress among New Zealand general practitioners. *The New Zealand Medical Journal*, 113(1113), 269–272.
8. Geurts, S. A., & Sonnentag, S. (2006). Recovery as an explanatory mechanism in the relation between acute stress reactions and chronic health impairment. *Scandinavian Journal of Work, Environment & Health*, 32(6), 482–492.
9. Ciciolla, L., & Luthar, S. S. (2019). Invisible household labor and ramifications for adjustment: mothers as captains of households. *Sex Roles*, 81(7–8), 467–486.
10. Irwin, A., Vikman, J., & Ellis, H. (2019). 'No-one knows where you are': veterinary perceptions regarding safety and risk when alone and on-call. *The Veterinary Record*, 185(23), 728.
11. Rubin, R., Orris, P., Lau, S. L., Hryhorczuk, D. O., Furner, S., & Letz, R. (1991). Neurobehavioral effects of the on-call experience in housestaff physicians. *Journal of Occupational Medicine*, 33(1), 13–18.
12. Lingenfelser, T., Kaschel, R., Weber, A., Zaiser-Kaschel, H., Jakober, B., & Küper, J. (1994). Young hospital doctors after night duty: their task-specific cognitive status and emotional condition. *Medical Education*, 28(6), 566–572.
13. Saxena, A. D., & George, C. F. (2005). Sleep and motor performance in on-call internal medicine residents. *Sleep*, 28(11), 1386–1391.
14. Scharf, V. F., McPhetridge, J. B., & Dickson, R. (2022). Sleep patterns, fatigue, and working hours among veterinary house officers: a cross-sectional survey study. *Journal of the American Veterinary Medical Association*, 260(11), 1377–1385.
15. Boudreaux, B., & Hill, T. (2022). Factors associated with successful passage of the American College of Veterinary Internal Medicine general examination. *Journal of Veterinary Internal Medicine*, 36(3), 1113–1118.
16. Adin, C. A., Fogle, C. A., & Marks, S. L. (2018). Duty hours restriction for our surgical trainees: An ethical obligation or a bad idea? *Veterinary Surgery*, 47(3), 327–332.

CHAPTER 20

1. Merck Animal Health. (2024). Improving Wellbeing and Mental Health. https://www .merck-animal-health-usa.com/offload-downloads/2023-vet-wellbeing-presentation (accessed June 10, 2024).
2. Razai, M. S., Kooner, P., & Majeed, A. (2023). Strategies and Interventions to Improve Healthcare Professionals' Well-Being and Reduce Burnout. *Journal of Primary Care & Community Health*, 14, 21501319231178641.
3. Armitage-Chan, E., & May, S. A. (2018). Identity, environment and mental wellbeing in the veterinary profession. *The Veterinary record*, 183(2), 68.
4. Armitage-Chan, E. (2020). 'I wish I was someone else': complexities in identity formation and professional wellbeing in veterinary surgeons. *The Veterinary Record*, 187(3), 113.
5. Armitage-Chan, E., & May, S. A. (2018). Developing a professional studies curriculum to support veterinary professional identity formation. *Journal of Veterinary Medical Education*, 45(4), 489–501.

CHAPTER 21

1. Bhandari, S. (2024). What Is a Martyr Complex? WebMD. https://www.webmd.com/ mental-health/what-is-a-martyr-complex (accessed June 10, 2024).
2. Volk, J. O., Schimmack, U., Strand, E. B., Reinhard, A., Vasconcelos, J., Hahn, J., Stiefelmeyer, K., & Probyn-Smith, K. (2022). Executive summary of the Merck Animal Health Veterinarian Wellbeing Study III and Veterinary Support Staff Study. *Journal of the American Veterinary Medical Association*, 260(12), 1547–1553.

CHAPTER 22

1. Merriam-Webster. (2024). Definition - perfectionism. Merriam-Webster.com. https://www.merriam-webster.com/dictionary/perfectionism#:~:text=Medical %20Definition-,perfectionism,short%20of%20perfection%20as%20unacceptable (accessed June 10, 2024).
2. Lo, A. & Abbott, M. J. (2019). Self-concept certainty in adaptive and maladaptive perfectionists. *Journal of Experimental Psychopathology*, 10(2), 2043808719843455.
3. Lewis, E. G., & Cardwell, J. M. (2020). The big five personality traits, perfectionism and their association with mental health among UK students on professional degree programmes. *BMC Psychology*, 8(1), 54.
4. Holden, C. L. (2020). Characteristics of Veterinary Students: Perfectionism, Personality Factors, and Resilience. *Journal of Veterinary Medical Education*, 47(4), 488–496.
5. Hewitt, P. L., Flett, G. L., Turnbull-Donovan, W., & Mikail, S. F. (1991). The Multidimensional Perfectionism Scale: Reliability, validity, and psychometric properties in psychiatric samples. *Psychological Assessment: A Journal of Consulting and Clinical Psychology*, 3(3), 464–468.

6. Wikipedia. (2024). Big Five personality traits. https://en.wikipedia.org/wiki/Big _Five_personality_traits (accessed June 10, 2024).
7. O'Connor, E. (2019). Sources of work stress in veterinary practice in the UK. *The Veterinary Record*, 184(19), 588.
8. Crane, M. F., Phillips, J. K., & Karin, E. (2015). Trait perfectionism strengthens the negative effects of moral stressors occurring in veterinary practice. *Australian Veterinary Journal*, 93(10), 354–360.
9. Kogan, L. R., Schoenfeld-Tacher, R., Hellyer, P., Grigg, E. K., & Kramer, E. (2020). Veterinarians and impostor syndrome: an exploratory study. *The Veterinary Record*, 187(7), 271.
10. Gottlieb, M., Chung, A., Battaglioli, N., Sebok-Syer, S. S., & Kalantari, A. (2020). Impostor syndrome among physicians and physicians in training: A scoping review. *Medical Education*, 54(2), 116–124.

CHAPTER 23

1. White, S.C. (2018). Veterinarians' emotional reactions and coping strategies for adverse events in spay-neuter surgical practice. *Anthrozoös* 31, 117-31.
2. Kogan, L. R., Rishniw, M., Hellyer, P. W., & Schoenfeld-Tacher, R. M. (2018). Veterinarians' experiences with near misses and adverse events. *Journal of the American Veterinary Medical Association*, 252(5), 586–595.
3. Wallis, J., Fletcher, D., Bentley, A., & Ludders, J. (2019). Medical errors cause harm in veterinary hospitals. *Frontiers in Veterinary Science*, 6, 12.

CHAPTER 24

1. U.S. Department of Health & Human Services. (2024). About Mental Health. CDC. https://www.cdc.gov/mentalhealth/learn/index.htm (accessed June 10, 2024).
2. CAMH. (2024). Mental Illness and Addiction: Facts and Statistics. https://www.camh .ca/en/driving-change/the-crisis-is-real/mental-health-statistics (accessed June 10, 2024).
3. Kedrowicz, A. A., & Royal, K. D. (2020). A comparison of public perceptions of physicians and veterinarians in the United States. *Veterinary Sciences*, 7(2), 50.
4. Reisbig, A. M., Danielson, J. A., Wu, T. F., Hafen Jr., M., Krienert, A., Girard, D., & Garlock, J. (2012). A study of depression and anxiety, general health, and academic performance in three cohorts of veterinary medical students across the first three semesters of veterinary school. *Journal of Veterinary Medical Education*, 39(4), 341–358.
5. Killinger, S. L., Flanagan, S., Castine, E., & Howard, K. A. (2017). Stress and depression among veterinary medical students. *Journal of Veterinary Medical Education*, 44(1), 3–8.
6. Cardwell, J. M., Lewis, E. G., Smith, K. C., Holt, E. R., Baillie, S., Allister, R., & Adams, V. J. (2013). A cross-sectional study of mental health in UK veterinary undergraduates. *The Veterinary Record*, 173(11), 266.

7. Humer, E., Neubauer, V., Brühl, D., Dale, R., Pieh, C., & Probst, T. (2023). Prevalence of mental health symptoms and potential risk factors among Austrian veterinary medicine students. *Scientific Reports*, 13(1), 13764.

8. Schunter, N., Glaesmer, H., Lucht, L., & Bahramsoltani, M. (2022). Depression, suicidal ideation and suicide risk in German veterinary medical students compared to the German general population. *PloS One*, 17(8), e0270912.

9. Bartram, D. J., Yadegarfar, G., & Baldwin, D. S. (2009). A cross-sectional study of mental health and well-being and their associations in the UK veterinary profession. *Social Psychiatry and Psychiatric Epidemiology*, 44(12), 1075–1085.

10. Perret, J. L., Best, C. O., Coe, J. B., Greer, A. L., Khosa, D. K., & Jones-Bitton, A. (2020). Prevalence of mental health outcomes among Canadian veterinarians. *Journal of the American Veterinary Medical Association*, 256(3), 365–375.

11. Fritschi, L., Morrison, D., Shirangi, A., & Day, L. (2009). Psychological well-being of Australian veterinarians. *Australian Veterinary Journal*, 87(3), 76–81.

12. Seedat, S., Scott, K. M., Angermeyer, M. C., Berglund, P., Bromet, E. J., Brugha, T. S., Demyttenaere, K., de Girolamo, G., Haro, J. M., Jin, R., Karam, E. G., Kovess-Masfety, V., Levinson, D., Medina Mora, M. E., Ono, Y., Ormel, J., Pennell, B. E., Posada-Villa, J., Sampson, N. A., Williams, D., … Kessler, R. C. (2009). Cross-national associations between gender and mental disorders in the World Health Organization World Mental Health Surveys. *Archives of General Psychiatry*, 66(7), 785–795.

13. Russon, J. M., Bland, K., Ravi-Caldwell, N., Haak, P. P., Kryda, K. T., Codecá, L., Darby, B. J., Bissett, C. J., Murphy, J., & Hungerford, L. (2023). Career stage differences in mental health symptom burden and help seeking among veterinarians during COVID-19. *Journal of the American Veterinary Medical Association*, 261(6), 898–906.

14. Volk, J. O., Schimmack, U., Strand, E. B., Reinhard, A., Vasconcelos, J., Hahn, J., Stiefelmeyer, K., & Probyn-Smith, K. (2022). Executive summary of the Merck Animal Health Veterinarian Wellbeing Study III and Veterinary Support Staff Study. *Journal of the American Veterinary Medical Association*, 260(12), 1547–1553.

15. Hilton, K. R., Burke, K. J., & Signal, T. (2023). Mental health in the veterinary profession: an individual or organisational focus? *Australian Veterinary Journal*, 101(1–2), 41–48.

16. Shirangi, A., Fritschi, L., Holman, C. D., & Morrison, D. (2013). Mental health in female veterinarians: effects of working hours and having children. *Australian Veterinary Journal*, 91(4), 123–130.

17. Strand, E. B., Brandt, J., Rogers, K., Fonken, L., Chun, R., Conlon, P., & Lord, L. (2017). Adverse Childhood Experiences among Veterinary Medical Students: A Multi-Site Study. *Journal of Veterinary Medical Education*, 44(2), 260–267.

18. CDC. (2024). About Adverse Childhood Experiences. https://www.cdc.gov/violenceprevention/aces/fastfact.html (accessed June 10, 2024).

19. Witte, T. K., Kramper, S., Carmichael, K. P., Chaddock, M., & Gorczyca, K. (2020). A survey of negative mental health outcomes, workplace and school climate, and identity disclosure for lesbian, gay, bisexual, transgender, queer, questioning, and asexual veterinary professionals and students in the United States and United

Kingdom. *Journal of the American Veterinary Medical Association*, 257(4), 417–431.

20. Perret, J. L., Best, C. O., Coe, J. B., Greer, A. L., Khosa, D. K., & Jones-Bitton, A. (2020). The complex relationship between veterinarian mental health and client satisfaction. *Frontiers in Veterinary Science*, 7, 92.

21. Campbell, M., Hagen, B. N. M., Gohar, B., Wichtel, J., & Jones-Bitton, A. (2023). A qualitative study exploring the perceived effects of veterinarians' mental health on provision of care. *Frontiers in Veterinary Science*, 10, 1064932.

CHAPTER 25

1. Bartram, D. J., & Baldwin, D. S. (2010). Veterinary surgeons and suicide: a structured review of possible influences on increased risk. *The Veterinary Record*, 166(13), 388–397.

2. Kassem, A. M., Witte, T. K., Nett, R. J., & Carter, K. K. (2019). Characteristics associated with negative attitudes toward mental illness among US veterinarians. *Journal of the American Veterinary Medical Association*, 254(8), 979–985.

3. Dalum, H. S., Tyssen, R., Moum, T., Thoresen, M., & Hem, E. (2022). Professional help-seeking behaviour for mental health problems among veterinarians in Norway: a nationwide, cross-sectional study (The NORVET study). *BMC Public Health*, 22(1), 1308.

4. Connolly, C. E., Norris, K., Dawkins, S., & Martin, A. (2022). Barriers to mental health help-seeking in veterinary professionals working in Australia and New Zealand: A preliminary cross-sectional analysis. *Frontiers in Veterinary Science*, 9, 1051571.

5. Russon, J. M., Bland, K., Ravi-Caldwell, N., Haak, P. P., Kryda, K. T., Codecá, L., Darby, B. J., Bissett, C. J., Murphy, J., & Hungerford, L. (2023). Career stage differences in mental health symptom burden and help seeking among veterinarians during COVID-19. *Journal of the American Veterinary Medical Association*, 261(6), 898–906.

6. Hancock, T. S., & Karaffa, K. M. (2022). "Obligated to Keep Things Under Control": Sociocultural Barriers to Seeking Mental Health Services Among Veterinary Medical Students. *Journal of Veterinary Medical Education*, 49(5), 662–677.

7. McArthur, M. L., Matthew, S. M., Brand, C. P. B., Andrews, J., Fawcett, A., & Hazel, S. (2019). Cross-sectional analysis of veterinary student coping strategies and stigma in seeking psychological help. *The Veterinary Record*, 184(23), 709.

8. Wikipedia. (2024). Sad clown paradox. https://en.wikipedia.org/wiki/Sad_clown_paradox (accessed June 10, 2024).

9. Lokhee, S., & Hogg, R. C. (2021). Depression, stress and self-stigma towards seeking psychological help in veterinary students. *Australian Veterinary Journal*, 99(7), 309–317.

10. Karaffa, K. M., & Hancock, T. S. (2019). Mental Health Stigma and Veterinary Medical Students' Attitudes Toward Seeking Professional Psychological Help. *Journal of Veterinary Medical Education*, 46(4), 459–469.

11. Drake, A. A., Hafen Jr., M., & Rush, B. R. (2017). A Decade of Counseling Services in One College of Veterinary Medicine: Veterinary Medical Students' Psychological

Distress and Help-Seeking Trends. *Journal of Veterinary Medical Education*, 44(1), 157–165.

12. University of Saskatchewan Western College of Veterinary Medicine. (2024). Veterinary Social Work. https://vmc.usask.ca/services/veterinary-social-work.php #About (accessed June 10, 2024).

CHAPTER 26

1. Figley, C. (2022). The Compassion Fatigue Awareness Project. http://www.compassionfatigue.org/ (accessed June 10, 2024).
2. Figley, C. R. & Roop, R. G. (2006). *Compassion fatigue in the animal-care community*. Humane Society Press.
3. VetLife. (2024). Compassion fatigue. https://www.vetlife.org.uk/mental-health/compassion-fatigue/ (accessed June 10, 2024).
4. Stoewen, D. L. (2020). Moving from compassion fatigue to compassion resilience Part 4: Signs and consequences of compassion fatigue. *The Canadian Veterinary Journal*, 61(11), 1207–1209.
5. American Veterinary Medical Association. (2023). Compassion fatigue. https://www.avma.org/resources-tools/wellbeing/work-and-compassion-fatigue (accessed March 29, 2022).
6. The Center for Victims of Torture. (2021). Professional Quality of Life. https://proqol.org/ (accessed June 10, 2024).
7. Perret, J. L., Best, C. O., Coe, J. B., Greer, A. L., Khosa, D. K., & Jones-Bitton, A. (2020). Prevalence of mental health outcomes among Canadian veterinarians. *Journal of the American Veterinary Medical Association*, 256(3), 365–375.
8. Ouedraogo, F. B., Lefebvre, S. L., Hansen, C. R., & Brorsen, B. W. (2021). Compassion satisfaction, burnout, and secondary traumatic stress among full-time veterinarians in the United States (2016–2018). *Journal of the American Veterinary Medical Association*, 258(11), 1259–1270.
9. Polachek, A. J., & Wallace, J. E. (2018). The paradox of compassionate work: a mixed-methods study of satisfying and fatiguing experiences of animal health care providers. *Anxiety, Stress, and Coping*, 31(2), 228–243.
10. Reif-Stice, C., Smith-Frigerio, S., Lawson, C. A., & Venette, S. (2023). Discerning the effect of the relationship between disclosure and responsiveness on depression, anxiety, and compassion fatigue among veterinarians. *Journal of the American Veterinary Medical Association*, 261(4), 551–558.
11. Dowling, T. (2018). Compassion does not fatigue!. *The Canadian Veterinary Journal*, 59(7), 749–750.

CHAPTER 27

1. Heinemann, L. V., & Heinemann, T. (2017). Burnout Research: Emergence and Scientific Investigation of a Contested Diagnosis. *Sage Open*, 7(1), 2158244017697154.

2. González, Á. S. M., González, P. S. M., Míguez-Santiyán, M. P., Rodríguez, F. S., & Pérez-López, M. (2023). Prevalence of burnout syndrome among veterinarians in Spain. *Journal of the American Veterinary Medical Association*, 261(5), 1–8.

3. Jones-Bitton, A., Gillis, D., Peterson, M., & McKee, H. (2023). Latent burnout profiles of veterinarians in Canada: Findings from a cross-sectional study. *The Veterinary Record*, 192(2), e2281.

4. Rohlf, V. I., Scotney, R., Monaghan, H., & Bennett, P. (2022). Predictors of Professional Quality of Life in Veterinary Professionals. *Journal of Veterinary Medical Education*, 49(3), 372–381.

5. Ouedraogo, F. B., Lefebvre, S. L., Hansen, C. R., & Brorsen, B. W. (2021). Compassion satisfaction, burnout, and secondary traumatic stress among full-time veterinarians in the United States (2016-2018). *Journal of the American Veterinary Medical Association*, 258(11), 1259–1270.

6. Perret, J. L., Best, C. O., Coe, J. B., Greer, A. L., Khosa, D. K., & Jones-Bitton, A. (2020). Prevalence of mental health outcomes among Canadian veterinarians. *Journal of the American Veterinary Medical Association*, 256(3), 365–375.

7. Mastenbroek, N. J., Jaarsma, A. D., Demerouti, E., Muijtjens, A. M., Scherpbier, A. J., & van Beukelen, P. (2014). Burnout and engagement, and its predictors in young veterinary professionals: the influence of gender. *The Veterinary Record*, 174(6), 144.

8. Hatch, P. H., Winefield, H. R., Christie, B. A., & Lievaart, J. J. (2011). Workplace stress, mental health, and burnout of veterinarians in Australia. *Australian Veterinary Journal*, 89(11), 460–468.

9. Volk, J. O., Schimmack, U., Strand, E. B., Reinhard, A., Vasconcelos, J., Hahn, J., Stiefelmeyer, K., & Probyn-Smith, K. (2022). Executive summary of the Merck Animal Health Veterinarian Wellbeing Study III and Veterinary Support Staff Study. *Journal of the American Veterinary Medical Association*, 260(12), 1547–1553.

10. Moore, I. C., Coe, J. B., Adams, C. L., Conlon, P. D., & Sargeant, J. M. (2014). The role of veterinary team effectiveness in job satisfaction and burnout in companion animal veterinary clinics. *Journal of the American Veterinary Medical Association*, 245(5), 513–524.

11. Steffey, M. A., Griffon, D. J., Risselada, M., Scharf, V. F., Buote, N. J., Zamprogno, H., & Winter, A. L. (2023). Veterinarian burnout demographics and organizational impacts: a narrative review. *Frontiers in Veterinary Science*, 10, 1184526.

12. Holowaychuk, M. K., & Lamb, K. E. (2023). Burnout symptoms and workplace satisfaction among veterinary emergency care providers. *Journal of Veterinary Emergency and Critical Care*, 33(2), 180–191.

13. Steffey, M. A., Griffon, D. J., Risselada, M., Buote, N. J., Scharf, V. F., Zamprogno, H., & Winter, A. L. (2023). A narrative review of the physiology and health effects of burnout associated with veterinarian-pertinent occupational stressors. *Frontiers in Veterinary Science*, 10, 1184525.

14. Neill, C. L., Hansen, C. R., & Salois, M. (2022). The Economic Cost of Burnout in Veterinary Medicine. *Frontiers in Veterinary Science*, 9, 814104.

15. Perret, J. L., Best, C. O., Coe, J. B., Greer, A. L., Khosa, D. K., & Jones-Bitton, A. (2020). Association of demographic, career, and lifestyle factors with resilience and

association of resilience with mental health outcomes in veterinarians in Canada. *Journal of the American Veterinary Medical Association*, 257(10), 1057–1068.

16. Darby, B. J., Watkins, S. T., Haak, P. P., Ravi-Caldwell, N., Bland, K., Bissett, C. J., Kryda, K. T., Murphy, J., Hungerford, L., & Russon, J. (2023). Veterinarians show resilience during COVID-19: challenges faced and successful coping strategies. *Journal of the American Veterinary Medical Association*, 261(6), 888–897.

CHAPTER 28

1. Google Trends. (2024). What are professional boundaries? https://trends.google.com /trends/explore?q=what%20are%20professional%20boundaries&date=2013-06-10 %202023-07-10 (accessed June 10, 2024).

2. Vande Griek, O. H., Clark, M. A., Witte, T. K., Nett, R. J., Moeller, A. N., & Stabler, M. E. (2018). Development of a taxonomy of practice-related stressors experienced by veterinarians in the United States. *Journal of the American Veterinary Medical Association*, 252(2), 227–233.

3. Kogan, L., Hellyer, P. W., Ruch-Gallie, R., Rishniw, M., & Schoenfeld-Tacher, R. (2016). Veterinarians' use and perceptions of information and communication technologies. *Medical Research Archives*, 4(2), 1–29.

4. Hashizume, C. T., Woloschuk, W., & Hecker, K. G. (2015). Changes in Veterinary Students' Attitudes Toward the Rural Environment and Rural Veterinary Practice: A Longitudinal Cohort Study. *Journal of Veterinary Medical Education*, 42(2), 112–119.

5. Schultz, K., Delva, D., & Kerr, J. (2012). Emotional effects of continuity of care on family physicians and the therapeutic relationship. *Canadian family physician Medecin de famille canadien*, 58(2), 178–185.

6. Maresca, G., Corallo, F., Catanese, G., Formica, C., & Lo Buono, V. (2022). Coping Strategies of Healthcare Professionals with Burnout Syndrome: A Systematic Review. *Medicina (Kaunas, Lithuania)*, 58(2), 327.

7. Swetz, K. M., Harrington, S. E., Matsuyama, R. K., Shanafelt, T. D., & Lyckholm, L. J. (2009). Strategies for avoiding burnout in hospice and palliative medicine: peer advice for physicians on achieving longevity and fulfillment. *Journal of Palliative Medicine*, 12(9), 773–777.

8. Zwack, J., & Schweitzer, J. (2013). If every fifth physician is affected by burnout, what about the other four? Resilience strategies of experienced physicians. *Academic medicine*, 88(3), 382–389.

9. Koh, M. Y., Chong, P. H., Neo, P. S., Ong, Y. J., Yong, W. C., Ong, W. Y., Shen, M. L., & Hum, A. Y. (2015). Burnout, psychological morbidity and use of coping mechanisms among palliative care practitioners: A multi-centre cross-sectional study. *Palliative Medicine*, 29(7), 633–642.

10. Cake, M. A., McArthur, M. M., Matthew, S. M., & Mansfield, C. F. (2017). Finding the Balance: Uncovering Resilience in the Veterinary Literature. *Journal of Veterinary Medical Education*, 44(1), 95–105.

11. Ward-Griffin, C., Brown, J. B., Vandervoort, A., McNair, S., & Dashnay, I. (2005). Double-Duty Caregiving: Women in the Health Professions. *Canadian Journal on Aging/ La Revue Canadienne Du Vieillissement*, 24(4), 379–394.

CHAPTER 29

1. Halliwell, R. E., & Hoskin, B. D. (2005). Reducing the suicide rate among veterinary surgeons: how the profession can help. *The Veterinary record*, 157(14), 397–398.
2. Platt, B., Hawton, K., Simkin, S., & Mellanby, R. J. (2010). Systematic review of the prevalence of suicide in veterinary surgeons. *Occupational Medicine*, 60(6), 436–446.
3. Tomasi, S. E., Fechter-Leggett, E. D., Edwards, N. T., Reddish, A. D., Crosby, A. E., & Nett, R. J. (2019). Suicide among veterinarians in the United States from 1979 through 2015. *Journal of the American Veterinary Medical Association*, 254(1), 104–112.
4. Milner, A. J., Niven, H., Page, K., & LaMontagne, A. D. (2015). Suicide in veterinarians and veterinary nurses in Australia: 2001-2012. *Australian Veterinary Journal*, 93(9), 308–310.
5. Perret, J. L., Best, C. O., Coe, J. B., Greer, A. L., Khosa, D. K., & Jones-Bitton, A. (2020). Prevalence of mental health outcomes among Canadian veterinarians. *Journal of the American Veterinary Medical Association*, 256(3), 365–375.
6. Schwerdtfeger, K. A., Bahramsoltani, M., Spangenberg, L., Hallensleben, N., & Glaesmer, H. (2020). Depression, suicidal ideation and suicide risk in German veterinarians compared with the general German population. *The Veterinary record*, 186(15), e2.
7. Dalum, H. S., Tyssen, R., & Hem, E. (2022). Prevalence and individual and work-related factors associated with suicidal thoughts and behaviours among veterinarians in Norway: a cross-sectional, nationwide survey-based study (the NORVET study). *BMJ Open*, 12(1), e055827.
8. Meltzer, H., Griffiths, C., Brock, A., Rooney, C., & Jenkins, R. (2008). Patterns of suicide by occupation in England and Wales: 2001-2005. *The British Journal of Psychiatry*, 193(1), 73–76.
9. Roberts, S. E., Jaremin, B., & Lloyd, K. (2013). High-risk occupations for suicide. *Psychological medicine*, 43(6), 1231–1240.
10. Zimmermann, C., Strohmaier, S., Niederkrotenthaler, T., Thau, K., & Schernhammer, E. (2023). Suicide mortality among physicians, dentists, veterinarians, and pharmacists as well as other high-skilled occupations in Austria from 1986 through 2020. *Psychiatry Research*, 323, 115170.
11. Peterson, C., Sussell, A., Li, J., Schumacher, P.K., Yeoman, K., & Stone, D.M. (2016). Suicide Rates by Industry and Occupation — National Violent Death Reporting System, 32 States. *Morbidity and Mortality Weekly Report*, 69,57–62.
12. Milner, A., Witt, K., Maheen, H., & LaMontagne, A. D. (2017). Access to means of suicide, occupation and the risk of suicide: a national study over 12 years of coronial data. *BMC Psychiatry*, 17(1), 125.

13. Witte, T. K., Spitzer, E. G., Edwards, N., Fowler, K. A., & Nett, R. J. (2019). Suicides and deaths of undetermined intent among veterinary professionals from 2003 through 2014. *Journal of the American Veterinary Medical Association*, 255(5), 595–608.

14. Houtsma, C., Bond, A. E., & Anestis, M. D. (2023). Practical Capability Among Veterinarians: Preliminary Evidence of the Importance of Access to Lethal Medications in the Workplace. *Archives of Suicide Research*, 27(4), 1351–1362.

15. Waitz-Kudla, S. N., Kramper, S., Roark, A., Mani, I., & Witte, T. K. (2023). Securing lethal means for suicide: a focus group study exploring perceptions and barriers among practicing veterinarians. *Journal of the American Veterinary Medical Association*, 261(11), 1683–1693.

16. American Foundation for Suicide Prevention. (2024). Suicide Statistics. https://afsp .org/suicide-statistics/ (accessed June 10, 2024).

17. Royal Canin. (2022). Vet Mental Health Under the Spotlight. https://www.royalcanin .com/au/about-us/news/love-your-pet-love-your-vet-survey (accessed November 1, 2024).

18. American Foundation for Suicide Prevention. (2024). Risk factors, protective factors, and warning signs. https://afsp.org/risk-factors-protective-factors-and-warning -signs/ (accessed June 10, 2024).

19. Platt, B., Hawton, K., Simkin, S., & Mellanby, R. J. (2012). Suicidal behaviour and psychosocial problems in veterinary surgeons: a systematic review. *Social Psychiatry and Psychiatric Epidemiology*, 47(2), 223–240.

20. Platt, B., Hawton, K., Simkin, S., Dean, R., & Mellanby, R. J. (2012). Suicidality in the veterinary profession: interview study of veterinarians with a history of suicidal ideation or behavior. *Crisis*, 33(5), 280–289.

21. Glaesmer, H., Bahramsoltani, M., Schwerdtfeger, K., & Spangenberg, L. (2021). Euthanasia Distress and Fearlessness About Death in German Veterinarians. *Crisis*, 42(1), 71–77.

22. Ogden, U., Kinnison, T., & May, S. A. (2012). Attitudes to animal euthanasia do not correlate with acceptance of human euthanasia or suicide. *The Veterinary Record*, 171(7), 174.

23. Tran, L., Crane, M. F., & Phillips, J. K. (2014). The distinct role of performing euthanasia on depression and suicide in veterinarians. *Journal of Occupational Health Psychology*, 19(2), 123–132.

24. Crane, M. F., Phillips, J. K., & Karin, E. (2017). "I've been a long time leaving": the role of limited skill transferability in increasing suicide-related cognitions and behavior in veterinarians. *Suicide & Life-Threatening Behavior*, 47(3), 309–320.

25. Allister, R. (2021). It's good to talk, but it matters how we do it. *The Veterinary Record*, 188(6), 235.

26. Wikipedia. (2024). Copycat suicide. https://en.wikipedia.org/wiki/Copycat_suicide (accessed June 10, 2024).

27. American Veterinary Medical Association. (2022). Preventing suicide: New guide free to profession. https://www.avma.org/blog/preventing-suicide-new-guide-free -profession (accessed June 10, 2024).

28. American Veterinary Medical Association. (2024). QPR suicide prevention training. https://www.avma.org/resources-tools/wellbeing/qpr-suicide-prevention-training (accessed June 10, 2024).

29. Westgate, J. (2022). Vetlife launches resource for veterinary workplaces affected by suicide. VetTimes. https://www.vettimes.co.uk/news/vetlife-launches-resource-for-veterinary-workplaces-affected-by-suicide/ (accessed June 10, 2024).

CHAPTER 30

1. Quain, A., Mullan, S., & Ward, M. P. (2022). Low and No-Contact Euthanasia: Associated Ethical Challenges Experienced by Veterinary Team Members during the Early Months of the COVID-19 Pandemic. *Animals*, 12(5), 560.

2. Quain, A., Mullan, S., McGreevy, P. D., & Ward, M. P. (2021). Frequency, Stressfulness and Type of Ethically Challenging Situations Encountered by Veterinary Team Members During the COVID-19 Pandemic. *Frontiers in Veterinary Science*, 8, 647108.

3. Quain, A., Mullan, S., & Ward, M. P. (2021). Risk Factors Associated With Increased Ethically Challenging Situations Encountered by Veterinary Team Members During the COVID-19 Pandemic. *Frontiers in Veterinary Science*, 8, 752388.

4. Rowe, Z. C., Drewery, M. L., Anderson, R. G., & Russo, C. M. (2022). Challenges Faced by U.S. Veterinary Technicians in the Workplace During COVID-19. *Frontiers in Veterinary Science*, 9, 831127.

5. Chalabi, M. (2022). Pets prove to be the pandemic's cute, furry growth area. The Guardian. https://www.theguardian.com/news/datablog/2022/jan/21/pets-ownership-pandemic-dogs-cats (accessed June 10, 2024).

6. Volk, J. O., Schimmack, U., Strand, E. B., Reinhard, A., Vasconcelos, J., Hahn, J., Stiefelmeyer, K., & Probyn-Smith, K. (2022). Executive summary of the Merck Animal Health Veterinarian Wellbeing Study III and Veterinary Support Staff Study. *Journal of the American Veterinary Medical Association*, 260(12), 1547–1553.

7. McKee, H., Gohar, B., Appleby, R., Nowrouzi-Kia, B., Hagen, B. N. M., & Jones-Bitton, A. (2021). High Psychosocial Work Demands, Decreased Well-Being, and Perceived Well-Being Needs Within Veterinary Academia During the COVID-19 Pandemic. *Frontiers in Veterinary Science*, 8, 746716.

8. Carney, K., & Thompson, R. R. (2021). Grief in Response to Uncertainty Distress Among Veterinary Students During the Early Stages of the COVID-19 Pandemic. *Frontiers in Veterinary Science*, 8, 662198.

9. Sacchettino, L., Gatta, C., Chirico, A., Avallone, L., Napolitano, F., & d'Angelo, D. (2023). Puppies Raised during the COVID-19 Lockdown Showed Fearful and Aggressive Behaviors in Adulthood: An Italian Survey. *Veterinary Sciences*, 10(3), 198.

10. Chopik, W. J., Oh, J., Weidmann, R., Weaver, J. R., Balzarini, R. N., Zoppolat, G., & Slatcher, R. B. (2023). The perks of pet ownership? The effects of pet ownership on well-being during the COVID-19 pandemic. *Personality & Social Psychology Bulletin*, 1461672231203417

11. Phillipou, A., Tan, E. J., Toh, W. L., Van Rheenen, T. E., Meyer, D., Neill, E., Sumner, P. J., & Rossell, S. L. (2021). Pet ownership and mental health during COVID-19 lockdown. *Australian Veterinary Journal*, 99(10), 423–426.

12. Amiot, C. E., Gagné, C., & Bastian, B. (2022). Pet ownership and psychological well-being during the COVID-19 pandemic. *Scientific Reports*, 12(1), 6091.

CHAPTER 31

1. Kogan, L. R., & Rishniw, M. (2023). Differences in perceptions and satisfaction exist among veterinarians employed at corporate versus privately owned veterinary clinics. *Journal of the American Veterinary Medical Association*, 261(12), 1838–1846.

2. VBJ 182. (2018). Big 6: rising corporatisation. VetTimes. https://www.vettimes.co.uk/article/big-6-rising-corporatisation/ (accessed June 10, 2024).

3. Business Sale Report. (2024). M&A in the Veterinary Sector – Mass Consolidation. https://www.business-sale.com/insights/for-buyers/ma-in-the-veterinary-sector-mass-consolidation-220585 (accessed June 10, 2024).

4. Loeb, J. (2023). Competition watchdog launches major review of vet services. https://bvajournals.onlinelibrary.wiley.com/do/10.1002/vetr.00200009 (accessed June 10, 2024).

5. Kelly, R. (2021). British, Canadian veterinary giants merge. VIN News. https://news.vin.com/default.aspx?pid=210&Id=10464850&f5=1 (accessed June 10, 2024).

6. Osborne, D. (2023). The corporatization of veterinary medicine. *The Canadian Veterinary Journal*, 64(5), 483–488.

7. Kelly, R. (2020). NVA, now top dog in Australia, sizes up more practices. VIN News. https://news.vin.com/default.aspx?pid=210&Id=9569758&f5=1 (accessed June 10, 2024).

8. Kelly, R. (2022). Froth subsiding from veterinary deals, Australian execs say. VIN News. https://news.vin.com/default.aspx?pid=210&Id=10983750&f5=1 (accessed June 10, 2024).

9. Mandow, N. (2023). Is your 'local' vet owned by German billionaires? News Room. https://newsroom.co.nz/2023/03/16/is-your-local-vet-owned-by-german-billionaires/ (accessed June 10, 2024).

10. Jelinski, M. D., Schreiner, B., Neale, A., & Townsend, H. G. G. (2022). Demographic survey of private veterinary practices in western Canada. *The Canadian Veterinary Journal*, 63(1), 27–30.

11. Ouedraogo, F. B., Bain, B., Hansen, C., & Salois, M. (2019). A census of veterinarians in the United States. *Journal of the American Veterinary Medical Association*, 255(2), 183–191.

12. Ouedraogo, F. B., & Lefebvre, S. L. (2022). Benefits of practice ownership among US private practice veterinarians extend to professional quality of life. *Journal of the American Veterinary Medical Association*, 260(15), 1971–1978.

13. Royal College of Veterinary Surgeons. (2020). The 2019 Survey of the Veterinary Profession. https://www.rcvs.org.uk/news-and-views/publications/the-2019-survey-of-the-veterinary-profession/ (accessed June 10, 2024).

14. Makortoff, K. (2024). UK watchdog plans formal investigation into vet pricing. The Guardian. https://www.theguardian.com/business/2024/mar/12/uk-vet-pricing-competition-and-markets-authority-cma (accessed June 10, 2024).

15. Vetspanel. (2024). Why are stress levels in corporate practices so high? https://www.vetspanel.com/why-are-stress-levels-in-corporate-practices-so-high/ (accessed June 10, 2024).

CHAPTER 32

1. Stephens, J. L. (1999). The future for third-party payment in veterinary medicine. *Journal of the American Veterinary Medical Association*, 214(7), 1010–1012.

2. Stowe, J. D. (2000). Pet insurance--essential option? *The Canadian Veterinary Journal*, 41(8), 639–644.

3. Burns, K. (2007). Pet health insurance gains ground in North America. *Journal of the American Veterinary Medical Association*, 230(5), 634–637.

4. American Veterinary Medical Association. (2024). Pet health insurance. https://www.avma.org/resources-tools/avma-policies/pet-health-insurance (accessed June 10, 2024).

5. Holowaychuk, M. (2017). How pet insurance can help the mental health of veterinarians. https://marieholowaychuk.com/2017/12/27/pet-insurance-can-help-mental-health-veterinarians/ (accessed June 10, 2024).

6. Kipperman, B. S., Kass, P. H., & Rishniw, M. (2017). Factors that influence small animal veterinarians' opinions and actions regarding cost of care and effects of economic limitations on patient care and outcome and professional career satisfaction and burnout. *Journal of the American Veterinary Medical Association*, 250(7), 785–794.

7. The Dog People. (2024). The Cost of Dog Parenthood in 2024. Rover.com. https://www.rover.com/ca/blog/cost-of-dog-parenthood/ (accessed June 10, 2024).

8. Chiu, L. J. V., Li, J., Lhermie, G., & Cazer, C. (2021). Analysis of the demand for pet insurance among uninsured pet owners in the United States. *The Veterinary Record*, 189(1), e243.

9. Chaumet, A. C. S. G., Rossi, T. A., Murphy, L. A., & Nakamura, R. K. (2021). Evaluation of owners' attitudes towards veterinary insurance in a specialty hospital. *The Journal of Small Animal Practice*, 62(9), 805–809.

10. Boller, M., Nemanic, T. S., Anthonisz, J. D., Awad, M., Selinger, J., Boller, E. M., & Stevenson, M. A. (2020). The effect of pet insurance on presurgical euthanasia of dogs with gastric dilatation-volvulus: a novel approach to quantifying economic euthanasia in veterinary emergency medicine. *Frontiers in Veterinary Science*, 7, 590615.

11. Becker, M., Volk, H., & Kunzmann, P. (2022). Is pet health insurance able to improve veterinary care? Why pet health insurance for dogs and cats has limits: an ethical consideration on pet health insurance. *Animals*, 12(13), 1728.

12. Springer, S., Lund, T. B., Grimm, H., Kristensen, A. T., Corr, S. A., & Sandøe, P. (2022). Comparing veterinarians' attitudes to and the potential influence of pet health insurance in Austria, Denmark and the UK. *The Veterinary Record*, 190(10), e1266.

13. Sandøe, P., Palmer, C., Corr, S. A., Springer, S., & Lund, T. B. (2023). Do people really care less about their cats than about their dogs? A comparative study in three European countries. *Frontiers in Veterinary Science*, 10, 1237547.

14. Metz, J. (2024). Pet Insurance Statistics 2024. https://www.forbes.com/advisor/pet-insurance/pet-insurance-statistics/#sources_section (accessed June 10, 2024).

15. North American Pet Health Insurance Association. (2024). Pet Insurance in North America. https://naphia.org/industry-data/ (accessed June 10, 2024).

16. Fernyhough, J. (2019). Pet insurance market looks to rise of the 'fur baby'. Financial Review. https://www.afr.com/companies/financial-services/pet-insurance-market-looks-to-rise-of-the-fur-baby-20190215-h1baml (accessed June 10, 2024).

17. Klir, K.-B. (2024). How Many People Have Pet Insurance in the UK in 2024? Statistics & FAQ. PetKeen. https://petkeen.com/how-many-people-have-pet-insurance-uk/ (accessed June 10, 2024).

18. Burns, K. (2014). Pet health insurance helping more pet owners afford optimal care. *Journal of the American Veterinary Medical Association*, 244(12), 1348–1353.

CHAPTER 33

1. Dubin, R. J., Angliss, G., Eng, C., Cisneros, T., & Griffon, D. (2021). Veterinarians' perceptions of COVID-19 pandemic-related influences on veterinary telehealth and on pet owners' attitudes toward cats and dogs. *Journal of the American Veterinary Medical Association*, 259(10), 1140–1147.

2. Springer, S., Lund, T. B., Corr, S. A., & Sandøe, P. (2024). Seeing the benefits, but not taking advantage of them: Dog and cat owners' beliefs about veterinary telemedicine. *The Veterinary Record*, 194(5), e3312.

3. Sigesmund, D., Coe, J. B., Moore, I. C., & Khosa, D. (2023). Pet owners prefer face-to-face consultations, with many being open to considering virtual consultations with veterinarians. *Journal of the American Veterinary Medical Association*, 262(1), 100–108.

4. Widmar, N. O., Bir, C., Slipchenko, N., Wolf, C., Hansen, C., & Ouedraogo, F. (2020). Online procurement of pet supplies and willingness to pay for veterinary telemedicine. *Preventive Veterinary Medicine*, 181, 105073.

5. Caney, S. M. A., Robinson, N. J., Gunn-Moore, D. A., & Dean, R. S. (2022). Veterinary surgeons', veterinary nurses' and owners' experiences of feline telemedicine consultations during the 2020 COVID-19 pandemic. *The Veterinary Record*, 191(5), e1738.

6. Larkin, M. (2024). Eliminating in-person VCPR requirement for telemedicine, proposed midlevel position discussed at information forum. AVMA News. https://www.avma.org/news/eliminating-person-vcpr-requirement-telemedicine-proposed-midlevel-position-discussed (accessed June 10, 2024).

7. Lundahl, L., Powell, L., Reinhard, C. L., Healey, E., & Watson, B. (2022). A Pilot Study Examining the Experience of Veterinary Telehealth in an Underserved Population Through a University Program Integrating Veterinary Students. *Frontiers in Veterinary Science*, 9, 871928.

8. Ireifej, S. J., & Krol, J. (2023). Case studies of fifteen novel species successfully aided with the use of a veterinary teletriage service. *Frontiers in Veterinary Science*, 10, 1225724.

9. Lubbers, B. V., Fajt, V. R., Teller, L. M., Apley, M. D., & Stillisano, J. (2023). Using telehealth clinical case vignettes to enhance clinical confidence and competence in veterinary students. *Frontiers in Veterinary Science*, 9, 1075752.

10. Fejzić, N., Muftić, A., Šerić-Haračić, S., & Muftić, E. (2023). The impact of digital presence and use of information technology on business performance of veterinary practices: a case study of Bosnia and Herzegovina. *Frontiers in Veterinary Science*, 10, 1208654.

11. Smith, A., Carroll, P. W., Aravamuthan, S., Walleser, E., Lin, H., Anklam, K., Döpfer, D., & Apostolopoulos, N. (2024). Computer vision model for the detection of canine pododermatitis and neoplasia of the paw. *Veterinary Dermatology*, 35(2), 138–147.

CHAPTER 34

1. Ortman, J. M. & Guarneri, C. E. (2009). United States Population Projections: 2000 to 2050. http://www.census.gov/population/www/projections/analytical-document09 .pdf (accessed April 6, 2022).

2. Zippia. (2024). Doctoral Student Demographics and Statistics in the US. https://www .zippia.com/doctoral-student-jobs/demographics/ (accessed June 10, 2024).

3. National Center for Science and Engineering Statistics (NCSES). (2023). Report Science and Engineering Degrees Earned. National Science Foundation. https://ncses .nsf.gov/pubs/nsf23315/report/science-and-engineering-degrees-earned (accessed June 10, 2024).

4. Thompson, D. (2013). The 33 whitest jobs in America. *Forbes*. https://www.theatlantic .com/business/archive/2013/11/the-33-whitest-jobs-in-america/281180/ (accessed February 4, 2022).

5. Bureau of Labor Statistics. (2022). Household data annual averages. https://www.bls .gov/cps/cpsaat11.pdf (accessed February 16, 2022).

6. Association of American Veterinary Medical Colleges. (2020). Annual AAVMC data report 2019–2020. https://public.tableau.com/profile/aavmc.research#!/vizhome/202 0AAVMCAnnualDataReport/Introduction (accessed February 4, 2022).

7. Greenhill, L. M., Cipriani Davis, K., Lowrie, P. M., & Amass, S. A. eds. (2013). Navigating Diversity and Inclusion in Veterinary Medicine. https://library.oapen.org /handle/20.500.12657/64185?show=full (accessed February 4, 2022).

8. YouTube. (2020). A profession in crisis: Discrimination in veterinary medicine. https://www.youtube.com/watch?v=j7Pl4YX_QNc (accessed February 4, 2022).

9. American Veterinary Medical Association. (2023). COE accreditation policies and procedures: requirements. https://www.avma.org/education/accreditation-policies -and-procedures-avma-council-education-coe/coe-accreditation-policies-and -procedures-requirements (accessed June 10, 2024).

10. Burkhard, M. J., Dawkins, S., Knoblaugh, S. E., El-Khoury, C., Coble, D., Malbrue, R. A., Read, E. K., Greenhill, L. M., & Moore, R. M. (2022). Supporting diversity, equity, inclusion, and belonging to strengthen and position the veterinary profession for

service, sustainability, excellence, and impact. *Journal of the American Veterinary Medical Association*, 260(11), 1283–1290.

11. Hammond, S., & Runion, K. (2022). Development of a 1-week intensive course on diversity and equity in veterinary medicine. *Journal of Veterinary Medical Education*, 49(1), 8–15. https://doi.org/10.3138/jvme-2020-0072

12. Milstein, M. S., Gilbertson, M. L. J., Bernstein, L. A., & Hsue, W. (2022). Integrating the Multicultural Veterinary Medical Association actionables into diversity, equity, and inclusion curricula in United States veterinary colleges. *Journal of the American Veterinary Medical Association*, 260(10), 1145–1152.

13. Royal College of Veterinary Surgeons. (2021). RCVS Diversity and Inclusion Group Strategy. https://www.rcvs.org.uk/news-and-views/publications/rcvs-diversity-and-inclusion-group-strategy/ (accessed June 10, 2024).

14. American Veterinary Medical Association. (2022). AVMA names first-ever chief DEI officer. https://www.avma.org/blog/avma-names-first-ever-chief-dei-officer (accessed June 10, 2024).

15. Odunayo, A., Alwood, A., Asokan, V., Balakrishnan, A., Berkowitz, S., Buckley, G., Chih, A., Claus, K., Cottam, E., Gonzalez, A., Hoareau, G. L., Holowaychuk, M., Johnson, P., Kielb, J., Ngwenyama, T., Pardo, M., Rutter, C., Sharpe, S., & Whitehead, K. (2022). Our quest for creating a space that is welcoming to all: A commentary from the American College of Veterinary Emergency and Critical Care Diversity, Equity, and Inclusion Committee. *Journal of Veterinary Emergency and Critical Care*, 32(2), 165–167.

16. ACVECC DEI Committee. (2024). Critically Diverse. https://www.linkedin.com/in/critically-diverse-544048256/ (accessed June 10, 2024).

17. American College of Veterinary Emergency and Critical Care. (2024). ACVECC Diversity, Equity, and Inclusion Links. https://www.acvecc.org/ACVECC-Diversity-Equity-and-Inclusion-Links (accessed June 10, 2024).

18. Chun, R., Davis, E., Frank, N., Green, H. W., Greenhill, L., Jandrey, K. E., Johannes, C. M., Levine, J., Marks, S. L., Polisetti, S., Rogers, K. S., & Sanchez, L. C. (2022). Can veterinary medicine improve diversity in post-graduate training programs? Current state of academic veterinary medicine and recommendations on best practices. *Journal of the American Veterinary Medical Association*, 261(3), 417–423.

19. Women Veterinary Leadership Development Initiative. (2023). Toolkits for Success: Pay Equity. https://wvldi.org/wp-content/uploads/2023/07/FINAL_Pay-Equity-Toolkit.pdf (accessed June 10, 2024).

20. Green Seymour, K. (2023). The Gender Pay Gap - Why More Women in Vet Med Does Not Equal Gender Equality. AAHA Trends. https://www.aaha.org/publications/trends-magazine/trends-articles/2023/march-2023/f1-gender-pay-gap/ (accessed June 10, 2024).

21. Yankowicz, S. (2024). Study finds shortage of women in leadership positions. DVM360. https://www.dvm360.com/view/study-finds-shortage-of-women-in-leadership-positions (accessed June 10, 2024).

CHAPTER 35

1. Brown, J. P., & Silverman, J. D. (1999). The current and future market for veterinarians and veterinary medical services in the United States. *Journal of the American Veterinary Medical Association*, 215(2), 161–183.
2. Englar, R. E. (2019). Tracking veterinary students' acquisition of communication skills and clinical communication confidence by comparing student performance in the first and twenty-seventh standardized client encounters. *Journal of Veterinary Medical Education*, 46(2), 235–257.
3. McDermott, M. P., Tischler, V. A., Cobb, M. A., Robbé, I. J., & Dean, R. S. (2015). Veterinarian-Client Communication Skills: Current State, Relevance, and Opportunities for Improvement. *Journal of Veterinary Medical Education*, 42(4), 305–314.
4. North American Veterinary Medical Education Consortium Board of Directors. (2020). Roadmap for Veterinary Medical Education in the 21st Century: Responsive, Collaborative, Flexible. https://www.aavmc.org/assets/data-new/files/NAVMEC/navmec_roadmapreport_web_single.pdf (accessed May 30, 2024).
5. Walsh, D. A., Klosterman, E. S., & Kass, P. H. (2009). Approaches to veterinary education--tracking versus a final year broad clinical experience. Part two: instilled values. *Revue scientifique et technique (International Office of Epizootics)*, 28(2), 811–822.
6. Densen, P. (2011). Challenges and opportunities facing medical education. *Transactions of the American Clinical and Climatological Association*, 122, 48–58.
7. Warren, A. L., & Donnon, T. (2013). Optimizing biomedical science learning in a veterinary curriculum: a review. *Journal of Veterinary Medical Education*, 40(3), 210–222.
8. Dowling, T. (2012). Course teaches mindfulness to students. WCVM Today. https://wcvmtoday.usask.ca/articles/2012/mindful-veterinary-practice.php (accessed May 30, 2024).
9. Correia, H. M., Smith, A. D., Murray, S., Polak, L. S., Williams, B., & Cake, M. A. (2017). The Impact of a Brief Embedded Mindfulness-Based Program for Veterinary Students. *Journal of Veterinary Medical Education*, 44(1), 125–133.
10. The Ohio State University College of Veterinary Medicine. (2024). Wellbeing Initiative. https://vet.osu.edu/about/be-well (accessed May 30, 2024).

CHAPTER 36

1. Vogelsang, J. (2016). 37 ways to use a DVM degree. DVM360. https://www.dvm360.com/view/37-ways-use-dvm-degree (accessed May 30, 2024).
2. American Veterinary Medical Association. (2024). Veterinarians: Protecting the health of animals and people. https://www.avma.org/resources/pet-owners/yourvet/veterinarians-protecting-health-animals-and-people (accessed August 23, 2024).
3. Widmar, N., Bir, C., Lai, J., & Wolf, C. (2020). Public Perceptions of Veterinarians from Social and Online Media Listening. *Veterinary Sciences*, 7(2), 75.

4. DVMoms: GAIN Facebook Grouphttps://www.facebook.com/groups/472561733321854/ (accessed May 30, 2024).
5. Vets Stay, Go, Diversify Facebook Group. https://www.facebook.com/groups/VetsSGD/members (accessed May 30, 2024).
6. Vets Stay, Go, Diversify. https://vsgd.co/ (accessed May 30, 2024).
7. Cornell University College of Veterinary Medicine. (2024). Leadership Program for Veterinary Students at Cornell University. https://www.vet.cornell.edu/education/other-educational-opportunities/leadership-program-veterinary-students-cornell-university (accessed May 30, 2024).
8. McGregor, D. D., Fraser, D. R., & Parker, J. S. L. (2020). Tracking. *Journal of Veterinary Medical Education*, 47(1), 100–105.

CHAPTER 37

1. U.S. Bureau of Statistics. (2024). Fastest Growing Occupations. https://www.bls.gov/ooh/fastest-growing.htm (accessed June 10, 2024).
2. U.S. Bureau of Statistics. (2024). Veterinary Technologists and Technicians. https://www.bls.gov/ooh/healthcare/veterinary-technologists-and-technicians.htm (accessed June 10, 2024).
3. Zimlich, R. (2018). RNs fight veterinary technicians over the word 'nurse'. DVM360. https://www.dvm360.com/view/rns-fight-veterinary-technicians-over-word-nurse (accessed June 10, 2024).
4. NAVTA. (2024). VTS - The NAVTA Committee on Veterinary Technician Specialties. https://navta.net/veterinary-technician-specialties/ (accessed June 10, 2024).
5. American Animal Hospital Association. (2024). Stay, Please. https://www.aaha.org/resources/white-paper-factors-that-support-retentionand-drive-attrition-in-the-veterinary-profession/ (accessed June 10, 2024).
6. Witte, T. K., Spitzer, E. G., Edwards, N., Fowler, K. A., & Nett, R. J. (2019). Suicides and deaths of undetermined intent among veterinary professionals from 2003 through 2014. *Journal of the American Veterinary Medical Association*, 255(5), 595–608.
7. Milner, A. J., Niven, H., Page, K., & LaMontagne, A. D. (2015). Suicide in veterinarians and veterinary nurses in Australia: 2001-2012. *Australian Veterinary Journal*, 93(9), 308–310.
8. van Soest, E. M., & Fritschi, L. (2004). Occupational health risks in veterinary nursing: an exploratory study. *Australian Veterinary Journal*, 82(6), 346–350.
9. Seagren, K. E., Sommerich, C. M., & Lavender, S. A. (2022). Musculoskeletal discomfort in veterinary healthcare professions. *Work*, 71(4), 1007–1027.
10. Rogers, C. W., Murphy, L. A., Murphy, R. A., Malouf, K. A., Natsume, R. E., Ward, B. D., Tansey, C., & Nakamura, R. K. (2022). An analysis of client complaints and their effects on veterinary support staff. *Veterinary medicine and science*, 8(2), 925–934.
11. Yukawa, S., & Yukawa, M. (2022). A survey assessing the prevalence of in-hospital violence against veterinary nurses working in small animal hospitals. *Open Veterinary Journal*, 12(4), 430–433.
12. Volk, J. O., Schimmack, U., Strand, E. B., Reinhard, A., Vasconcelos, J., Hahn, J., Stiefelmeyer, K., & Probyn-Smith, K. (2022). Executive summary of the Merck

Animal Health Veterinarian Wellbeing Study III and Veterinary Support Staff Study. *Journal of the American Veterinary Medical Association*, 260(12), 1547–1553.

13. Ho, N. T., Santoro, F., Palacios Jimenez, C., & Pelligand, L. (2023). Cross-sectional survey of sleep, fatigue and mental health in veterinary anaesthesia personnel. *Veterinary Anaesthesia and Analgesia*, 50(4), 315–324.

14. Kimber, S., & Gardner, D. H. (2016). Relationships between workplace well-being, job demands and resources in a sample of veterinary nurses in New Zealand. *New Zealand Veterinary Journal*, 64(4), 224–229.

15. Kogan, L. R., Wallace, J. E., Schoenfeld-Tacher, R., Hellyer, P. W., & Richards, M. (2020). Veterinary Technicians and Occupational Burnout. *Frontiers in Veterinary Science*, 7, 328.

16. Hayes, G. M., LaLonde-Paul, D. F., Perret, J. L., Steele, A., McConkey, M., Lane, W. G., Kopp, R. J., Stone, H. K., Miller, M., & Jones-Bitton, A. (2020). Investigation of burnout syndrome and job-related risk factors in veterinary technicians in specialty teaching hospitals: a multicenter cross-sectional study. *Journal of Veterinary Emergency and Critical Care*, 30(1), 18–27.

17. Larkin, M. (2016). Technician shortage may be a problem of turnover instead - Income, wellness issues plague veterinary technicians, too, survey says. American Veterinary Medical Association. https://www.avma.org/javma-news/2016-10-15/technician-shortage-may-be-problem-turnover-instead (accessed June 10, 2024).

18. Imrie, P. (2022). Vet group introduces £30k pay rate for RVNs. VetTimes. https://www.vettimes.co.uk/news/vet-group-introduces-30k-pay-rate-for-rvns/ (accessed June 10, 2024).

19. Doherty, C. (2020). Widening the lead: Non-DVM wages and inflation. *The Canadian Veterinary Journal*, 61(11), 1211–1214.

20. Veterinary Emergency Group. (2024). Be a VEG Nurse. https://careers.veterinaryemergencygroup.com/nurses-2/ (accessed June 10, 2024).

CHAPTER 38

1. Global Animal Health Association. (2022). Global State of Pet Care: Stats, Facts and Trends. Health For Animals. https://healthforanimals.org/reports/pet-care-report/global-trends-in-the-pet-population/ (accessed June 10, 2024).

2. American Association of Veterinary Medical Colleges. (2024). AAVMC Statement on U.S. Veterinary Workforce. https://www.aavmc.org/resources/aavmc-statement-on-u-s-veterinary-workforce/ (accessed August 23, 2024).

3. Canadian Veterinary Medical Association. (2024). https://www.canadianveterinarians.net/policy-and-outreach/priority-areas/veterinary-workforce-shortage/ (accessed June 10, 2024).

4. American Veterinary Medical Association. (2023). Straight talk about veterinary workforce issues - Dispelling misinformation and disinformation in the post-COVID era. https://www.avma.org/news/straight-talk-about-veterinary-workforce-issues (accessed June 10, 2024).

5. American Association of Veterinary Medical Colleges. (2022). AAVMC Statement on U.S. Veterinary Workforce. https://www.aavmc.org/wp-content/uploads/2022/07/AAVMC-Statement-on-Workforce-July-2022.pdf (accessed June 10, 2024).

6. University of Saskatchewan Western College of Veterinary Medicine. (2022). Small animal ER closed overnight on June 22 due to staff shortage. https://vmc.usask.ca/referring-veterinarians/rdvm/small-animal-er-closed-overnight-on-june-22-due-to-staff-shortage.php (accessed June 10, 2024).

7. Ross, S. (2023). Atlantic Vet College will no longer offer overnight emergency care. CBC News. https://www.cbc.ca/news/canada/prince-edward-island/pei-atlantic-veterinary-hospital-reduced-hours-1.6827971 (accessed June 10, 2024).

8. Smith, M. (2023). Alberta seeing 'crisis' in veterinarian staff shortages, emergency animal care. CBC News. https://www.cbc.ca/news/canada/edmonton/alberta-seeing-crisis-in-veterinarian-staff-shortages-emergency-animal-care-1.6902128 (accessed June 10, 2024).

9. Lloyd, J.W. (2022). Pet Healthcare in the US: Are There Enough Veterinary Specialists? Is There Adequate Training Capacity? Mars Veterinary. https://www.marsveterinary.com/wp-content/uploads/2022/03/Characterizing%20the%20Need%20-%20Specialists%20-%20FINAL_2.24.pdf (accessed June 10, 2024).

10. Mars Veterinary Health. (2023). Tackling the Veterinary Professional Shortage. https://www.marsveterinary.com/tackling-the-veterinary-professional-shortage/ (accessed June 10, 2024).

11. American Association of Veterinary Medical Colleges. (2024). AAVMC Response: Demand for and Supply of Veterinarians in the U.S. to 2032. https://www.aavmc.org/wp-content/uploads/2024/03/Demand-for-and-Supply-of-Veterinarians-in-the-U.S.-to-2032-1.pdf (accessed June 10, 2024).

12. Webb, A. (2022). 12 mins to readStaff shortages leave vet sector facing ticking time bomb. VetTimes. https://www.vettimes.co.uk/news/staff-shortages-leave-vet-sector-facing-ticking-time-bomb/ (accessed June 10, 2024).

13. Australia Veterinary Association. (2024). Planning an effective veterinary workforce. https://www.ava.com.au/policy-advocacy/advocacy/workforce/ (accessed June 10, 2024).

14. American Animal Hospital Association. (2024). Stay, Please. https://www.aaha.org/resources/white-paper-factors-that-support-retentionand-drive-attrition-in-the-veterinary-profession/ (accessed June 10, 2024).

15. Prescott-Clements, L., Soreskog-Turp, J., Crawford, B., & Williams, K. (2022). The Development and Implementation of a National Veterinary Graduate Development Programme (VetGDP) to Support Veterinarians Entering the UK Workforce. *Journal of Veterinary Medical Education*, e20220112.

16. American Veterinary Medical Association. (2024). Mentoring for early-career veterinarians. https://www.avma.org/education/veterinary-career-center/mentoring-new-veterinarians (accessed June 10, 2024).

17. MentorVet. (2023). Impact Report. https://www.mentorvet.net/impactreport (accessed June 10, 2024).

CHAPTER 39

1. Green Cross Academy of Traumatology. (2024). Standards of Care. https://greencross .org/about-gc/standards-of-care-guidelines/ (accessed June 10, 2024).
2. Stoewen, D. L. (2021). Moving from compassion fatigue to compassion resilience Part 5: Building personal resilience. *The Canadian Veterinary Journal*, 62(11), 1229–1231.
3. Holowaychuk, M. K., Atilla, A., Archer, R. M., & Kwong, G. P. S. (2023). Self-care practices and depression, anxiety, and stress scores in veterinary students during a semester. *The Canadian Veterinary Journal*, 64(6), 571–578.
4. Drake, A. S., Hafen Jr., M., Davis, E. G., & Rush, B. R. (2022). Authentic Conversations about Self-Care with Fourth-Year Veterinary Medical Students. *Journal of Veterinary Medical Education*, 49(6), 679–685.
5. Neff, K. (2015). *Self-Compassion: The Proven Power of Being Kind to Yourself.* William Morrow Paperbacks.
6. Neff, K. (2024). Instruments for Researchers. Self-Compassion.org. https://self -compassion.org/self-compassion-scales-for-researchers/ (accessed June 10, 2024).
7. McArthur, M., Mansfield, C., Matthew, S., Zaki, S., Brand, C., Andrews, J., & Hazel, S. (2017). Resilience in veterinary students and the predictive role of mindfulness and self-compassion. *Journal of Veterinary Medical Education*, 44(1), 106–115.
8. Smith, B. W., Dalen, J., Wiggins, K., Tooley, E., Christopher, P., & Bernard, J. (2008). The brief resilience scale: assessing the ability to bounce back. *International Journal of Behavioral Medicine*, 15(3), 194–200.
9. Mills, J., Wand, T., & Fraser, J. A. (2018). Examining self-care, self-compassion and compassion for others: a cross-sectional survey of palliative care nurses and doctors. *International Journal of Palliative Nursing*, 24(1), 4–11.

CHAPTER 40

1. Students of the Canadian Veterinary Medical Association. (2023). SCVMA New Graduate Report - Class of 2022. https://www.canadianveterinarians.net/media/ qnkmyla3/2022-scvma-grad-report_final_en.pdf (accessed June 10, 2024).
2. Students of the Canadian Veterinary Medical Association. (2021). SCVMA New Graduate Report - Class of 2020. *The Canadian Veterinary Journal,* 62(3), 334–339.
3. National Association of Veterinary Technicians in America. (2022). NAVTA 2022 Demographic Survey Results: Pay & Education Have Increased; Burnout & Debt Are Still Issues. https://navta.website/2022DemographicSurvey (accessed June 10, 2024).
4. Volk, J. O., Schimmack, U., Strand, E. B., Reinhard, A., Vasconcelos, J., Hahn, J., Stiefelmeyer, K., & Probyn-Smith, K. (2022). Executive summary of the Merck Animal Health Veterinarian Wellbeing Study III and Veterinary Support Staff Study. *Journal of the American Veterinary Medical Association*, 260(12), 1547–1553.
5. Merck Animal Health. (2024). Creating a Positive, More Energized Veterinary Team. https://www.merck-animal-health-usa.com/offload-downloads/2023-vet-team -wellbeing-presentation (accessed June 10, 2024).

6. Lederhouse, C. (2022). Exploring employee assistance programs for veterinary practices: Are they a bother or benefit? AVMA News. https://www.avma.org/news/exploring-employee-assistance-programs-veterinary-practices-are-they-bother-or-benefit (accessed June 10, 2024).

7. Vet Mind Matters. (2024). Help When You Need It. https://vetmindmatters.org/help-links/ (accessed June 10, 2024).

8. Silverwood, J. (2022). Vetlife Helpline celebrates 30th anniversary. VetTimes. https://www.vettimes.co.uk/news/vetlife-helpline-celebrates-30th-anniversary/ (accessed June 10, 2024).

9. American Veterinary Medical Association. (2024). Wellbeing resources for veterinary professionals. https://www.avma.org/resources-tools/wellbeing (accessed June 10, 2024).

10. Australia Veterinary Association. (2024). THRIVE programs and events. https://www.ava.com.au/Thrive/thrive-programs/ (accessed June 10, 2024).

11. Canadian Veterinary Medical Association. (2024). Veterinary Health and Wellness Resources. https://www.canadianveterinarians.net/veterinary-resources/veterinary-health-and-wellness-resources/ (accessed June 10, 2024).

12. Cima, G. (2020). Social work expands in veterinary hospitals - Emergency, specialty practices hiring to counsel staff members, clients. JAVMA News. https://www.avma.org/javma-news/2020-06-15/social-work-expands-veterinary-hospitals (accessed June 10, 2024).

13. The University of Tennessee Knoxville College of Social Work. (2024). Veterinary Social Work Certificate Program. https://csw.utk.edu/veterinary-social-work-certificate-program/ (accessed June 10, 2024).

14. American Veterinary Medical Association. (2024). AVMA and Royal College of Veterinary Surgeons Joint Statement on Veterinary Mental Health and Wellbeing. https://www.avma.org/sites/default/files/resources/Joint-RCVS-statement.pdf (accessed June 10, 2024).

About the Author

Marie Holowaychuk, DVM, Dipl. ACVECC

Veterinarian, Mental Health and Wellness Advocate, Speaker, and Author

Dr. Marie Holowaychuk is a veterinarian, speaker, and wellness advocate dedicated to improving mental health and wellbeing in the veterinary profession. A board-certified emergency and critical care specialist, she brings over 20 years of clinical, academic, and consulting experience, combined with a passion for fostering sustainable, fulfilling careers.

After completing veterinary school in Canada and advanced training in the United States, Marie spent five years as a faculty member at the Ontario Veterinary College, followed by relief work across North America. During her career, she not only witnessed but personally experienced the emotional and mental toll of veterinary practice, including burnout and compassion fatigue. These challenges led her to focus on wellness, burnout prevention, and workplace culture.

As the founder of Reviving Veterinary Medicine, Marie provides evidence-based resources to support self-care, effective communication, and professional resilience. She is a certified coach, yoga and meditation teacher, and wellbeing facilitator. A sought-after speaker, she has delivered keynotes, workshops, and seminars worldwide, inspiring veterinary teams to prioritize their wellbeing.

Marie is also an accomplished writer, having published numerous articles and book chapters on veterinary medicine and mental health. She hosts the Reviving Vet Med Podcast, where she explores workplace challenges, personal growth, and strategies for creating a healthier profession.

Through her writing, speaking, and coaching, Marie is committed to fostering a culture of compassion, resilience, and support in veterinary medicine, helping professionals build careers—and lives—that are both meaningful and sustainable.

For Product Safety Concerns and Information please contact our EU
representative GPSR@taylorandfrancis.com Taylor & Francis Verlag GmbH,
Kaufingerstraße 24, 80331 München,

Printed and bound by CPI Group (UK),   R0 4YY
05/12/2025
02013038-0015